DATE DUE

CANCER TREATMENT AND SURVIVAL

Gann Monograph on Cancer Research

The "Gann Monograph on Cancer Research" series is promoted by the Japanese Cancer Association. This semiannual series of monographs was initiated in 1966 by the late Dr. Tomizo Yoshida (1903–1973) and is now published jointly by Japan Scientific Societies Press, Tokyo and CRC Press, Boca Raton. Each volume consists of collected contributions on current topics in cancer problems and allied research fields. The planning for each volume is done by the Monograph Committee of the Japanese Cancer Association, with the final approval of the Board of Directors. It is hoped that the series will serve as an important source of information in the field of cancer research.

The publication of these monographs owes much to the financial support given by the late Professor Kazushige Higuchi, the Jikei University School of Medicine.

Japanese Cancer Association

Monograph Committee of the Japanese Cancer Association

Hiroyasu Esumi	Yoshiyuki Hashimoto	Nobuyuki Ito
Masaaki Terada	Shigeru Tsukagoshi	Takashi Tsuruo
Tadashi Utakoji		

Tomoyuki Kitagawa (Executive Secretary)

JAPANESE CANCER ASSOCIATION
Gann Monograph on Cancer Research No. 43

CANCER TREATMENT AND SURVIVAL

SITE-SPECIFIC REGISTRIES IN JAPAN

Edited by   SHAW WATANABE
SUKETAMI TOMINAGA
TADAO KAKIZOE

JAPAN SCIENTIFIC SOCIETIES PRESS, Tokyo
CRC PRESS, Boca Raton New York London Tokyo

© JAPAN SCIENTIFIC SOCIETIES PRESS, 1995
All rights reserved. No part of this publication may be reproduced or transmitted in any form or by any means, electronic or mechanical, including photocopy, recording, or any information storage and retrieval system, without permission in writing from the publisher.

August 1995

Published jointly by
JAPAN SCIENTIFIC SOCIETIES PRESS
2-10 Hongo, 6-chome, Bunkyo-ku, Tokyo 113, Japan
ISBN 4-7622-8796-2

and

CRC PRESS
2000 Corporate Blvd., N.W., Boca Raton, FL 33431, U.S.A.
ISBN 0-8493-7778-1

Library of Congress Cataloging-in-Publication Data

Cancer treatment and survival: site-specific registries in Japan/
  edited by Shaw Watanabe, Suketami Tominaga, Tadao Kakizoe.
     p. cm. — (Gann monograph on cancer research; no. 43)
  Includes bibliographical references and indexes.
  ISBN 0-8493-7778-1 (alk. paper)
  1. Cancer — Japan — Statistics. I. Watanabe, Shaw, 1941– .
II. Tominaga, Suketami. III. Kakizoe, Tadao. IV. Series.
[DNLM: 1. Registries — Japan. 2. Neoplasms — epidemiology — Japan. 3. Neoplasms — therapy — Japan — statistics. 4. Neoplasms — mortality — Japan. 5. Survival Rate — Japan.
W3 GA163 no. 43 1995/QZ 200/C2187 1995]
RC279. J3C367   1995
614. 5'999—dc20
DNLM/DLC
for Library of Congress   95/33187
                                                                                     CIP

Distributed in all areas outside Japan and Asia between Pakistan and Korea by CRC Press.

Printed in Japan

PREFACE

Site-specific cancer registries developed in Japan before the population-based cancer registry to evaluate the effects of diagnosis and treatment of this disease. Gastric carcinoma was the most frequent cancer, so the registration of gastric cancer patients first began in 1965 with the collaboration of interested surgeons. Following its success other site-specific cancer registries were established. These registries usually involve a research group or association of expert doctors whose enthusiasm has provided stimulation and has resulted in many improvements in diagnostic and surgical techniques. A grant-in-aid for cancer research from the Ministry of Health and Welfare has partially supported the registries for nearly 30 years.

The present number of organ- or site-specific cancer registries is 18, and several others are planned. Since these registries usually contain detailed clinical information concerning diagnosis, treatment and survival, they have also contributed to the creation and revision of the TNM classification by presenting various prognostic factors. In the liver cancer registry the registration form sometimes involves etiological information, *e.g.*, HBV and HCV infection, Family histories are described in the breast cancer registry, and complete family pedigrees offered in the familial polyposis registry. This allows the changing pattern of etiological factors in Japan to be followed in some types of cancers.

For this monograph each site-specific registration committee was requested to describe the history, organization, number of patients and their clinical characteristics, survival rates by TNM stage and their time trends in relation to the development of diagnostic methods, and to elaborate on new treatment. The member institutes of registry are leading hospitals which cover 10–40% of all cancer patients in Japan.

The editors deeply appreciate the efforts made by the contributing committee members from each registry in writing the chapters, and the warm support of the Japanese Cancer Association for publishing this book, We hope the information contained herein may contribute to an understanding of the historical background, current diagnostic and therapeutic results of Japan's cancer patients.

June 1995

Shaw WATANABE
Suketami TOMINAGA
Tadao KAKIZOE

CONTENTS

Preface v

History and Overview of the Site-specific Cancer Registries in Japan ....
.... Shaw Watanabe, Naohito Yamaguchi, and Yoshihide Kinjo   1

Head and Neck Cancer Registry .... The Japanese Joint Committee   9

Carcinoma of the Major Salivary Glands ....
.... The Japanese Joint Committee on TNM Classification,
        the Head and Neck Subcommittee, the Salivary Gland Division   21

Thyroid Cancer Registry .... Japan Society of Thyroid Surgery   29

Statistics of Esophageal Cancer Registry ....
        Japanese Committee for Registration of Esophageal Cancer, Japanese
.... Society for Esophageal Diseases   39

Treatment Results of Gastric Cancer Patients: An Analysis of Nationwide
    Database .... The Japanese Research Society for Gastric Cancer   47

A General View of Large Bowel Cancer in Japan ....
.... Registry Committee, Japanese Society for
                            Cancer of the Colon and Rectum   57

Registry of Familial Adenomatous Polyposis
    .... The Polyposis Committee of the Japanese Research Society for
                            Cancer of the Colon and Rectum   69

Primary Liver Cancer in Japan ...... The Liver Cancer Study Group of Japan   81

Statistics Registry of Biliary Tract Cancer ....
.... Japanese Society of Biliary Surgery   97

The Present Status of Pancreatic Cancer Registration ....
.... The Pancreatic Cancer Registration Committee of
                            the Japan Pancreas Society   107

Time Trends and Survival Rate of Lung Cancer ....
.... Lung Cancer Registration Committee   119

Bone Tumor Registration .... Musculoskeletal Tumor Committee of
.... the Japanese Orthopaedic Association 129

Statistics of Malignant Melanoma .... The Japanese Skin Cancer Society 147

Clinical Statistics on Registered Breast Cancer Patients in Japan ....
.... Registration Committee of the Japanese Breast Cancer Society 159

Registration of Gynecologic Malignancies ....
.... The Japan Society of Obstetrics and Gynecology 169

Statistics of Bladder Cancer Registry, 1982–1987 ....
.... Bladder Cancer Registry, Japanese Urological Association 181

Statistics of Brain Tumors, 1969–1987: General Features ....
.... The Committee of the Brain Tumor Registry of Japan 191

The Japan Children's Cancer Registry: Outline, Results, and Perspectives ....
.... The Committee of the Japan Children's Cancer Registry 203

Appendix: List of Hospitals Participating to the Registries 213

Subject Index 237

HISTORY AND OVERVIEW OF THE SITE-SPECIFIC CANCER REGISTRIES IN JAPAN

Shaw WATANABE, Naohito YAMAGUCHI, and Yoshihide KINJO

Cancer Information and Epidemiology Division,
National Cancer Center Research Institute*

The organ- or site-specific cancer registries were organized in Japan to obtain precise clinical information on cancer patients. The gastric cancer registry began in 1965, and the uterine cancer registry, soft part and bone tumor registry followed. The number of site-specific registries is now more than 18, and each has specific characteristics as shown in each chapter of this book.

Hospitals participating with the registries are over two thirds of those with more than 600 beds, about half those with 400–599 beds, and about 10% of those with less than 200 beds. On average, 23–30% of all cancer patients in the country are estimated to be listed in one of these registries by expert clinicians. The rate of pediatric tumor registration is high and estimated to be about half of all cases of that type. Historical and characteristic features of site-specific cancer registries are overviewed.

Although mortality rates in Japan are accurately recorded by the Ministry of Health and Welfare (4), improved survival rates of cancer patients make it impossible to estimate cancer incidence from the mortality data (13). Population-based cancer registries are therefore maintained by the local government, mainly at the prefectural level, and a research group gathers these data to estimate cancer incidence in Japan (1, 11). The organ- or site-specific cancer registries have been developed through the efforts of the scientific community and associations of clinical doctors. Their purpose is to determine the current status of diagnosis and treatment with the aim of improving patient survival rate. They are thus more research oriented than the population-based registry for public health services.

Characteristics of Site-specific Cancer Registry

There are various types of cancer registries according to the different purposes (Table I). A cancer registry is mandatory to evaluate the effects of diagnosis and treatment by maintaining complete follow-up information on the patients. If more detailed clinical data are required, however, the size of registry should be made smaller. The registry of patients in a clinical trial is such an example. The number of patients in each trial may reach a few hundred, but patient information is biased by

---

* 5-1-1 Tsukiji, Chuo-ku, Tokyo 104, Japan

TABLE I. Characteristics of Various Cancer Registries in Japan

Record	Annual No. of patients	Clinical trial	Organ-specific registry	Hospital registry	District registry	Death registry
No. patients	300,000	10–100	60,000	100,000	120,000	210,000
Criteria		Present	Present	None	None	None
ID		Yes	Yes	Yes	Yes	Yes
Histology	–50%	–100%	80–100%	–90%	–70%	None
Stage	None	TNM	TNM	Various	Simple	None
Diagnosis	None	Yes	Precise	Various	Simple	None
Treatment	None	Precise	Precise	Various	Simple	None
Others		End point Side effect	Survival Side effect Prognosis Etiology Precancerous lesion Basic disease Family history	Survival	Incidence rates	Mortality rates

ID: identification of patients.

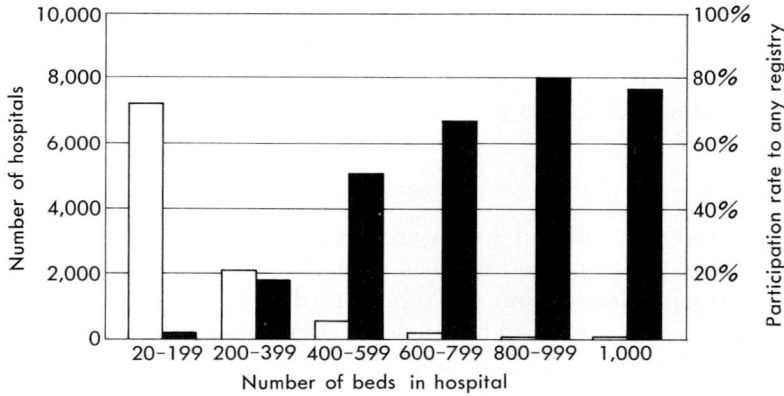

FIG. 1. Number of hospitals in Japan and their participation in the site-specific cancer registry

firm eligibility criteria of the study. After evaluation of treatment effects over a relatively short period, it is better to transfer these patients to the site-specific cancer registry to compare their clinical characteristics with other patients. Standardization of the treatment regimen and longer follow-up results are beneficial to learn of any late adverse effects, such as a second primary cancer.

Organization of the site-specific cancer registries depends on the purpose of the registry. It is basically based upon the voluntary participation of doctors in leading hospitals, so it does not represent data on all patients in Japan. On average, it covers one fourth to one third of all incident cases each year. The hospitals participating in the registries represent more than two thirds of large hospitals with more than 600 beds, about half of those with 400–599 beds, and less than 10% of those with less than 200 beds (Fig. 1).

The site-specific cancer registries require more precise and abundant clinical data than the population-based registry. Questions about cancer etiology such as probable cancer causes, precancerous lesions, and family history are sometimes included in the organ-specific registry. These data are available for clinical epidemiology. Site-specific cancer registry should be linked to the hospital patients' registry, but the latter is insufficiently developed in most hospitals. Alert clinicians who participate in the cancer registry promote establishment of the hospital patients' registry. We collected about 100,000 discharge summaries per year for 6 years from 18 national hospitals, and the contents were improved every year according to widened recognition of the role of the intrahospital registry.

The population-based cancer registry is useful for developing a cancer strategy in a region because it usually covers 70–80% of the incident cases; however, it is hard to get detailed information such as TNM classification, histology, *etc*. It is also difficult to get precise information about diagnostic methods and treatment procedure, because the standardization of clinical data is very difficult among reluctant doctors. In addition, many active doctors in the university hospitals, which have a central role in clinical research in most districts, are reluctant to register their patients with the regional cancer registry. A complimentary linkage between the regional cancer registry and site-specific cancer registry is therefore needed for the current status of cancer patients to be known.

Benefits of Site-specific Registry and Its History

Benefits of the site-specific cancer registry are as follows: (a) to know the current method of diagnosis, treatment, and result of therapy; (b) to determine the biological characteristics of cancer; (c) to learn the cause of cancer and precancerous lesions; and (d) to know of late adverse effects such as multiple primary cancers. (b) and (c) could be used in cancer prevention and early detection.

The first systematic site-specific cancer registry in Japan was started in 1963 when Dr. Kiyoshi Miwa began the registry of gastric cancer patients. Gastric cancer was the primary cause of cancer death at that time. Dr. Miwa, a gastroenterology surgeon in the National Cancer Center Hospital became the chief investigator, starting the registry in 1970 with support by a grant-in-aid for cancer research from the Ministry of Health and Welfare. The first 6 years of the research group, however, concerned only gastric cancer. The uterine cervical cancer registry started in 1965, and that of uterine body cancer in 1966, ovarian cancer and lung cancer in 1967, esophageal cancer in 1969, hematopoietic cancer in 1972, colorectal cancer in 1974, breast cancer in 1975, thyroid cancer in 1979, and bile duct cancer in 1987 (Table II). Registries of colorectal cancer, breast cancer, and thyroid cancer joined the research group during the 1979–1984 period under Dr. Teruo Sakano, the second chief investigator of the group. Between the 1985 and 1990 period, Dr. Keiichi Maruyama, subsequent chief investigator called on the registry of bile duct cancer to join the research group. Since 1991, Dr. Shaw Watanabe, successor to the program, has expanded the group to include registries on pancreatic cancer, liver tumor, and childhood cancer. There is now also collaboration with the TNM committee. The TNM committee in Japan partly supports various of the site-specific registries, the brain tumor, bladder cancer, and soft part and bone tumor registries. The bone tumor

TABLE II. History and Organization of Site-specific Cancer Registries

1.	Head & neck	TNM Committee, Japan Head & Neck Tumor Association
2.	Esophagus	Japanese Committee for Registration of Esophageal Cancer, Japanese Society for Esophageal Diseases
3.	Stomach	The Japanese Research Society for Gastric Cancer
4.	Large intestine	Registry Committee, Japanese Research Society for Cancer of the Colon and Rectum
	Polyposis coli	The Polyposis Committee, Japanese Research Society for Cancer of the Colon and Rectum
5.	Liver	The Liver Cancer Study Group of Japan
6.	Bile duct	The Japanese Society of Biliary Surgery
7.	Pancreas	The Pancreatic Cancer Registration Committee of the Japan Pancreas Study
8.	Lung	Japanese Lung Cancer Registration
9.	Bone	Musculoskeletal Tumor Committee of the Japanese Orthopaedic Association
10.	Skin	Japanese Skin Cancer Society
11.	Breast	Registration Committee of the Japanese Breast Cancer Society
12.	Uterine cervix	The Japan Society of Obstetrics and Gynecology
13.	Uterine body	The Japan Society of Obstetrics and Gynecology
14.	Ovary	The Japan Society of Obstetrics and Gynecology
15.	Bladder	Bladder Cancer Registry, Japanese Urological Association
16.	Brain	The Committee of the Brain Tumor Registry of Japan
17.	Thyroid	Japan Society of Thyroid Surgery
18.	Childhood cancer	The Registration Committee for Childhood Cancer
19.	Retinoblastoma	The Committee for the National Registry of Retinoblastoma

TABLE III. Number of Patients in Each Registry and Estimated Coverage Rates in 1992

		Year	Total No. registered patients	Annual No. registered	Estimated No. of patients	Coverage rate
1.	Head & neck	1979–present	18,416	1,000	7,000	14.2%
2.	Esophagus	1969–present	21,402	1,500	8,000	18.8
3.	Stomach	1963–present	253,382	12,000	78,000	15.4
4.	Large intestine	1974–present	24,234	4,000	57,000	7.0
5.	Liver	1965–present	46,952	10,000	25,000	40.0
6.	Bile duct	1987–present	5,293	1,000	19,000	5.3
7.	Pancreas	1981–present	13,498	1,300	15,000	8.7
8.	Lung	1967–1984	33,989	2,100	62,000	3.4
		1989–present	5,000			
9.	Bone, soft tissue[a]	1964–present	49,000	3,000		
10.	Skin[b]	1987–1993	9,439			
11.	Breast	1975–present	45,885	4,000	24,000	16.7
12.	Uterine cervix	1965–present	122,000	2,100	10,400	20.2
13.	Uterine body	1966–present	2,600			
14.	Ovary	1967–present	1,954			
15.	Bladder	1982–present	10,600	2,000	8,000	25.0
16.	Brain[c]	1969–present	46,002	4,500	13,000	34.6
17.	Thyroid	1979–present	19,446	1,500		
18.	Childhood cancer	1975–present	29,804	1,500	2,000	75.0
Total			758,896	51,500	328,400	15.4

[a] Including benign tumor.
[b] Periodic survey.
[c] Including metastatic brain tumor.

registry was established in 1964, the liver tumor registry in 1965, the brain tumor registry in 1969, the childhood cancer registry in 1975, and the pancreatic cancer registry in 1981. Duration of these site-specific registries and their funding organizations are listed in Tables II and III. To date, 18 registries are collecting information on cancer patients, and several others have also carried out *ad hoc* collection of patient data. A joint workshop was held in the National Cancer Center in 1993 to compare and standardize results of all these registries, and this was the trigger for publishing this book.

The number of registered patients, estimated number of total cancer patients, and coverage rate of each registry is shown in Table III. The average number of registered cases is about 800 for the head and neck, 1,500 for the esophagus, 12,000 for the stomach, 4,000 for the colon and rectum, 10,000 for the liver, 1,000 for the bile duct, 1,300 for the pancreas, 2,100 for the lung, 3,000 for the bone and soft tissue, 4,000 for the breast, 2,100 for the ovary, 2,000 for the urinary bladder, 4,500 for the brain, 1,500 for the thyroid, and 1,500 for childhood. The rate of coverage would be 15.4% based on the estimated 346,000 cancer patients in 1990.

Results of the Registries and Their Application for Clinical Study

Some of the benefits of the registry are: (a) to show improvements in diagnostic and treatment procedures, (b) to transfer better methods to other hospitals, (c) to identify patients at high risk, and (d) to determine annual trends in cancer diagnosis and treatment. These data would not be obtainable, especially on rare cancers, because of the small number of cases in individual hospitals. A few examples of clinical research using registry data are shown below (*6, 7*). The death rate within 30 days after an operation for gastric cancer by different surgical procedures from 1969–1973 to 1974–1978 is shown in Table IV. The total operative death rate decreased from 2.3% to 1.7%. In total gastrectomy, it decreased 1.2%, and in pyloric resection it decreased 1.6% from 4.6% to 3.0%. Five-year survival rates in these two surgical procedures increased 5% in contrast to the small improvement from 56.3% to 57.8% in all patients (Table IV).

Long registration of many cases can show changes in the etiologic factors. Comparison of the past histories of the patients registered between 1978–1979 and 1984–1985 in the Liver Tumor Registry revealed many interesting features (*9*). Histology was 919 hepatocellular carcinoma, 94 cholangiogenic carcinoma and 10 mixed type in

TABLE IV. Changes in Operative Death Rates and 5-Year Survival Rates by Surgical Procedure

	1969–1973			1974–1978		
	No.	Operative death	5-Year	No.	Operative death	5-Year
Total gastrectomy	2,291	4.1	30.1	4,760	2.9	35.3
Pyloric subtotal gastrectomy	234	4.7	39.0	257	3.1	44.1
Pyloric resection	393	4.6	46.3	679	3.0	51.2
Cardiac subtotal gastrectomy	4,157	2.0	60.1	6,944	1.4	63.9
Cardiac resection	4,672	1.3	67.2	9,027	1.2	66.9
Total	11,747	2.3	56.3	21,667	1.7	57.8

TABLE V. Past History of Patients with Intractable Cancer

Site	Bile duct	Gallbladder	Papilla Vater	Pancreas
No. of patients	415	457	128	11,317
Male: female	2.1:1	1:1.9	1:1	1.6:1
Diabetes mellitus	6.7%	6.1%	7.8%	15.7%
Pancreatitis	0.5	0.9	1.7	4.6
Peptic ulcer	5.5	7.0	4.7	8.1
Gallstone	6.5	9.2	6.3	6.0
Bile stone	1.0	0.7	1.7	–
Cholecystitis	2.2	4.4	–	–
Hepatitis	2.4	3.1	–	–
Drinking	40.4	20.7	78.4	na
Smoking	43.6	24.3	21.6	na

na: not applicable.

TABLE VI. Second Primary Cancers from Retinoblastoma Patients

Observation period (years)	Number of patients			Incidence of 2nd cancer	Cumulative incidence	p
	At risk	Died	2nd cancer			
0–1	514	7	2	0.004	0.004	0.006
1–4	452	29	0	0	0.004	0.006
5–9	366	15	10	0.046	0.049	0.027
10–14	139	1	5	0.056	0.101	0.053
15–19	40	1	2	0.064	0.158	0.090

1978–1979, but these numbers were 2,292, 137, and 18, respectively, in 1984–1985. The proportion of hepatocellular carcinoma doubled during this short period. Seropositive rate of surface antigen of hepatitis B virus dropped from 34.1% to 24.6%, and positive rate of hepatitis C virus antibody increased from 61.2% to 68.6% during this 6-year period. Longer data accumulation revealed obvious risk factors in past history: chronic hepatitis, hepatic cirrhosis, blood transfusion, and heavy drinking of alcoholic beverages.

It is required to identify a high risk group for prevention or early detection of intractable cancer, such as bile duct and pancreas cancer. Past history of the patients with bile duct, gallbladder, papilla Vater, and pancreas cancers gives some hints for further epidemiological study (8, 10). Diabetes mellitus, pancreatitis, and peptic ulcer were common in the past history of pancreatic cancer patients, gallstone in gallbladder cancer patients, and the drinking of alcohol in patients with carcinoma of the papilla Vater (Table V).

Studies on the risk of multiple primary cancers become more important according to the increase in cancer survivors. Interaction of exposure to carcinogenic treatment and predisposition to cancer is one focus of cancer biology. The long-term retinoblastoma registry shows the risk of second primary cancer (Table VI). It indicates that 16% of retinoblastoma survivors had a second primary cancer: osteosarcoma, pinealoma, squamous cell carcinoma, Meibomian carcinoma, malignant fibrous histiocytoma, or leukemia during the 20 years after initial treatment (5).

The site-specific cancer registries can further contribute to: (a) upgrading the intra-hospital cancer registry, (b) revising TNM and AJC classifications, (c) introducing linkage to the local population-based registry, and (d) analyzing prognostic factors. The TNM Committee in UICC accepted the Japanese classification of gastric cancer; stage classification of lung cancer and brain tumors are also under review. For brain tumor, prognostic factors could not be properly analyzed by the Cox regression model; rather, the non-linear tree regression model could more properly distinguish 13 groups according to the prognosis (2) (see Nomura's chapter, p. 191).

Future of Site-specific Cancer Registry

As described above, organ- or site-specific cancer registries have contributed much to clinical cancer research, even though they have operated with limited human resources and insufficient funds. More comprehensive registration systems should be established to develop communication among registries using standardized procedures. Establishment of a common service system is mandatory to make summary reports, calculate survivals and analyze prognostic factors, and proper support from the government is also necessary for an efficient system. The supercomputer project which started in 1994 in the National Cancer Center may aid this effort in the near future (*12*).

Acknowledgments

The authors acknowledge the many organizations handling site-specific cancer registries. Drs. Kiyoshi Miwa, Teruo Sakano, and Keiichi Maruyama are appreciated for their help in the historical review and the Misses Hiroko Arimoto, Yasuko Ishida, Ikumi Isogai, and Hamako Kato for their help in the central office for site-specific cancer registry. Messrs. Kazuo Kobayashi and Hisaji Eto, Chief of the Investigation Office in the Administrative Office of the National Cancer Center assisted with computer facilities and communication with the Biostatistics Bureau in the Ministry of Health and Welfare. Dr. Masaaki Terada, Director of our Research Institute supported and encouraged the authors in the preparation of this book.

REFERENCES

1. Kakizoe, T. and Watanabe, S. (eds.). "Medical Informatics in Cancer Research," (1992) (in Japanese). Kyowa-Kikaku, Tokyo.
2. Nomura, K., Yamaguchi, N., and Watanabe, S. Results of the statistical analysis of prognostic factors for brain tumors. *WHO*, in press.
3. Tominaga, S., Aoki, K., Fujimoto, I., and Kurihara, M. (eds.). "Cancer Mortality and Morbidity Statistics: Japan and the World-1994," Gann Monograph on Cancer Research No. 41 (1994). Japan Sci. Soc. Press, Tokyo.
4. The Bureau of Vital Statistics. Vital Statistics of the Nation. Ministry of Health and Welfare, Tokyo (1993).
5. The Committee for the National Registry of Retinoblastoma. Survival rate and risk factors for patients with retinoblastoma in Japan. *Jpn. J. Ophthalmol.*, **36**, 121–131 (1992).
6. The Japanese Research Society for Gastric Cancer. Report of the National Gastric Cancer Registry, Vol. 14, National Cancer Center (1983) (in Japanese).
7. The Japanese Research Society for Gastric Cancer. Report of the National Gastric Cancer Registry, Vol. 25, National Cancer Center (1986) (in Japanese).
8. The Japanese Society of Biliary Surgery. Report of the National Biliary Cancer Regis-

try of Patients in 1989, The Japanese Society of Biliary Surgery, Kanazawa (1992) (in Japanese).
9. The Liver Cancer Study Group of Japan. Eighth Report of a Follow-up Study on Primary Liver Cancer. The Liver Cancer Study Group, Kyoto (1988) (in Japanese).
10. The Pancreatic Cancer Registration Committee. Report of the National Pancreas Cancer Registry of Patients in 1990; Summary of 10-Year Registration. The Pancreatic Cancer Registration Committee (1991) (in Japanese).
11. Tominaga, S., Aoki, K. Fujimoto, I., and Kurihara, M. (eds.). "Cancer Mortality Statistics: Japan and the World-1994," Gann Monograph on Cancer Research No. 41 (1994). Japan. Sci. Soc. Press, Tokyo.
12. Watanabe, S. Why do we need cancer information? *Jpn. J. Clin. Oncol.,* **20**, 7–15 (1990).
13. Watanabe, S., Oshima, A. Fujimoto, I. *et al.* Workshop for the evaluation of survival trends for cancer patients. *Jpn. J. Clin. Oncol.,* **19**, 178–180 (1989).

HEAD AND NECK CANCER REGISTRY

The Japanese Joint Committee*

The head and neck cancer registry has recorded 16,518 cases treated between 1979 and 1991 in major Japanese institutions for head and neck cancer treatment. Each year 1,000 to 1,500 patients have been registered with the cooperation of about 30 institutions. The registry covers 14.2% of the estimated total number of laryngeal cancer cases in Japan.

Several analyses have been made of the registered cases. The male-to-female ratio was 3.37:1 and the peak of the age distribution was in the seventh decade. Tumors were most frequently detected in the oral cavity, followed by the larynx, maxillary sinus, hypopharynx, and mesopharynx in this order. The percentage of maxillary sinus carcinoma dropped significantly from 19.0% to 6.7% during the 13 year period. Squamous cell carcinoma was the most common histologic type, accounting for 93.2% of all cases.

Radiotherapy alone was the most common treatment method for the primary lesion. Although the percentage of patients with radiotherapy alone decreased in later years from 29.5% to 24.0%, that of surgically treated patients increased markedly from 15.0% to 23.2%. The annual number of patients who received microsurgical transfer of a free flap increased dramatically from 5 to 246 during the study period. Cumulative survival rates calculated by the registered data were too high compared to reported figures and are not totally reliable because of insufficient follow-up of the registered cases.

In 1977 the Japanese Joint Committee (JJC) began several studies to evaluate the third edition of the TNM Classification of the International Union Against Cancer (UICC) (1). Included in these studies was an evaluation of the TNM classification of head and neck cancer. In 1978 the Subcommittee for Head and Neck Cancer of the JJC performed a trial registration of head and neck cancer cases treated between 1970 and 1973 with the cooperation of 18 major hospitals and universities in Japan. Documentation was made of 2,809 cases and nationwide statistics were presented on all head and neck tumors, including information on the TNM classification, for the first time in Japan.

On the basis of this study, the Subcommittee planned an annual registration program for head and neck carcinoma. The collected data were to be analyzed to formulate Japanese proposals for the TNM classification of head and neck cancer. The first registration took place in 1981 for head and neck cancer patients treated in

---

* Manuscript was prepared by Masahisa Saikawa, Department of Surgical Oncology, National Cancer Center Hospital, 5-1-1 Tsukiji, Chuo-ku, Tokyo 104, Japan

the year 1979. Since then the registration has been repeated every year, and after 13 years of data collection, the registry contains 16,518 cases. This vast registry has contributed greatly to the understanding of the statistics and treatment of head and neck cancer in Japan, as well as to the formation of Japanese proposals for TNM classification. The data in this registry formed the basis of several publications (*3–5*).

Data Collection

Head and neck cancer is a collection of several distinct tumors, each of which arises in a distinct portion of the head and neck area and has a particular biological behavior, treatment indication, treatment method, and curability distinct from other head and neck tumors. To register each tumor precisely in spite of the complex anatomy of the head and neck region, we use five registration forms: the first for carcinomas of the oral cavity and mesopharynx, the second for carcinomas of the larynx and hypopharynx, the third for carcinoma of the maxillary sinus, the fourth for carcinomas of the nasopharynx, nasal cavity, and paranasal sinuses excluding the maxillary sinus, and the last for carcinoma of the major salivary glands.

The first four registration forms are sent every year to cooperating institutions by the secretariat of the head and neck cancer registry in the National Cancer Center. The completed registration forms are returned, checked by assistants, and stored in a computerized data file. Each year a detailed analysis of new entries is performed and the results are distributed in a booklet form to the cooperating institutions. The registration of major salivary gland carcinoma cases is performed by another secretariat in Chiba University and will be reported in a separate chapter of this volume.

Registration is restricted to new clinical cases of head and neck cancer. Each case is registered in the year of the first clinical consultation.

At present the head and neck cancer registry is supported by grants-in-aid for cancer research from the Ministry of Health and Welfare with the cooperation of major institutions for head and neck cancer treatment in Japan. This registry is not supported by any societies, and therefore the data in the registry is not totally public and is available only to researchers in the cooperating institutions.

Basic Data on Registered Patients

Table I shows the number of registered patients and cooperating institutions in each registration year. About 1,000 to 1,500 patients are registered annually, and there has been a slight increasing tendency in later years. The annual number of cooperating institutions varies between 28 and 36.

Head and neck carcinoma was more common in male patients (Table II). The male-to-female ratio (M/F ratio) was 3.37:1, and was almost constant throughout the study period (Table III).

Tumors were observed most frequently in the seventh decade in both male and female patients (Table II). The percentage of patients in the ninth decade increased from 3.9% to 6.6% during the 13 year period, while that of patients in the third and fourth decades decreased from 5.3% to 3.6% (Table IV).

Table V illustrates annual change in the distribution of primary site. Head and neck cancer was most frequently detected in the oral cavity (35.2%), followed by the

TABLE I. Number of Registered Patients and Cooperating Institutions by Year

Year	Number of registered patients	Number of cooperating institutions
1979	1,176	33
1980	1,105	28
1981	1,349	35
1982	1,139	31
1983	1,240	35
1984	1,115	32
1985	1,353	34
1986	1,334	34
1987	1,093	30
1988	1,286	36
1989	1,315	28
1990	1,539	31
1991	1,474	30
Total	16,518	

TABLE II. Distribution of Gender by Age[a]

Age	Male	Female	Total	M/F ratio
0–9	10	1	11	10.00:1
10–19	45	20	65	2.25:1
20–29	91	83	174	1.10:1
30–39	375	211	586	1.78:1
40–49	1,423	455	1,878	3.13:1
50–59	3,595	836	4,431	4.30:1
60–69	3,933	1,051	4,984	3.74:1
70–79	2,560	813	3,373	3.15:1
80–89	597	273	870	2.19:1
90–	20	6	26	3.33:1
Total	12,649	3,749	16,398	3.37:1

[a] One hundred and twenty cases of unknown age or gender were omitted.

TABLE III. Distribution of Gender by Year[a]

Year	Male	Female	Total	M/F ratio
1979	872	284	1,156	3.07:1
1980	856	249	1,105	3.44:1
1981	1,035	314	1,349	3.30:1
1982	882	257	1,139	3.43:1
1983	977	263	1,240	3.71:1
1984	882	233	1,115	3.79:1
1985	1,051	302	1,353	3.48:1
1986	1,030	304	1,334	3.39:1
1987	829	264	1,093	3.14:1
1988	976	308	1,284	3.17:1
1989	990	324	1,314	3.06:1
1990	1,205	334	1,539	3.61:1
1991	1,131	342	1,473	3.31:1
Total	12,716	3,778	16,494	3.37:1

[a] Twenty-four cases of unknown gender were omitted.

TABLE IV. Age Distribution by Four-year Period[a]

Age	1979–1983	1984–1987	1988–1991	Total
0–9	2 (0.0%)	0 (0.0%)	9 (0.2%)	11 (0.1%)
10–19	23 (0.4)	20 (0.4)	22 (0.4)	65 (0.4)
20–29	70 (1.2)	54 (1.1)	50 (0.9)	174 (1.1)
30–39	246 (4.1)	191 (3.9)	149 (2.7)	586 (3.6)
40–49	725 (12.1)	530 (10.8)	623 (11.3)	1,878 (11.5)
50–59	1,664 (27.8)	1,370 (28.0)	1,398 (25.3)	4,432 (27.0)
60–69	1,782 (29.8)	1,441 (29.4)	1,761 (31.9)	4,984 (30.4)
70–79	1,237 (20.7)	1,006 (20.6)	1,130 (20.5)	3,373 (20.6)
80–89	233 (3.9)	275 (5.6)	362 (6.6)	870 (5.3)
90–	6 (0.1)	8 (0.2)	12 (0.2)	26 (0.2)
Total	5,988 (100.0)	4,895 (100.0)	5,516 (100.0)	16,399 (100.0)

[a] One hundred and nineteen cases of unknown age were omitted.

TABLE V. Distribution of Primary Site by Year

Year	Oral cavity	Larynx	Hypopharynx	Mesopharynx	Nasopharynx	Nasal cavity, etc.	Maxillary sinus	Total
1979	403 (34.3%)	326 (27.7%)	62 (5.3%)	86 (7.3%)	55 (4.7%)	20 (1.7%)	224 (19.0%)	1,176 (100.0%)
1980	407 (36.8)	308 (27.9)	82 (7.4)	106 (9.6)	45 (4.1)	0 (0.0)	157 (14.2)	1,105 (100.0)
1981	421 (31.2)	474 (35.1)	120 (8.9)	103 (7.6)	84 (6.2)	0 (0.0)	147 (10.9)	1,349 (100.0)
1982	362 (31.8)	346 (30.4)	104 (9.1)	66 (5.8)	78 (6.8)	22 (1.9)	161 (14.1)	1,139 (100.0)
1983	372 (30.0)	412 (33.2)	109 (8.8)	114 (9.2)	78 (6.3)	22 (1.8)	133 (10.7)	1,240 (100.0)
1984	428 (38.4)	333 (29.9)	91 (8.2)	90 (8.1)	49 (4.4)	15 (1.3)	109 (9.8)	1,115 (100.0)
1985	458 (33.9)	411 (30.4)	124 (9.2)	125 (9.2)	56 (4.1)	26 (1.9)	153 (11.3)	1,353 (100.0)
1986	449 (33.7)	422 (31.6)	147 (11.0)	103 (7.7)	69 (5.2)	26 (1.9)	118 (8.8)	1,334 (100.0)
1987	350 (32.0)	365 (33.4)	122 (11.2)	91 (8.3)	61 (5.6)	16 (1.5)	88 (8.1)	1,093 (100.0)
1988	482 (37.5)	374 (29.1)	136 (10.6)	108 (8.4)	57 (4.4)	25 (1.9)	104 (8.1)	1,286 (100.0)
1989	479 (36.4)	361 (27.5)	148 (11.3)	124 (9.4)	75 (5.7)	27 (2.1)	101 (7.7)	1,315 (100.0)
1990	616 (40.0)	402 (26.1)	161 (10.5)	155 (10.1)	72 (4.7)	27 (1.8)	106 (6.9)	1,539 (100.0)
1991	580 (39.3)	425 (28.8)	162 (11.0)	120 (8.1)	58 (3.9)	30 (2.0)	99 (6.7)	1,474 (100.0)
Total	5,807 (35.2)	4,959 (30.0)	1,568 (9.5)	1,391 (8.4)	837 (5.1)	256 (1.5)	1,700 (10.3)	16,518 (100.0)

Nasal cavity, *etc.*: nasal cavity and paranasal sinuses excluding the maxillary sinus.

TABLE VI. Distribution of Gender by Primary Site[a]

Primary site	Male	Female	Total	M/F ratio
Oral cavity	3,869	1,936	5,805	2.00:1
Larynx	4,595	363	4,958	12.66:1
Hypopharynx	1,228	340	1,568	3.61:1
Mesopharynx	1,153	238	1,391	4.84:1
Nasopharynx	582	255	837	2.28:1
Nasal cavity, *etc.*	143	93	236	1.54:1
Maxillary sinus	1,146	553	1,699	2.07:1
Total	12,716	3,778	16,494	3.37:1

[a] Twenty-four cases of unknown gender were omitted.

larynx (30.0%), maxillary sinus (10.3%), hypopharynx (9.5%), and mesopharynx (8.4%) in this order. During the study period, the percentage of maxillary sinus carcinoma dropped significantly from 19.0% to 6.7%, while that of hypopharyngeal

TABLE VII. Age Distribution by Primary Site[a]

Primary site	0–9	10–19	20–29	30–39	40–49	50–59	60–69	70–79	80–89	90–	Total
Oral cavity	1 (0.0%)	21 (0.4%)	107 (1.9%)	343 (5.9%)	805 (14.0%)	1,579 (27.4%)	1,541 (26.7%)	1,032 (17.9%)	323 (5.6%)	15 (0.3%)	5,767 (100.0%)
Larynx	4 (0.1)	2 (0.0)	4 (0.1)	32 (0.6)	333 (6.7)	1,310 (26.5)	1,739 (35.2)	1,260 (25.5)	246 (5.0)	7 (0.1)	4,937 (100.0)
Hypopharynx	2 (0.1)	1 (0.1)	0 (0.0)	14 (0.9)	143 (9.2)	417 (26.8)	532 (34.1)	349 (22.4)	100 (6.4)	0 (0.0)	1,558 (100.0)
Mesopharynx	2 (0.1)	4 (0.3)	9 (0.7)	23 (1.7)	174 (12.6)	393 (28.5)	436 (31.6)	270 (19.6)	69 (5.0)	1 (0.1)	1,381 (100.0)
Nasopharynx	0 (0.0)	27 (3.3)	43 (5.2)	75 (9.1)	177 (21.4)	218 (26.3)	187 (22.6)	84 (10.1)	17 (2.1)	0 (0.0)	828 (100.0)
Nasal cavity, etc.	1 (0.4)	1 (0.4)	6 (2.6)	17 (7.2)	26 (11.1)	62 (26.4)	63 (26.8)	47 (20.0)	11 (4.7)	1 (0.4)	235 (100.0)
Maxillary sinus	1 (0.1)	9 (0.5)	5 (0.3)	82 (4.8)	220 (13.0)	453 (26.8)	486 (28.7)	331 (19.6)	104 (6.1)	2 (0.1)	1,693 (100.0)
Total	11 (0.1)	65 (0.4)	174 (1.1)	586 (3.6)	1,878 (11.5)	4,432 (27.0)	4,984 (30.4)	3,373 (20.6)	870 (5.3)	26 (0.2)	16,399 (100.0)

[a] One hundred and nineteen cases of unknown age were omitted.

carcinoma increased from 5.3% to 11.0%. This registry covered 14.2% of the estimated total number of laryngeal carcinoma patients based on the incidence of laryngeal cancer between 1984 and 1988 in Japan.

The M/F ratio was the highest (12.66:1) in cases of laryngeal cancer (Table VI). Cancers of the oral cavity, nasopharynx, nasal cavity, and paranasal sinuses showed M/F ratios lower than the average (1.54:1 to 2.28:1). The peak of the age distribution was observed in the sixth decade with carcinomas of the oral cavity and nasopharynx, and in the seventh decade with other tumors (Table VII).

As shown in Table VIII, squamous cell carcinoma was the most common histologic type. Including its several histologic variants, squamous cell carcinoma accounted for 93.2% of all cases. This was followed by undifferentiated carcinoma (1.8%), adenoid cystic carcinoma (1.5%), malignant neoplasm (0.9%), mucoepidermoid carcinoma (0.8%), and adenocarcinoma (0.7%) in this order.

Table IX indicates that the most frequent subsite of oral cancer was the tongue (54.0%), followed by the gingiva (16.5%), floor of the mouth (13.7%), and buccal mucosa (8.0%).

Glottic and supraglottic carcinomas accounted for 61.8% and 30.0% of laryngeal cancer cases, respectively (Table X). The percentage of each subsite did not change greatly during the study period.

Clinical Stage

Table XI shows the percentage distribution of clinical stage. In later years the percentage of stage III cases decreased and that of stage IV cases increased, which is explained by the change in the UICC TNM classification from the third (*1*) to the fourth edition (*2*). Some cases classified as N1, or stage III, in the third edition are classified as N2, or stage IV, in the fourth edition. The percentage of early cases (stages I and II) increased from 41.7% to 46.8% in later years.

TABLE VIII. Histological Distribution by Primary Site

Histologic type	Oral cavity	Larynx	Hypo-pharynx	Meso-pharynx	Naso-pharynx	Nasal cavity, etc.	Maxillary sinus	Total
Neoplasm, malig.	36	4	3	26	19	28	36	152
Carcinoma, NOS	22	5	1	11	8	7	11	65
Ca., undiff., NOS	21	11	11	24	159	24	52	302
Giant cell and spindle cell ca.	0	1	0	0	0	0	0	1
Small cell ca., NOS	2	0	0	0	0	0	0	2
Verrucous ca., NOS	49	14	0	4	0	0	1	68
Papillary S.C.C.	10	11	3	3	1	0	6	34
S.C.C. in situ, NOS	46	94	2	8	1	0	7	158
S.C.C., NOS	2,618	2,325	768	646	308	65	742	7,472
S.C.C., kerat., NOS	2,615	2,170	642	470	56	38	549	6,540
S.C.C., large cell, non-kerat.	85	230	93	91	185	13	132	829
S.C.C., small cell, non-kerat.	20	52	33	11	43	9	30	198
S.C.C., spindle cell	9	26	7	4	14	2	8	70
S.C.C. in situ with ques. str. invasion	4	2	1	2	2	0	2	13
Lymphoepithelial ca.	0	0	0	0	4	0	0	4
Basal cell ca., NOS	1	2	0	1	1	0	0	5
Multicentric basal cell ca.	0	0	0	0	0	0	1	1
Transitional cell ca., NOS	0	0	0	0	1	0	2	3
Transitional cell ca., spindle cell	0	0	0	0	0	0	1	1
Adenocarcinoma, NOS	34	6	3	14	7	11	34	109
Scirrhous adenocarcinoma	0	0	0	0	1	0	0	1
Adenoid cystic ca.	100	1	1	41	18	26	57	244
Carcinoid tumor, NOS	0	1	0	0	0	0	0	1
Clear cell adenocarcinoma, NOS	1	0	0	1	0	0	0	2
Mucoepidermoid ca.	96	2	0	24	2	0	15	139
Acinar cell ca.	5	0	0	6	0	4	1	16
Adenosquamous ca.	2	0	0	0	1	1	2	6
Malig. melanoma, NOS	9	0	0	0	0	7	2	18
Fibrosarcoma, NOS	0	0	0	0	0	0	1	1
Mixed tumor, malig., NOS	12	1	0	4	2	0	3	22
Carcinosarcoma, NOS	1	0	0	0	0	0	0	1
Osteosarcoma, NOS	2	0	0	0	0	0	0	2
Ameloblastoma, malig.	0	0	0	0	0	0	2	2
Malig. lymphoma, NOS	0	0	0	0	1	1	0	2
Burkitt's lymphoma, NOS	1	0	0	0	0	0	0	1
Unknown	6	1	0	0	3	20	3	33
Total	5,807	4,959	1,568	1,391	837	256	1,700	16,518

malig.: malignant. NOS: not otherwise specified. Ca., ca.: carcinoma. undiff.: undifferentiated.
S.C.C.: squamous cell carcinoma. kerat.: keratinizing. ques. str. invasion: questionable stromal invasion.

Treatment Method

Radiotherapy alone was the most common treatment method for the primary lesion (Table XII). Its use, however, decreased in later years from 29.5% to 24.0%. The three modality therapy (radiotherapy with surgery and chemotherapy) and radiotherapy plus chemotherapy also tended to decrease in percentage. Instead, the percentage of surgically treated cases increased markedly from 15.0% to 23.2%. The increase in percentage of cases classified as "Others" reflects the increase in those treated with a combination of surgery and chemotherapy.

TABLE IX. Subsite of Carcinoma of the Oral Cavity by Four-year Period

Subsite	1979–1983	1984–1987	1988–1991	Total
Lip	36 (1.8%)	28 (1.7%)	33 (1.5%)	97 (1.7%)
Buccal mucosa	155 (7.9)	128 (7.6)	182 (8.4)	465 (8.0)
Retromolar area	38 (1.9)	36 (2.1)	45 (2.1)	119 (2.0)
Gingiva	329 (16.7)	260 (15.4)	372 (17.2)	961 (16.5)
Hard palate	95 (4.8)	64 (3.8)	61 (2.8)	220 (3.8)
Floor of the mouth	232 (11.8)	248 (14.7)	315 (14.6)	795 (13.7)
Tongue	1,071 (54.5)	919 (54.5)	1,145 (53.1)	3,135 (54.0)
Oral cavity, NOS	9 (0.5)	2 (0.1)	4 (0.2)	15 (0.3)
Total	1,965 (100.0)	1,685 (100.0)	2,157 (100.0)	5,807 (100.0)

TABLE X. Subsite of Carcinoma of the Larynx by Four-year Period

Subsite	1979–1983	1984–1987	1988–1991	Total
Glottis	1,142 (61.2%)	995 (65.0%)	926 (59.3%)	3,063 (61.8%)
Supraglottis	570 (30.5)	472 (30.8)	444 (28.4)	1,486 (30.0)
Subglottis	36 (1.9)	33 (2.2)	31 (2.0)	100 (2.0)
Larynx, NOS	118 (6.3)	31 (2.0)	161 (10.3)	310 (6.3)
Total	1,866 (100.0)	1,531 (100.0)	1,562 (100.0)	4,959 (100.0)

TABLE XI. Percentage Distribution of Clinical Stage[a] by Four-year Period[b]

Period	No. of patients	Stage 0	Stage I	Stage II	Stage III	Stage IV
1979–1983	5,401 (100.0%)	0.2%	21.1%	20.6%	30.3%	27.8%
1984–1987	4,638 (100.0)	0.2	21.2	22.3	28.2	28.2
1988–1991	5,156 (100.0)	0.2	22.4	24.4	21.2	31.8
Total	15,195 (100.0)	0.2	21.6	22.4	26.5	29.3

[a] Clinical stage was determined according to the UICC TNM classification, 3rd ed. (1), for cases between 1979 and 1985, and according to the UICC TNM classification, 4th ed. (2), for cases between 1986 and 1991. Cases with carcinoma of the maxillary sinus between 1979 and 1985 were classified according to the TNM classification of the Japanese Joint Committee.
[b] Cases with insufficient information were omitted.

The treatment method for the primary lesion differed greatly among primary sites (Table XIII). The most common method for maxillary sinus carcinoma was the three modality therapy, used in 70.9% of the cases. Patients with nasopharyngeal and mesopharyngeal carcinomas were most frequently treated with radiotherapy alone or radiotherapy plus chemotherapy. The most common treatment modality in laryngeal cancer was radiotherapy, while it was surgery in oral cancer.

Patients with radical or conservative neck dissection later increased in percentage, while those without neck dissection or with enucleation only decreased (Table XIV). Neck dissection was performed most frequently in patients with hypopharyngeal carcinoma (Table XV).

The method of reconstruction changed dramatically during the study period (Table XVI). Although in 1981 microsurgical transfer of a free flap was performed in

TABLE XII. Treatment Method for the Primary Lesion by Four-year Period[a]

Treatment method	1979–1983	1984–1987	1988–1991	Total
No treatment	91 (1.5%)	92 (1.9%)	110 (2.0%)	293 (1.8%)
Rad. alone	1,755 (29.5)	1,188 (24.3)	1,345 (24.0)	4,288 (26.1)
Surg. alone	895 (15.0)	964 (19.7)	1,301 (23.2)	3,160 (19.2)
Preop. rad.	463 (7.8)	404 (8.3)	520 (9.3)	1,387 (8.4)
Postop. rad.	222 (3.7)	250 (5.1)	180 (3.2)	652 (4.0)
Preop. & postop. rad.	118 (2.0)	60 (1.2)	88 (1.6)	266 (1.6)
Rad. → salvage	214 (3.6)	120 (2.5)	103 (1.8)	437 (2.7)
Rad.+chem.+surg.	1,066 (17.9)	867 (17.7)	850 (15.1)	2,783 (16.9)
Rad.+chem.	762 (12.8)	618 (12.6)	575 (10.2)	1,955 (11.9)
Others	362 (6.1)	325 (6.6)	541 (9.6)	1,228 (7.5)
Total	5,948 (100.0)	4,888 (100.0)	5,613 (100.0)	16,449 (100.0)

Rad.: radiation. Surg.: surgery. Preop.: preoperative. Postop.: postoperative. Chem.: chemotherapy.
[a] Sixty-nine cases with insufficient information were omitted.

TABLE XIII. Treatment Method for the Primary Lesion by Primary Site[a]

Treatment method	Oral cavity	Larynx	Hypopharynx	Mesopharynx	Nasopharynx	Nasal cavity, etc.	Maxillary sinus	Total
No treatment	99	71	35	39	21	8	20	293
	(1.7%)	(1.4%)	(2.2%)	(2.8%)	(2.5%)	(3.1%)	(1.2%)	(1.8%)
Rad. alone	1,120	1,997	315	416	353	29	58	4,288
	(19.4)	(40.4)	(20.2)	(30.1)	(42.6)	(11.3)	(3.4)	(26.1)
Surg. alone	1,435	1,232	267	144	9	32	41	3,160
	(24.8)	(24.9)	(17.1)	(10.4)	(1.1)	(12.5)	(2.4)	(19.2)
Preop. rad.	634	326	237	117	6	18	49	1,387
	(11.0)	(6.6)	(15.2)	(8.5)	(0.7)	(7.0)	(2.9)	(8.4)
Postop. rad.	219	211	103	43	7	22	47	652
	(3.8)	(4.3)	(6.6)	(3.1)	(0.8)	(8.6)	(2.8)	(4.0)
Preop. & postop. rad.	66	46	33	26	7	12	76	266
	(1.1)	(2.3)	(2.1)	(1.9)	(0.8)	(4.7)	(4.5)	(1.6)
Rad. → salvage	131	194	44	42	3	6	17	437
	(2.3)	(3.9)	(2.8)	(3.0)	(0.4)	(2.3)	(1.0)	(2.7)
Rad.+chem.+surg.	869	279	190	156	20	66	1,203	2,783
	(15.0)	(5.6)	(12.2)	(11.3)	(2.4)	(25.8)	(70.9)	(16.9)
Rad.+chem.	574	385	208	285	352	36	115	1,955
	(9.9)	(7.8)	(13.3)	(20.7)	(42.5)	(14.1)	(6.8)	(11.9)
Others	641	198	129	112	51	27	70	1,228
	(11.1)	(4.0)	(8.3)	(8.1)	(6.2)	(10.5)	(4.1)	(7.5)
Total	5,788	4,939	1,561	1,380	829	256	1,696	16,449
	(100.0)	(100.0)	(100.0)	(100.0)	(100.0)	(100.0)	(100.0)	(100.0)

[a] Sixty-nine cases with insufficient information were omitted.

only five cases, it was the most common reconstructive method in 1991. In 1990 and 1991, free flap transfer was performed in 246 and 195 patients, respectively. The number of cases with vascularized bone graft also increased. Reconstructive surgery was performed most commonly in patients with carcinomas of the hypopharynx, oral cavity, and mesopharynx (Table XVII).

TABLE XIV. Neck Dissection by Four-year Period[a]

Period	No dissection	Radical N.D.	Conservative N.D.	Partial N.D.	Enucleation	Total
1979–1983	4,007 (67.8%)	1,247 (21.1%)	298 (5.0%)	227 (3.8%)	127 (2.2%)	5,906 (100.0%)
1984–1987	2,975 (60.9)	1,219 (25.0)	387 (7.9)	253 (5.2)	49 (1.0)	4,883 (100.0)
1988–1991	3,238 (58.6)	1,491 (27.0)	471 (8.5)	280 (5.1)	44 (0.8)	5,524 (100.0)
Total	10,220 (62.6)	3,957 (24.3)	1,156 (7.1)	760 (4.7)	220 (1.3)	16,313 (100.0)

N.D.: neck dissection.
[a] Two hundred and five cases with insufficient information were omitted.

TABLE XV. Neck Dissection by Primary Site[a]

Primary site	No dissection	Radical N.D.	Conservative N.D.	Partial N.D.	Enucleation	Total
Oral cavity	2,960 (51.4%)	1,827 (31.8%)	384 (6.7%)	478 (8.3%)	105 (1.8%)	5,754 (100.0%)
Larynx	3,453 (70.5)	777 (15.9)	503 (10.3)	123 (2.5)	40 (0.8)	4,896 (100.0)
Hypopharynx	603 (39.0)	713 (46.1)	160 (10.3)	53 (3.4)	17 (1.1)	1,546 (100.0)
Mesopharynx	818 (59.8)	431 (31.5)	51 (3.7)	49 (3.6)	18 (1.3)	1,367 (100.0)
Nasopharynx	735 (89.7)	50 (6.1)	16 (2.0)	6 (0.7)	12 (1.5)	819 (100.0)
Nasal cavity, etc.	224 (89.2)	15 (6.0)	5 (2.0)	4 (1.6)	3 (1.2)	251 (100.0)
Maxillary sinus	1,427 (84.9)	144 (8.6)	37 (2.2)	47 (2.8)	25 (1.5)	1,680 (100.0)
Total	10,220 (62.6)	3,957 (24.3)	1,156 (7.1)	760 (4.7)	220 (1.3)	16,313 (100.0)

[a] Two hundred and five cases with insufficient information were omitted.

TABLE XVI. Reconstructive Surgery by Year[a]

Year	No reconstruction	Pedicled flap (A)	Free flap (B)	Free bone graft (C)	Vascularized bone graft (D)	(A)+(B)	(A)+(C)	(B)+(C)	(B)+(D)	Others	Total
1981	1,113 (85.0%)	141 (10.8%)	5 (0.4%)	0 (0.0%)	0 (0.0%)	0 (0.0%)	0 (0.0%)	0 (0.0%)	0 (0.0%)	51 (3.9%)	1,310 (100.0%)
1982	969 (85.8)	98 (8.7)	5 (0.4)	0 (0.0)	0 (0.0)	0 (0.0)	0 (0.0)	0 (0.0)	0 (0.0)	57 (5.0)	1,129 (100.0)
1983	1,012 (81.7)	142 (11.5)	28 (2.3)	0 (0.0)	0 (0.0)	0 (0.0)	0 (0.0)	0 (0.0)	0 (0.0)	56 (4.5)	1,238 (100.0)
1984	902 (81.1)	103 (9.3)	28 (2.5)	0 (0.0)	0 (0.0)	0 (0.0)	0 (0.0)	0 (0.0)	0 (0.0)	79 (7.1)	1,112 (100.0)
1985	1,088 (80.5)	130 (9.6)	60 (4.4)	0 (0.0)	0 (0.0)	0 (0.0)	0 (0.0)	0 (0.0)	0 (0.0)	73 (5.4)	1,351 (100.0)
1986	1,047 (78.5)	127 (9.5)	68 (5.1)	0 (0.0)	0 (0.0)	0 (0.0)	0 (0.0)	0 (0.0)	0 (0.0)	92 (6.9)	1,334 (100.0)
1987	902 (82.8)	98 (9.0)	34 (3.1)	0 (0.0)	0 (0.0)	0 (0.0)	0 (0.0)	0 (0.0)	0 (0.0)	56 (5.1)	1,090 (100.0)
1988	987 (78.0)	97 (7.7)	82 (6.5)	26 (2.1)	4 (0.3)	14 (1.1)	1 (0.1)	2 (0.2)	0 (0.0)	52 (4.1)	1,265 (100.0)
1989	939 (72.0)	87 (6.7)	194 (14.9)	7 (0.5)	1 (0.1)	5 (0.4)	1 (0.1)	4 (0.3)	10 (0.8)	57 (4.4)	1,305 (100.0)
1990	1,109 (73.2)	109 (7.2)	218 (14.4)	10 (0.7)	6 (0.4)	6 (0.4)	5 (0.3)	5 (0.3)	11 (0.7)	35 (2.3)	1,514 (100.0)
1991	1,076 (74.9)	116 (8.1)	174 (12.1)	9 (0.6)	5 (0.3)	3 (0.2)	8 (0.6)	3 (0.2)	10 (0.7)	33 (2.3)	1,437 (100.0)
Total	11,144 (79.1)	1,248 (8.9)	896 (6.4)	52 (0.4)	16 (0.1)	28 (0.2)	15 (0.1)	14 (0.1)	31 (0.2)	641 (4.6)	14,085 (100.0)

Information on reconstructive surgery was not available for cases of 1979 and 1980.
[a] Cases with insufficient information were omitted.

TABLE XVII. Reconstructive Surgery by Primary Site[a]

Primary site	No reconstruction	Pedicled flap (A)	Free flap (B)	Free bone graft (C)	Vascularized bone graft (D)	(A)+(B)	(A)+(C)	(B)+(C)	(B)+(D)	Others	Total
Oral cavity	3,429 (69.1%)	651 (13.1%)	412 (8.3%)	35 (0.7%)	12 (0.2%)	10 (0.2%)	8 (0.2%)	6 (0.1%)	27 (0.5%)	370 (7.5%)	4,960 (100.0%)
Larynx	4,105 (96.1)	109 (2.6)	11 (0.3)	4 (0.1)	3 (0.1)	1 (0.0)	2 (0.0)	0 (0.0)	0 (0.0)	38 (0.9)	4,273 (100.0)
Hypopharynx	697 (49.6)	270 (19.2)	291 (20.7)	0 (0.0)	0 (0.0)	11 (0.8)	0 (0.0)	0 (0.0)	0 (0.0)	137 (9.7)	1,406 (100.0)
Mesopharynx	863 (73.1)	135 (11.4)	124 (10.5)	6 (0.5)	1 (0.1)	3 (0.3)	0 (0.0)	0 (0.0)	4 (0.3)	44 (3.7)	1,180 (100.0)
Nasopharynx	722 (99.3)	2 (0.3)	0 (0.0)	0 (0.0)	0 (0.0)	0 (0.0)	0 (0.0)	0 (0.0)	0 (0.0)	3 (0.4)	727 (100.0)
Nasal cavity, etc.	203 (87.1)	10 (4.3)	0 (0.0)	1 (0.4)	0 (0.0)	0 (0.0)	0 (0.0)	0 (0.0)	0 (0.0)	19 (8.2)	233 (100.0)
Maxillary sinus	1,125 (86.1)	71 (5.4)	58 (4.4)	6 (0.5)	0 (0.0)	3 (0.2)	5 (0.4)	8 (0.6)	0 (0.0)	30 (2.3)	1,306 (100.0)
Total	11,144 (79.1)	1,248 (8.9)	896 (6.4)	52 (0.4)	16 (0.1)	28 (0.2)	15 (0.1)	14 (0.1)	31 (0.2)	641 (4.6)	14,085 (100.0)

[a] Cases with insufficient information were omitted.

TABLE XVIII. Cumulative Survival Rate by Clinical Stage[a,b]

Stage	No. of patients	Years				
		1	2	3	4	5
0	276	93.1%	81.6%	76.2%	72.6%	69.6%
I	2,011	98.0	93.3	90.9	88.8	86.5
II	2,146	95.4	86.3	81.8	80.2	77.4
III	2,953	90.5	79.3	74.2	71.0	69.2
IV	3,059	83.9	67.3	62.2	59.7	57.7

[a] Clinical stage was determined according to the UICC TNM classification, 3rd ed. (1), for cases between 1979 and 1985, and according to the UICC TNM classification, 4th ed. (2), for cases between 1986 and 1991. Cases with carcinoma of the maxillary sinus between 1979 and 1985 were classified according to the TNM classification of the Japanese Joint Committee.
[b] Cases with insufficient information were omitted.

TABLE XIX. Cumulative Survival Rate by Primary Site[a]

Primary site	No. of patients	Years				
		1	2	3	4	5
Oral cavity	3,496	90.9%	78.7%	74.8%	72.8%	70.5%
Larynx	3,171	96.5	89.5	85.3	82.5	80.1
Hypopharynx	935	82.0	67.5	62.8	60.3	58.9
Mesopharynx	839	88.6	74.3	69.8	66.8	65.1
Nasopharynx	543	88.9	77.4	72.2	69.2	64.9
Nasal cavity, etc.	166	87.8	83.4	79.5	76.7	76.0
Maxillary sinus	1,295	88.0	73.9	67.8	65.1	63.7

[a] Cases with insufficient information were omitted.

Survival

Tables XVIII and XIX indicate cumulative survival rates of the registered cases by clinical stage and by primary site, respectively. The five-year survival rates shown in these tables are higher than reported figures by 10% to 20%. For example, the reported five-year survival rate for hypopharyngeal carcinoma is about 35%, while that indicated in Table XIX is 58.9%. This is presumably explained by insufficient follow-up of the registered cases. As many as 59.7% of all cases were followed up less than five years. The rates shown in Tables XVIII and XIX need further confirmation.

Acknowledgment

This registry has been supported by grants-in-aid for cancer research from the Ministry of Health and Welfare, Japan.

REFERENCES

1. Harmer, M.H. "International Union Against Cancer; TNM Classification of Malignant Tumours, 3rd ed.," (1978). International Union Against Cancer, Geneva.
2. Hermanek, P. and Sobin, L.H. "International Union Against Cancer; TNM Classification of Malignant Tumors, 4th ed.," (1987). Springer-Verlag, Berlin.
3. Ono, I. Early detection of head and neck cancer. *KARKINOS*, 2(2), 221–226 (1989) (in Japanese).
4. Ono, I. An evaluation of surgical treatment of head and neck cancer. *KARKINOS*, 1(2), 27–33 (1988) (in Japanese).
5. Ono, I. The TNM classification of head and neck cancer (in Japanese). *In* "The Latest Therapy for Head and Neck Cancer," ed. M. Hirano, pp. 10–20 (1987). Igaku Kyoiku Shuppan Co. Ltd., Tokyo.

CARCINOMA OF THE MAJOR SALIVARY GLANDS

The Japanese Joint Committee on TNM Classification, the Head
and Neck Subcommittee, the Salivary Gland Division*

Between 1958 and 1993, a total of 1,898 patients with carcinoma of major salivary glands were documented by the Salivary Gland Division of the Head and Neck Subcommittee of the Japanese Joint Committee on TNM Classification. There were 1,106 males and 792 females, ranging in age from 3 to 95 years. The tumor arose in the parotid gland in 1,461 patients (77.0%), whereas 371 (19.5%) and 66 (3.5%) had submandibular or sublingual gland primary tumors, respectively. In the parotid gland carcinoma, the occurrence of facial nerve paralysis was about 30%. For patients with carcinoma of the parotid gland, the 5- and 10-year survival rates were 60.4% and 50.2%, respectively. With regard to primary site, the parotid gland had the best survival rate among the major salivary glands.

Malignant tumors of the major salivary glands are rare and account for just 6% of all head and neck cancers (15). Parotid tumors account for 73% of all salivary gland neoplasms, of which 15% are malignant (5). Between 1958 and 1993, a total of 1898 patients with carcinoma of major salivary glands were documented by the Salivary Gland Division of the Head and Neck Subcommittee of the Japanese Joint Committee on TNM Classification. Data were collected from Japanese university hospitals and cancer center hospitals.

Data Collection

A recordable case was defined as one that had no previous tumor-directed treatment or surgical intervention other than biopsy for a histologically confirmed carcinoma of the salivary gland. For each patient, information was taken on age, sex, histologic diagnosis (by ICD-O morphology code), TNM classification (UICC 1987, Geneva), physical findings, first definitive treatment, and follow-up findings.

Basic Data on Registered Patients

During the 1958–1993 period registration was made of 1,106 males and 792 females, ranging in age from 3 to 95 years. The tumor arose in the parotid gland in 1,461 patients (77.0%), whereas 371 (19.5%) and 66 (3.5%) had submandibular or

---

* Manuscript was prepared by Takeshi Hino, Haruhiko Suzuki, Tsutomu Numata, Minoru Nomoto, and Akiyosi Konno, Department of Otorhinolaryngology, School of Medicine, Chiba University, 1-8-1 Inohana, Chuo-ku, Chiba 280, Japan

TABLE I. Distribution of Site of Origin According to Sex

	Male	Female	Total
Parotid gland	867	594	1,461
Submandibular gland	210	161	371
Sublingual gland	29	37	66
Total	1,106	792	1,898

TABLE II. Distribution of Histologic Types According to Sex and Site of Origin

	PG		SMG		SLG	
	Male	Female	Male	Female	Male	Female
Squamous cell carcinoma	145	40	26	11	1	1
Adenoid cystic carcinoma	106	136	60	81	17	25
Acinic cell carcinoma	28	48	5	4	1	0
Adenocarcinoma	250	105	53	13	4	4
Mucoepidermoid carcinoma	177	147	30	26	4	7
Mixed tumor, malignant	76	76	17	16	1	0
Carcinoma, undifferentiated type	41	32	13	7	0	0
Carcinoma	22	9	5	3	0	0
Neoplasm, malignant	2	1	1	0	1	0
Total	867	594	210	161	29	37

PG: parotid gland, SMG: submandibular gland, SLG: sublingual gland.

TABLE III. Distribution of Histologic Types According to Facial Nerve Paralysis in Patients with Carcinoma of the Parotid Gland

	FNP + (%)	FNP − (%)	Total
Squamous cell carcinoma	71 (37)	114 (63)	185
Adenoid cystic carcinoma	65 (27)	177 (73)	242
Acinic cell carcinoma	12 (16)	64 (84)	76
Adenocarcinoma	134 (38)	221 (62)	355
Mucoepidermoid carcinoma	74 (23)	250 (77)	324
Mixed tumor, malignant	49 (28)	123 (72)	172
Carcinoma, undifferentiated type	27 (37)	46 (63)	73
Carcinoma	9 (29)	22 (71)	31
Neoplasm, malignant	1 (33)	2 (67)	3
Total	442 (30)	1,019 (70)	1,461

FNP: facial nerve paralysis.

sublingual gland primary tumors, respectively (Table I). Table II shows distribution of histologic types according to sex and site of origin. In patients with carcinoma of the parotid gland, adenocarcinoma was the most common histologic type (355 patients (24.3%)), followed by mucoepidermoid carcinoma (324 (22.2%)), adenoid cystic carcinoma (242 (16.6%)), squamous cell carcinoma (185 (12.7%)), malignant mixed tumor (152 (10.4%)), acinic cell carcinoma (76 (5.2%)), and undifferentiated carcinoma (73 (5.0%)). However, adenoid cystic carcinoma was the most common histologic type in the submandibular and sublingual gland tumors (141 (38.0%) and 42

(53.6%), respectively).

There is an intimate anatomical relationship between the parotid gland and facial nerve. Facial nerve paralysis is extremely rare in benign parotid gland lesions, while it is a rather common symptom in malignant tumors (11). Table III shows distribution of histologic types according to facial nerve paralysis in the parotid gland carcinoma. In patients with adenocarcinoma, epidermoid carcinoma, or undifferentiated carcinoma, the occurrence of facial nerve paralysis was about 40%.

Clinical Stage and Pathological Stage

Tables IV and V show TNM classification and stage grouping (UICC 1987, Geneva), respectively. When patients with carcinoma of the parotid gland were staged according to this criteria, 304 (20.8%), 436 (29.8%), 327 (22.4%), and 394 (27.0%) had stages I to IV of the disease, respectively (Table VI). In submandibular gland carcinoma, 143 out of 371 patients were stage IV (38.5%), and in sublingual gland carcinoma, 27 out of 66 were stage II (40.9%).

Tables VII–IX show T and N status. The incidence of regional lymph node involvement was higher in patients with carcinoma of the submandibular gland than in those with the parotid and sublingual gland carcinoma.

Table X demonstrates distribution of primary sites according to M status.

TABLE IV. TNM Clinical Classification

T-primary tumor:
TX Primary tumor cannot be assessed
T0 No evidence of primary tumor
T1 Tumor 2 cm or less in greatest dimension
T2 Tumor more than 2 cm but not more than 4 cm in greatest dimension
T3 Tumor more than 4 cm but not more than 6 cm in greatest dimension
T4 Tumor more than 6 cm in greatest dimension
Note: all categories are subdivided: (a) no local extension, (b) local extension. Local extension is clinical or macroscopic evidence of invasion of skin, soft tissues, bone, or nerve. Microscopic evidence alone is not local extension for classification purposes.

N-regional lymph nodes:
NX Regional lymph nodes cannot be assessed
N0 No regional lymph node metastasis
N1 Metastasis in a single ipsilateral lymph node, 3 cm or less in greatest dimension
N2 Metastasis in a single ipsilateral lymph node, more than 3 cm but not more than 6 cm in greatest dimension, or in multiple ipsilateral lymph nodes, none more than 6 cm in greatest dimension, or in bilateral or contralateral lymph nodes, none more than 6 cm in greatest dimension
   N2a Metastasis in a single ipsilateral lymph node, more than 3 cm but not more than 6 cm in greatest dimension
   N2b Metastasis in multiple ipsilateral lymph nodes, none more than 6 cm in greatest dimension
   N2c Metastasis in bilateral or contralateral lymph nodes, none more than 6 cm in greatest dimension
N3 Metastasis in a lymph node more than 6 cm in greatest dimension
Note: midline nodes are considered ipsilateral nodes.

M-distant metastasis:
MX Presence of distant metastasis cannot be assessed
M0 No distant metastasis
M1 Distant metastasis

TABLE V. Stage Grouping

Stage	I	T1a	N0	M0
		T2a	N0	M0
Stage	II	T1b	N0	M0
		T2b	N0	M0
		T3a	N0	M0
Stage	III	T3b	N0	M0
		T4a	N0	M0
		Any T (except T4a)	N1	M0
Stage	IV	T4b	Any N	M0
		Any T	N2, N3	M0
		Any T	Any N	M1

TABLE VI. Distribution of Stage According to Primary Site

Stage	PG	SMG	SLG	Total
I	304	74	18	394
II	436	77	27	540
III	327	77	10	414
IV	394	143	11	548
Total	1,461	391	66	1,898

TABLE VII. T and N Status (Parotid Gland Carcinoma)

	N0	N1	N2a	N2b	N2c	N3	Total
T1a	87	2	0	3	0	0	92
T1b	60	6	2	6	0	0	74
T2a	216	8	0	9	1	0	234
T2b	283	27	2	66	0	1	379
T3a	98	4	3	6	0	0	111
T3b	245	36	3	56	2	2	344
T4a	21	1	0	1	0	0	23
T4b	114	28	3	52	4	3	204
Total	1,124	112	13	199	7	6	1,461

TABLE VIII. T and N Status (Submandibular Gland Carcinoma)

	N0	N1	N2a	N2b	N2c	N3	Total
T1a	18	3	1	2	0	0	24
T1b	7	0	0	3	0	1	11
T2a	60	11	1	9	4	0	85
T2b	39	18	0	19	0	0	76
T3a	33	1	1	5	1	0	41
T3b	36	8	3	19	2	1	69
T4a	8	0	1	2	0	0	11
T4b	25	8	0	13	4	4	54
Total	226	49	7	72	11	6	371

TABLE IX. T and N Status (Sublingual Gland Carcinoma)

	N0	N1	N2a	N2b	N2c	N3	Total
T1a	7	1	0	0	0	0	8
T1b	6	0	0	0	0	0	6
T2a	11	0	0	3	1	0	15
T2b	19	2	0	3	1	0	25
T3a	4	0	0	0	0	0	4
T3b	6	1	0	0	0	0	7
T4a	0	0	0	0	0	0	0
T4b	1	0	0	0	0	0	1
Total	54	4	0	6	2	0	66

TABLE X. Distribution of Histologic Types According to Distant Metastasis

	PG		SMG		SLG	
	M0	M1	M0	M1	M0	M1
Squamous cell carcinoma	171	14	32	5	2	0
Adenoid cystic carcinoma	235	7	128	13	39	3
Acinic cell carcinoma	73	3	9	0	1	0
Adenocarcinoma	333	22	63	9	8	0
Mucoepidermoid carcinoma	321	3	53	5	11	0
Mixed tumor, malignant	165	7	34	7	1	0
Carcinoma, undifferentiated type	68	5	19	1	0	0
Carcinoma	30	1	6	2	0	0
Neoplasm, malignant	3	0	1	0	1	0

Survival

The 5- and 10-year survival rates were calculated by the life table method. Figure 1 shows survival curves for the three sites of primary tumor. For patients with carci-

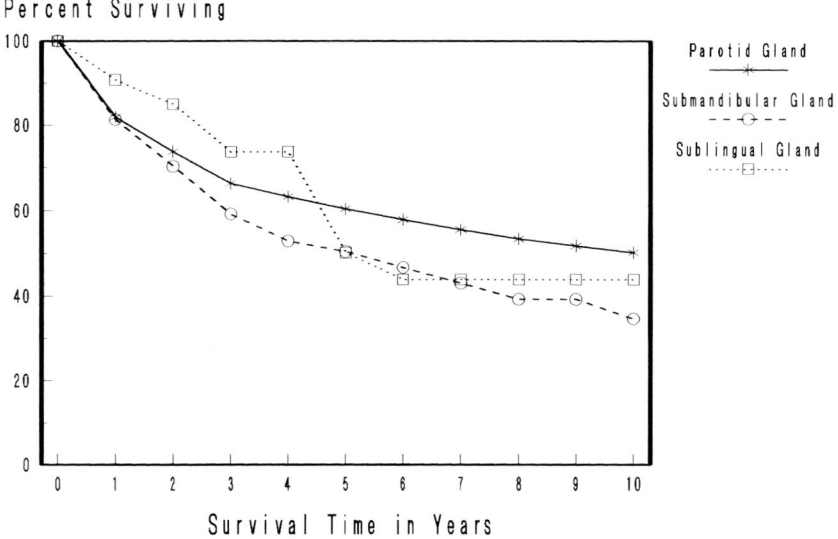

FIG. 1. Survival curves for the three sites of primary tumors

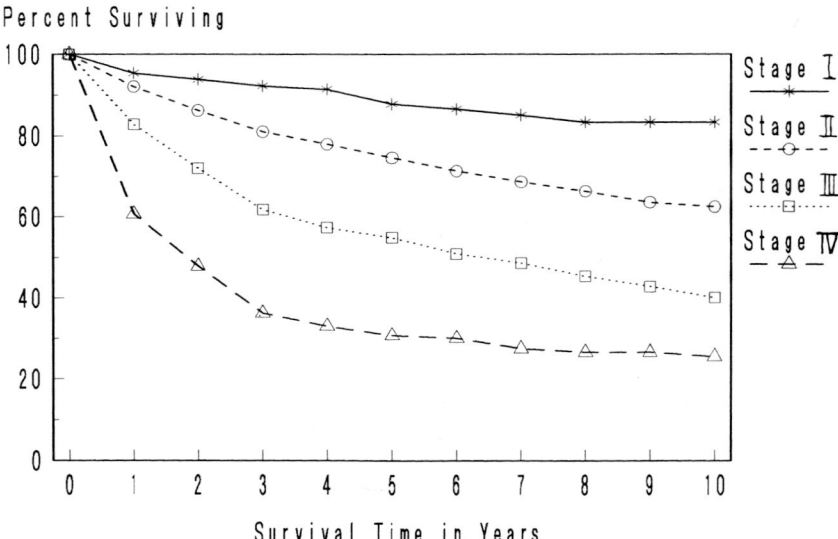

Fig. 2. Survival curves by staging system for carcinoma of the parotid gland

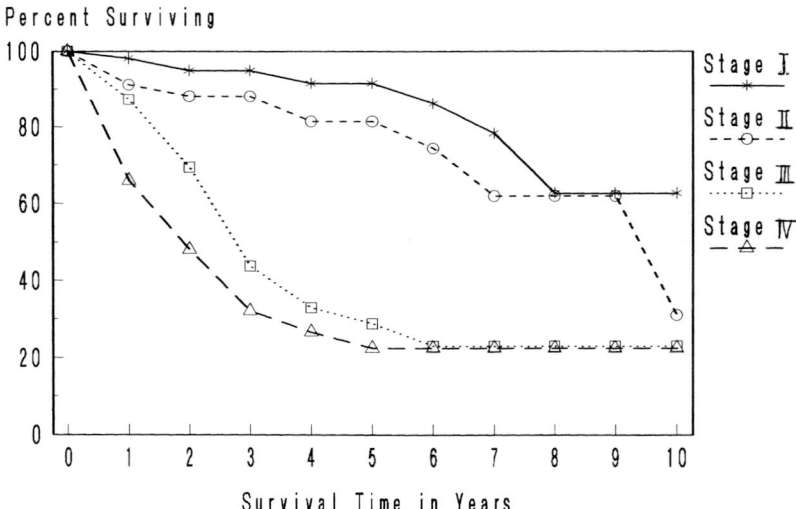

Fig. 3. Survival curves by staging system for carcinoma of the submandibular gland

noma of the parotid gland, the 5- and 10-year survival rates were 60.4% and 50.2%, respectively, for those with carcinoma of the submandibular gland, the survival rates were 50.4% and 34.6%, and for those with the sublingual gland, the survival rates were 50.1% and 43.8%. With regard to primary site, the parotid gland had the best survival rate among the major salivary glands. Figures 2 and 3 demonstrate the relationship between stage and survival for patients with parotid and submandibular gland carcinoma. A survival gradient from stage to stage is evident in the parotid gland carcinoma, while in submandibular gland carcinoma the gradient is not as

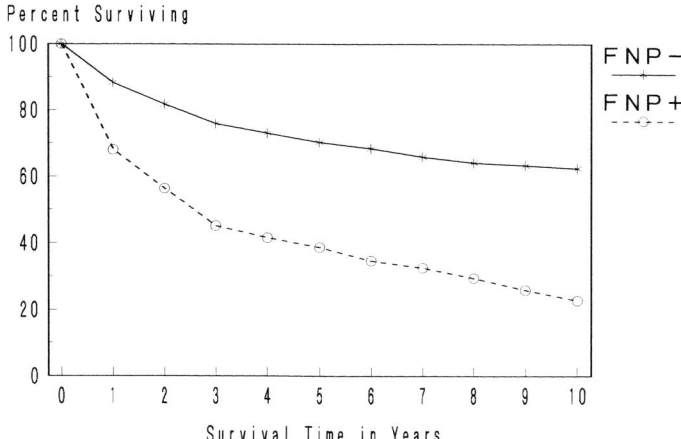

FIG. 4. Survival curves for the two groups of facial nerve paralysis for carcinoma of the parotid gland

TABLE XI. The Relationship of Histology to Survival in Parotid and Submandibular Gland Carcinoma

	PG		SMG	
	5 y (%)	10 y (%)	5 y (%)	10 y (%)
Squamous cell carcinoma	40.8	20.4	28.1	0
Adenoid cystic carcinoma	70.3	57.9	67.1	35.4
Acinic cell carcinoma	82.9	75.2	Low	Low
Adenocarcinoma	51.2	40.4	39.1	32.6
Mucoepidermoid carcinoma	73.2	66.9	28.6	22.3
Mixed tumor, malignant	63.8	58.6	53.6	53.6
Carcinoma, undifferentiated type	36.1	28.7	34.1	Rare

y: years.

good. As the number of cases with sublingual gland carcinoma was small, the relationship of stage to survival was not analyzed. Figure 4 indicates the relationship between facial nerve paralysis and survival in patients with parotid gland carcinoma. Survival was poor in those who presented facial nerve paralysis. The relationship of histology to the 5- and 10-year survivals is shown in Table XI. Survivals of squamous cell carcinoma, adenocarcinoma, and undifferentiated carcinoma were poor compared with those of other histologic types except mucoepidermoid carcinoma of submandibular gland carcinoma.

Acknowledgment

We are grateful to all the participating institutes that allow us to analyze their cases.

REFERENCES

1. Armstrong, J.G., Harrison, L.B., Spiro, R.H., Fass, D.E., Strong, E.W., and Fuks, Z.Y. Malignant tumors of major salivary gland origin. *Arch. Otolaryng. Head Neck Surg.*, **116**, 290–293 (1990).
2. Byers, R.M., Jesse, R.H., Guillamondegui, O.M., and Luna, M.A. Malignant tumors of the submaxillary gland. *Am. J. Surg.*, **126**, 458–463 (1973).
3. Conley, J., Myers, E., and Cole, R. Analysis of 115 patients with tumors of the submandibular gland. *Ann. Otol.*, **81**, 323–330 (1972).
4. Eneroth, C.M. Incidence and prognosis of salivary gland tumors at different sites: a study of parotid submandibular and palatal tumors in 2,632 patients. *Acta Otolaryng.*, **263**, 174–178 (1970).
5. Eveson, J.W. and Cawson, R.A. Salivary gland tumors: a review of 2,410 cases with particular reference to histological types, site, age and sex distribution. *J. Pathol.*, **146**, 51–58 (1985).
6. Friedman, M., Levin, B., Grybauskas, V., Strorigl, T., Manaligod, J., Hill, J.H., and Skolnik, E. Malignant tumors of the major salivary glands. *Otolaryng. Clin. North Am.*, **19**, 625–636 (1986).
7. Hayasaki, K., Kaneko, T., Suzuki, H., Ishige, T., and Sunami, S. A proposal of TNM classification system for cancer of the salivary gland — comprehensive retrospective study. *Otologia Fukuoka*, **31**, 1087–1090 (1985).
8. Ishige, T., Kaneko, T, Naitoh, J., and Hayasaki, K. TNM classification system for cancer of parotid gland — a comprehensive retrospective study of 1,004 primary cases. *J. Jpn. Soc. Somato-pharyng.*, **3**, 101–113 (1991).
9. Ishige, T., Kaneko, T., Konno, A., Naitoh, J., and Hayasaki, K. TNM classification system for cancer of the submandibular gland — a comprehensive retrospective study of 271 primary cases. *J. Otolaryng. Jpn.*, **95**, 32–40 (1992).
10. Ishige, T. and Kaneko, T. Carcinoma of major salivary glands: a study of parotid and submandibular gland carcinomas in 1,418 cases. *J. Jpn. Soc. Cancer Ther.*, **27**, 1890–1895 (1992).
11. Katoh, T., Ishige, T., Kasai, H., Naitoh, J., Kaneko, T., Kitamura, T., Nagao, K., and Matsuzaki, O. Malignant parotid gland tumors and facial nerve paralysis. *Arch. Otorhinolaryng.*, **240**, 139–144 (1984).
12. Levitt, S.H., McHugh, R.B., Gomez-Marin, O., Hyams, V.J., Soule, E.H., Strong, E.W., Sellers, A.H., Woods, J.E., and Guillamondegui, O.M. Clinical staging system for cancer of the salivary gland. *Cancer*, **47**, 2712–2724 (1981).
13. Reddy, S.P., Marks, J.E., and Hines, I.L. Treatment of locally advanced, high grade, malignant tumors of major salivary glands. *Laryngoscope*, **98**, 450–454 (1988).
14. Spilo, R.H., Huvos, A.G., and Strong, E.W. Cancer of the parotid gland: a clinicopathological study of 288 primary cases. *Am. J. Surg.*, **130**, 452–459 (1975).
15. Spiro, R.H. Salivary neoplasms: overview of a 35-year experience with 2,807 patients. *Head Neck Surg.*, **8**, 177–184 (1986).
16. Spiro, R.H., Armstrong, J., Harrison, L., Geller, N.L., Lin, S.Y., and Strong, E.W. Carcinoma of major salivary glands: recent trends. *Arch. Otolaryng. Head Neck Surg.*, **115**, 316–321 (1989).
17. Weber, R.S., Byers, R.M., Petit, B., Wolf, P., Ang, K., and Luna, M. Submandibular gland tumors. *Arch. Otolaryng. Head Neck Surg.*, **116**, 1055–1060 (1990).
18. Wyatt, M.G., Coleman, N., Eveson, J.W., and Webb, A.J. Management of high grade parotid carcinomas. *Br. J. Surg.*, **76**, 1275–1277 (1988).

THYROID CANCER REGISTRY

Japan Society of Thyroid Surgery*

The Japan Society of Thyroid Surgery implemented a nationwide registration of thyroid cancer cases in 1978. As of 1991 the registry had documented 19,446 patients treated between 1977 and that year in the member hospitals of the Society. Annually 1,500 to 2,000 cases were registered with the cooperation of about 75 hospitals, and the registry covered 28.4% of the estimated total number of thyroid cancer cases in Japan.

The female-to-male ratio of the registered cases was 6.07:1. The average age at first treatment was 48.8 years. Histologically, a high frequency of cases with papillary carcinoma (78.2%) was characteristic, with cases with follicular (14.0%) and anaplastic (1.9%) carcinomas being few in number. This discrepancy became larger in the later years. The peak of the age distribution was in the fifth and sixth decades with papillary, follicular, and medullary carcinomas, and in the seventh and eighth decades with anaplastic carcinoma, squamous cell carcinoma, and malignant lymphoma.

Clinical stage I cases were very frequent (46.4%) while stage IV cases were scarce (3.8%). The most common technique for diagnosis was palpation. Routine roentgenography of the neck and ultrasonography were also commonly used and 89.1% of the patients received a radical treatment for thyroid carcinoma. The five-year and ten-year cumulative survival rates were 91.5% and 86.3%, respectively. The five-year survival rate of stage IV cases was especially low (31.8%). Although the five-year survival rates of differentiated carcinomas were high (94.7% for papillary carcinoma and 93.4% for follicular carcinoma), that of anaplastic carcinoma was only 13.0%.

In 1976, the Japan Society of Thyroid Surgery formed the Thyroid Cancer Registration Committee with the charge of establishing a nationwide registry of thyroid carcinoma. The first registration took place in 1978 with the cooperation of 91 major Japanese hospitals offering thyroid cancer treatment, and 1,105 entries were recorded of patients treated in the year 1977.

Since that time the registration has continued annually, and at present the registry contains 15 years of data with 19,446 thyroid cancer patients registered. This registry has greatly contributed to the study of thyroid carcinoma in Japan, and several articles (*1–3, 9*) have been published based on the data contained.

---

* Manuscript was prepared by Masahisa Saikawa, Department of Surgical Oncology, National Cancer Center Hospital, 5-1-1 Tsukiji, Chuo-ku, Tokyo 104, Japan

Data Collection

Because the incidence of occult thyroid carcinoma is very high in Japan (*4*), there are a large number of patients whose thyroid cancer is discovered only at autopsy. Patients who are monitored a long time before their first treatment are also very common. To avoid confusion and to enhance the accuracy of the data, registration is restricted to patients with new clinical thyroid carcinoma which has been confirmed pathologically; thyroid cancers detected incidentally at autopsy have not been included. A patient is entered in the registry in the year of his/her first treatment rather than in the year of his/her first clinical consultation.

Each year the secretariat of the Japan Society of Thyroid Surgery sends registration forms to member hospitals of the Society, which are major Japanese hospitals for thyroid cancer treatment. The physicians in these hospitals complete the forms according to the General Rules for the Description of Thyroid Cancer, 4th edition (*8*), prepared and issued by the Japan Society of Thyroid Surgery. The first edition of the General Rules was based on the TNM (*7*) and World Health Organization (WHO) (*5*) classifications and several modifications have been made to describe each type of cancer more precisely. The completed registration forms are collected in the National Cancer Center, where each entry is checked by assistants and filed in a computerized form.

Pathological diagnoses made in individual hospitals are accepted without additional review. When a patient has more than one histologic type of thyroid carcinoma, the two dominant histologic types are registered.

Each year histological distribution of registered thyroid cancers, age and gender distribution by histologic type, and the TNM classification by histologic type are analyzed. The results are distributed to members of the Japan Society of Thyroid Surgery in an abstract volume at the annual meeting of the Society. A follow-up investigation on patients is performed every three years with the cooperation of the member hospitals.

A researcher can employ data of this registry with permission from the Japan Society of Thyroid Surgery, and each member hospital is free to utilize its own entries.

Basic Data on Registered Patients

Table I shows the annual change in the number of registered patients and participating hospitals. Although the number of hospitals has varied over the years (from 51 to 91), the number of registered patients has gradually increased. When compared with an estimated number of thyroid cancer cases calculated on the basis of overall cancer incidence in Japan between 1984 and 1988, the registered cases accounted for 28.4% of the latter. The average female-to-male ratio (F/M ratio) over the 15 year period was 6.07:1 (Table II), and tended to increase in later years.

The average age at first treatment was 48.8 years with a standard error of 14.7 years. The median was 49 years. The first treatment occurred most often in the sixth decade in males and in the fifth decade in females (Table III). The F/M ratio exceeded 6.00:1 from the third to sixth decades, although it was lower than that in the younger and older generations.

TABLE I. Number of Registered Patients and Participating Hospitals by Registration Year

Year	Number of registered patients	Number of participating hospitals
1977	1,105	91
1978	841	57
1979	857	51
1980	1,069	52
1981	1,143	69
1982	1,079	57
1983	1,175	56
1984	1,072	57
1985	1,233	69
1986	1,384	71
1987	1,528	74
1988	1,549	82
1989	1,471	75
1990	1,935	65
1991	2,005	76
Total	19,446	

TABLE II. Distribution of Gender by Registration Year[a]

Year	Male	Female	Total	F/M ratio
1977	163	942	1,105	5.78:1
1978	137	704	841	5.14:1
1979	131	726	857	5.54:1
1980	169	898	1,067	5.31:1
1981	163	980	1,143	6.01:1
1982	166	911	1,077	5.49:1
1983	162	1,013	1,175	6.25:1
1984	143	928	1,071	6.49:1
1985	168	1,065	1,233	6.34:1
1986	207	1,177	1,384	5.69:1
1987	220	1,308	1,528	5.95:1
1988	209	1,339	1,548	6.41:1
1989	216	1,255	1,471	5.81:1
1990	258	1,677	1,935	6.50:1
1991	239	1,766	2,005	7.39:1
Total	2,751	16,689	19,440	6.07:1

[a] Six cases of unknown gender were omitted.

Table IV indicates the change of age at first treatment by 5-year period. The percentage of patients in the third and fourth decades decreased while that of older patients increased. During the period between 1987 and 1991, 125 patients received their first treatment for thyroid carcinoma at the age of 80 or over.

Histology

Table V summarizes histological distribution of the registered cases. For patients with more than one histologic type, only the most predominant type is indicated.

A high frequency of cases with papillary carcinoma and few with follicular

TABLE III. Distribution of Age at Treatment by Gender[a]

Age[b]	Male	Female	Total	F/M ratio
0–9	6	7	13	1.17:1
10–19	64	305	369	4.77:1
20–29	217	1,382	1,599	6.37:1
30–39	414	3,024	3,438	7.30:1
40–49	529	4,077	4,606	7.71:1
50–59	609	3,942	4,551	6.47:1
60–69	556	2,524	3,080	4.54:1
70–79	282	1,180	1,462	4.18:1
80–89	50	179	229	3.58:1
90–	0	5	5	—
Total	2,727	16,625	19,352	6.07:1

[a] Ninety-four cases whose gender or age at treatment was unknown were omitted.
[b] Age at time of first treatment.

TABLE IV. Distribution of Age at Treatment by 5-Year Period[a]

Age[b]	1977–1981	1982–1986	1987–1991	Total
0–9	5 (0.1%)	2 (0.0%)	6 (0.1%)	13 (0.0%)
10–19	89 (1.8)	116 (2.0)	164 (1.9)	369 (1.9)
20–29	538 (10.8)	438 (7.4)	623 (7.4)	1,599 (8.3)
30–39	1,025 (20.6)	1,127 (19.1)	1,287 (15.2)	3,439 (17.8)
40–49	1,175 (23.7)	1,368 (23.2)	2,063 (24.3)	4,606 (23.8)
50–59	990 (19.9)	1,440 (24.3)	2,122 (25.0)	4,552 (23.5)
60–69	767 (15.4)	871 (14.7)	1,442 (17.0)	3,080 (15.9)
70–79	344 (6.9)	480 (8.1)	640 (7.6)	1,464 (7.6)
80–89	41 (0.8)	65 (1.1)	123 (1.5)	229 (1.2)
90–	0 (0.0)	3 (0.1)	2 (0.0)	5 (0.0)
Total	4,974 (100.0)	5,910 (100.0)	8,472 (100.0)	19,356 (100.0)

[a] Ninety cases whose age at treatment was unknown were omitted.
[b] Age at time of first treatment.

TABLE V. Histological Distribution of Registered Cases

Histologic type	No. of cases
Papillary carcinoma	15,196 (78.2%)
Follicular carcinoma	2,721 (14.0)
Medullary carcinoma	258 (1.3)
Anaplastic carcinoma	378 (1.9)
Squamous cell carcinoma	51 (0.3)
Malignant lymphoma, NOS	373 (1.9)
Others	469 (2.4)
Neoplasm, malignant	28 (0.1)
Carcinoma, NOS	241 (1.3)
Adenocarcinoma, NOS	182 (0.9)
Adenoid cystic carcinoma	10 (0.1)
Chromophobe carcinoma	6 (0.0)
Plasmacytoma, NOS	2 (0.0)
Total	19,446 (100.0)

NOS: not otherwise specified.

TABLE VI. Annual Change in Histological Distribution

Year	Papillary carcinoma	Follicular carcinoma	Medullary carcinoma	Anaplastic carcinoma	Squamous cell ca.	Malignant lymphoma	Others	Total
1977	829 (75.1%)	208 (18.8%)	20 (1.8%)	29 (2.6%)	1 (0.1%)	12 (1.1%)	6 (0.5%)	1,105 (100.0%)
1978	650 (77.4)	138 (16.4)	12 (1.4)	27 (3.2)	1 (0.1)	12 (1.4)	1 (0.1)	841 (100.0)
1979	620 (72.4)	164 (19.1)	15 (1.8)	35 (4.1)	3 (0.3)	15 (1.7)	5 (0.6)	857 (100.0)
1980	820 (76.7)	165 (15.4)	14 (1.3)	42 (3.9)	5 (0.5)	18 (1.7)	5 (0.5)	1,069 (100.0)
1981	892 (77.9)	187 (16.4)	24 (2.1)	20 (1.8)	6 (0.5)	11 (1.0)	3 (0.3)	1,143 (100.0)
1982	870 (80.5)	138 (12.8)	16 (1.5)	32 (3.0)	1 (0.1)	19 (1.8)	3 (0.3)	1,079 (100.0)
1983	929 (79.1)	174 (14.8)	13 (1.1)	25 (2.1)	7 (0.6)	21 (1.8)	6 (0.5)	1,175 (100.0)
1984	855 (79.8)	143 (13.3)	6 (0.6)	9 (0.8)	1 (0.1)	28 (2.6)	30 (2.8)	1,072 (100.0)
1985	896 (72.6)	252 (20.4)	17 (1.4)	17 (1.4)	1 (0.1)	26 (2.1)	24 (2.0)	1,233 (100.0)
1986	989 (71.4)	255 (18.4)	19 (1.4)	31 (2.2)	8 (0.6)	27 (2.0)	55 (4.0)	1,384 (100.0)
1987	1,174 (76.9)	231 (15.1)	26 (1.7)	22 (1.4)	2 (0.1)	36 (2.4)	37 (2.4)	1,528 (100.0)
1988	1,224 (79.0)	182 (11.8)	18 (1.2)	31 (2.0)	2 (0.1)	30 (1.9)	62 (4.0)	1,549 (100.0)
1989	1,194 (81.3)	155 (10.5)	16 (1.1)	21 (1.4)	6 (0.4)	27 (1.8)	52 (3.5)	1,471 (100.0)
1990	1,583 (81.8)	163 (8.4)	24 (1.2)	22 (1.1)	7 (0.4)	57 (3.0)	79 (4.1)	1,935 (100.0)
1991	1,671 (83.3)	166 (8.3)	18 (0.9)	15 (0.8)	0 (0.0)	34 (1.7)	101 (5.0)	2,005 (100.0)
Total	15,196 (78.2)	2,721 (14.0)	258 (1.3)	378 (1.9)	51 (0.3)	373 (1.9)	469 (2.4)	19,446 (100.0)

ca.: carcinoma.

TABLE VII. Histological Distribution by Gender[a]

Histologic type	Male	Female	Total	F/M ratio
Papillary carcinoma	1,999	13,194	15,193	6.60:1
Follicular carcinoma	394	2,326	2,720	5.90:1
Medullary carcinoma	67	191	258	2.85:1
Anaplastic carcinoma	113	264	377	2.34:1
Squamous cell carcinoma	18	33	51	1.83:1
Malignant lymphoma	97	275	372	2.84:1
Others	63	406	469	6.44:1
Total	2,751	16,689	19,940	6.07:1

[a] Six cases of unknown gender were omitted.

TABLE VIII. Histological Distribution by Age at Treatment[a]

Age[b]	Papillary carcinoma	Follicular carcinoma	Medullary carcinoma	Anaplastic carcinoma	Squamous cell ca.	Malignant lymphoma	Others	Total
0–9	11 (0.1%)	2 (0.1%)	0 (0.0%)	0 (0.0%)	0 (0.0%)	0 (0.0%)	0 (0.0%)	13 (0.0%)
10–19	284 (1.9)	60 (2.2)	13 (5.1)	0 (0.0)	0 (0.0)	0 (0.0)	12 (2.6)	369 (1.9)
20–29	1,309 (8.6)	204 (7.5)	29 (11.4)	7 (2.0)	0 (0.0)	3 (0.8)	47 (10.0)	1,599 (8.3)
30–39	2,802 (18.5)	493 (18.2)	43 (16.9)	5 (1.4)	1 (2.0)	4 (1.1)	91 (19.4)	3,439 (17.8)
40–49	3,754 (24.7)	638 (23.5)	63 (24.6)	22 (6.3)	3 (6.0)	30 (8.4)	96 (20.5)	4,606 (23.8)
50–59	3,595 (23.7)	622 (23.0)	58 (22.8)	54 (15.4)	11 (22.0)	65 (18.1)	147 (31.3)	4,552 (23.5)
60–69	2,290 (15.1)	469 (17.3)	33 (12.9)	110 (31.4)	16 (32.0)	108 (30.1)	54 (11.5)	3,080 (15.9)
70–79	969 (6.4)	196 (7.2)	16 (6.3)	123 (35.2)	13 (26.0)	126 (35.1)	21 (4.5)	1,464 (7.6)
80–89	146 (1.0)	26 (1.0)	0 (0.0)	28 (8.0)	5 (10.0)	23 (6.4)	1 (0.2)	229 (1.2)
90–	3 (0.0)	0 (0.0)	0 (0.0)	1 (0.3)	1 (2.0)	0 (0.0)	0 (0.0)	5 (0.0)
Total	15,163 (100.0)	2,710 (100.0)	255 (100.0)	350 (100.0)	50 (100.0)	359 (100.0)	469 (100.0)	19,356 (100.0)

[a] Ninety cases whose age at treatment was unknown were omitted.
[b] Age at time of first treatment.

carcinoma and anaplastic carcinomas are very characteristic of this distribution. According to Ezaki et al. (3), there was a tendency for Japanese pathologists to diagnose a follicular variant of papillary carcinoma as follicular carcinoma and atypical adenoma also as follicular carcinoma. The marked difference in incidence between papillary and follicular carcinomas could have been much larger if a pathological review had been made for each entry. Ezaki et al. (3) state this high papillary to follicular (P/F) ratio is a pattern seen in iodine-rich areas.

Observation of the annual change in histological distribution (Table VI) shows the percentage of cases with papillary carcinoma increased in later years, while cases with follicular or anaplastic carcinoma decreased.

The F/M ratio was high in differentiated carcinomas (6.60:1 for papillary carcinoma and 5.90:1 for follicular carcinoma, Table VII).

Table VIII illustrates histological distribution by age at first treatment. Cases with papillary, follicular, and medullary carcinomas were treated most frequently in the fifth and sixth decades, while those with anaplastic carcinoma, squamous cell carcinoma, and malignant lymphoma in the seventh and eighth decades.

Clinical and Pathological Stages

The clinical and pathological stages of the registered patients are summarized in Tables IX and X, respectively. Both stages of each entry were reclassified according to the latest UICC TNM classification (6). Clinical stage I cases were very frequent (46.4%) while stage IV cases were scarce (3.8%). The same tendency was recognized with pathological stage. The percentage of stage IV cases decreased both clinically and pathologically in later years. The percentage of small carcinomas has not increased in spite of recent developments in diagnostic techniques.

TABLE IX. Percent Distribution of Clinical Stage[a] by 5-Year Period[b]

Period	No. of patients	Stage I	Stage II	Stage III	Stage IV
1977–1981	4,449 (100.0%)	46.4%	27.6%	20.7%	5.3%
1982–1986	5,165 (100.0)	46.0	31.5	18.9	3.6
1987–1991	7,189 (100.0)	46.4	34.2	16.3	3.1
Total	16,803 (100.0)	46.4	31.6	18.2	3.8

[a] Clinical stage according to the UICC TNM Classification, 4th ed. (6).
[b] Cases whose clinical stage was unknown were omitted.

TABLE X. Percent Distribution of Pathological Stage[a] by 5-Year Period[b]

Period	No. of patients	Stage I	Stage II	Stage III	Stage IV
1977–1981	4,411 (100.0%)	48.2%	15.5%	30.9%	5.4%
1982–1986	5,287 (100.0)	47.0	16.9	32.6	3.5
1987–1991	7,234 (100.0)	45.5	14.9	36.5	3.1
Total	16,932 (100.0)	46.7	15.7	33.8	3.8

[a] Pathological stage according to the UICC TNM Classification, 4th ed. (6).
[b] Cases whose pathological stage was unknown were omitted.

Methods of Diagnosis

Table XI shows the change in utilization of several diagnostic methods. The most frequently used technique for diagnosis is palpation (97.9%), although its false negative rate was not negligible (31.4%). Routine roentgenography of the neck and ultrasonography are also commonly employed. Ultrasonography has become very popular with improvement of the devices used. Fine-needle aspiration cytology had only begun to spread in Japan in the period between 1987 and 1989. Its low false negative rate (21.5%) is very impressive.

Table XI. Methods of Diagnosis and Their False Negative Rates[a]

Method of diagnosis		1977–1980	1981–1983	1984–1986	1987–1989
Palpation	% of pts.	98.5%	98.7%	98.5%	97.9%
	FNR	29.4	33.0	35.8	31.4
Routine x-ray	% of pts.	46.6	79.2	90.9	92.3
	FNR	39.4	43.6	46.9	44.9
CT scan	% of pts.	83.3	63.0	34.3	39.5
	FNR	47.0	56.7	45.2	19.6
Fine-needle aspiration cytology	% of pts.	2.3	0.8	3.2	54.0
	FNR	19.7	16.7	28.3	21.5
Lymphography	% of pts.	9.0	6.2	4.3	2.1
	FNR	20.8	31.7	40.8	30.7
Radionuclide scanning	% of pts.	87.0	80.6	74.8	70.2
	FNR	28.0	35.3	41.0	38.0
Ultrasonography	% of pts.	49.0	68.8	83.5	89.4
	FNR	32.5	31.2	32.9	29.5

% of pts.: percentage of patients who underwent the particular diagnostic method.
FNR: false negative rate.
[a] Information on diagnostic methods for patients treated in 1990 and 1991 was not available.

Table XII. Percentage of Radically Treated Patients by 5-Year Period[a]

Period	No. of patients	Radical	Palliative
1977–1981	4,762 (100.0%)	86.3%	13.7%
1982–1986	5,588 (100.0)	89.0	11.0
1987–1991	8,152 (100.0)	90.8	9.2
Total	18,502 (100.0)	89.1	10.9

[a] Cases with insufficient information were omitted.

Table XIII. Operative Method for Primary Site by 5-Year Period[a]

Operative method	1977–1981	1982–1986	1987–1991	Total
Total thyroidectomy	661 (13.3%)	1,114 (18.8%)	1,934 (22.8%)	3,709 (19.1%)
Subtotal thyroidectomy	1,261 (25.3)	1,869 (31.5)	2,938 (34.7)	6,068 (31.3)
Lobectomy	2,325 (46.6)	2,287 (38.5)	2,919 (34.5)	7,531 (38.9)
Thyroidectomy less than lobectomy	607 (12.2)	505 (8.5)	526 (6.2)	1,638 (8.4)
Other operation	11 (0.2)	22 (0.4)	37 (0.4)	70 (0.4)
No operation	120 (2.4)	137 (2.3)	120 (1.4)	377 (1.9)
Total	4,985 (100.0)	5,934 (100.0)	8,474 (100.0)	19,393 (100.0)

[a] Cases with insufficient information were omitted.

TABLE XIV. Neck Dissection by 5-Year Period[a]

Neck dissection	1977–1981	1982–1986	1987–1991	Total
Radical neck dissection	234 (4.8%)	356 (6.1%)	505 (6.0%)	1,095 (5.8%)
Functional neck dissection	1,924 (39.4)	2,710 (46.7)	4,597 (55.0)	9,231 (48.4)
Partial neck dissection	1,081 (22.2)	977 (16.9)	1,060 (12.7)	3,118 (16.4)
Enucleation	170 (3.5)	121 (2.1)	151 (1.8)	442 (2.3)
No neck dissection	1,469 (30.1)	1,634 (28.2)	2,052 (24.5)	5,155 (27.1)
Total	4,878 (100.0)	5,798 (100.0)	8,365 (100.0)	19,041 (100.0)

[a] Cases with insufficient information were omitted.

TABLE XV. Cumulative Survival Rate by Clinical Stage[a,b]

Stage	No. of patients	Years									
		1	2	3	4	5	6	7	8	9	10
All cases	12,557	96.1%	94.2%	93.5%	92.4%	91.5%	90.5%	89.5%	88.6%	87.4%	86.3%
I	5,052	99.9	99.2	99.2	98.9	98.6	98.5	98.2	97.6	96.9	96.2
II	3,608	98.9	97.9	96.4	95.3	94.5	92.7	91.1	90.8	89.2	85.4
III	1,930	95.3	92.0	90.5	88.4	86.9	85.5	84.9	82.6	80.7	80.7
IV	508	50.0	39.3	37.5	34.4	31.8	28.3	23.9	22.7	19.9	19.9

[a] Clinical stage according to the UICC TNM Classification, 4th ed. (6).
[b] Cases with insufficient information were omitted.

TABLE XVI. Cumulative Survival Rate by Pathological Stage[a,b]

Stage	No. of patients	Years									
		1	2	3	4	5	6	7	8	9	10
I	5,043	99.8%	99.2%	99.2%	98.7%	98.4%	98.3%	98.0%	97.6%	96.9%	96.2%
II	1,543	99.1	98.4	97.6	95.7	94.8	94.1	92.6	92.6	91.2	91.2
III	3,939	97.5	94.8	93.6	92.3	91.1	89.1	88.5	86.4	85.1	83.6
IV	508	50.0	39.3	37.5	34.4	31.8	28.3	23.9	22.7	19.9	19.9

[a] Pathological stage according to the UICC TNM Classification, 4th ed. (6).
[b] Cases with insufficient information were omitted.

TABLE XVII. Cumulative Survival Rate by Histologic Type[a]

Histologic type	No. of patients	Years									
		1	2	3	4	5	6	7	8	9	10
Papillary ca.	9,912	98.5%	97.1%	96.3%	95.4%	94.7%	93.7%	93.0%	92.0%	91.2%	90.2%
Follicular ca.	1,648	98.7	96.9	96.3	94.8	93.4	92.6	91.9	90.7	87.7	86.0
Medullary ca.	187	95.9	93.2	89.7	89.7	89.7	89.7	87.3	87.3	87.3	87.3
Anaplastic ca.	304	25.4	16.3	15.6	13.7	13.0	11.6	9.1	9.1	9.1	9.1
Squamous cell ca.	45	35.7	23.8	—	—	—	—	—	—	—	—
Malignant lymphoma	251	80.6	74.8	74.8	74.8	72.1	69.2	59.9	59.9	59.9	—
Others	210	96.6	94.3	94.3	84.9	72.8	72.8	72.8%	72.8	—	—

[a] Cases with insufficient information were omitted.

With a wider acceptance of ultrasonography and fine-needle aspiration cytology, radionuclide scanning of the thyroid, CT scan, and lymphography of the thyroid have become less frequently utilized. The lowest false negative rate seen in the 1987–1989 period with CT scan is probably explained by the narrower indication of this diagnostic method and the selection of patients to which it was applied.

Treatment

The percentage of thyroid carcinoma patients who were treated radically was very high (89.1%, Table XII); it increased slightly in later years, but did not change significantly throughout the observation period.

Tables XIII and XIV describe the change in operative methods for the primary lesion and neck, respectively. For both the extent of resection seems to have become greater in later years.

Cumulative Survival Rates

The five-year and ten-year cumulative survival rates for all registered cases were 91.5% and 86.3%, respectively (Table XV). These rates are probably the best for patients treated for any carcinoma.

The five-year survival rate worsened with higher clinical stage. That of stage IV cases was especially low (31.8%) compared with the earlier stages. The difference in survival curves by clinical stage was statistically significant ($p = 0.0001$) by the log-rank test.

The above facts regarding clinical stage were also applicable to pathological stage (Table XVI). Survival rates were significantly different among various histologic types (Table XVII). Although the five-year survival rates of differentiated carcinomas were high (94.7% for papillary carcinoma and 93.4% for follicular carcinoma), that of anaplastic carcinoma was only 13.0%. No patient with squamous cell carcinoma survived more than 2 years. The difference in survival curves according to histologic type was statistically significant ($p = 0.0001$) by the log-rank test.

Acknowledgment

This registry has been supported by grants-in-aid for cancer research from the Ministry of Health and Welfare, Tokyo, and the Chiyou Fund of Matsumoto, Japan.

REFERENCES

1. Ebihara, S. Prognostic factors in papillary and follicular carcinomas of the thyroid. *KARKINOS*, **6**(5), 473–479 (1993) (in Japanese).
2. Ebihara, S. Prognostic factors in papillary and follicular carcinomas of the thyroid. *J. Jpn. Soc. Head and Neck Surg.*, **1**, 89–93 (1991) (in Japanese).
3. Ezaki, H., Ebihara, S., Fujimoto, Y. *et al.* Analysis of thyroid carcinoma based on material registered in Japan during 1977–1986 with special reference to predominance of papillary type. *Cancer*, **70**(4), 806–814 (1992).
4. Fukunaga, F.H. and Yatani, R. Geographic pathology of occult carcinomas. *Cancer*, **36**, 1095–1099 (1975).
5. Hedinger, Chr. and Sobin, L.H. Histological typing of thyroid tumours. International

Histological Classification of Tumours No. 11. (1974). World Health Organization, Geneva.
6. Hermanek, P. and Sobin, L.H. "International Union Against Cancer; TNM Classification of Malignant Tumours, 4th ed.," (1987). Springer-Verlag, Berlin.
7. International Union Against Cancer. "TNM Classification of Malignant Tumours, 2nd ed.," (1974). International Union Against Cancer, Geneva.
8. Japan Society of Thyroid Surgery. "General Rules for the Description of Thyroid Cancer, 4th ed.," (1991). Kanehara Shuppan, Tokyo.
9. Katayama, S. and Kuma, K. Multi-institutional analysis of anaplastic carcinoma and malignant lymphoma of the thyroid in Japan. *Endocr. Surg.,* **6**, 167–179 (1989) (in Japanese).

STATISTICS OF ESOPHAGEAL CANCER REGISTRY

Japanese Committee for Registration of Esophageal Cancer,
Japanese Society for Esophageal Diseases*

The Esophageal Cancer Registry began in 1965, and the total number of patients registered was 21,402 (males 17,824 and females 3,578) up to 1986. pT3, pN1, and M0 tumors were most common. Histologically, well and moderately differentiated squamous cell carcinoma accounted for nearly 70% of the cases. Double primary cancer of the esophagus with another organ increased to 10% after 1981.

The five year survival rate of all registered cases was 15.3%, and that of all resected cases was 23.6%. The five year survival rate of Stage I was 64.2%, Stage IIA 40.9%, Stage IIB 28.1%, Stage III 18.5%, and Stage IV 5.4%. Ten year survival rate of all surgical cases was 18.6%.

The Japanese Society for Esophageal Diseases (JSDE) was established in 1965; "Guidelines for Clinical and Pathologic Studies on Carcinoma of the Esophagus" was first published by JSDE in April 1969, and was revised eight times during the subsequent 23 years (5). Patients with esophageal carcinoma in Japan have been recorded according to these guidelines. In October 1976, the Committee for Registration of Esophageal Cancer was started as a task force of the JSDE with the intention of recording and analyzing patients from as many Japanese institutions as possible. Patients going back to 1969 were registered retrospectively, and new patients added; twelve reports have been published to date.

Data Collection

Registration cards were prepared using the criteria classifications set forth in the JSDE guidelines. The information was easily accessible from many Japanese institutions, since it had been recorded according to the guidelines since 1969. TNM classification made by the International Union Against Cancer was used on the registration forms because it had been included in the guidelines. The completed registration forms were sent to the secretariat of the Task Force, located in the National Cancer Center Hospital, Tokyo. Each category was input on a HITAC M 16-H (Hitachi, Ltd., Tokyo) and checked for accuracy. Registered patients were followed up periodically, and survival rates were computed according to the life-table method of Cutler and Ederer (2) with the computer.

---

* Manuscript was prepared by Toshifumi Iizuka, Segi Clinic, 1-7-1 Iwamoto-cho, Chiyoda-ku, Tokyo 102, Japan and Hoichi Kato, Department of Surgery, National Cancer Center Hospital, 5-1-1 Tsukiji, Chuo-ku, Tokyo 104, Japan

Basic Data of Registered Patients

Number of resected patients among registered cases from 1969 to 1986 is shown in Table I. The number increased from 505 in 1969 to 2,006 in 1984. Age-sex-year specific estimated number of cancer incidence in Japan was 7,255 in 1984, 7,706 in 1985, and 8,063 in 1986. The ratio of registered patients to estimated total number was 27.6% in 1984, 24.8% in 1985, and 24.8% in 1986. Thus, about one-fourth to one-fifth of the patients were covered in the registration.

Age distribution is shown in Table II. Mean age gradually rose from 61.6 in 1969 to 63.7 in 1986. The age of females was slightly higher than males, but the difference was slight. Number of patients with double primary carcinoma increased from 17 in 1969 to 184 in 1986 (Table III), and the frequency of double primary carcinoma increased from 3.6% in 1969 to 12.6% in 1986. Tumor locations each year are shown in Table IV. Middle esophageal carcinoma was most common each year.

T-classification is classified into four classes according to the depth of invasion following the fourth edition of TNM classification. T1 indicates a tumor limited to mucosa and submucosa. The number of p-T1 cases increased from 6 in 1969 to 210 in 1986 (Table V).

Esophagoscopic examination, including iodine staining, aided the detection of many p-T1 cancers in Japan in recent years. Frequency of p-T1 cases in registered patients increased ten-fold from 1.2% in 1969 to 12.6% in 1986.

TABLE I. Number of Patients by Sex (2-Year Increments)

	1969–1971	1972–1974	1975–1977	1978–1980	1981–1983	1984–1986	Total
Both sexes	1,639	2,374	2,610	3,872	5,383	5,524	21,402
Male	1,354	1,930	2,157	3,193	4,484	4,696	17,824
Female	285	444	443	679	899	828	3,578

TABLE II. Age Distribution

Age	1969–1971			1972–1974			1975–1977		
	All	Male	Female	All	Male	Female	All	Male	Female
–29	0	0	0	0	0	0	1	0	1
30–34	4	3	1	3	1	2	3	3	0
35–39	12	9	3	23	17	6	11	8	3
40–44	46	39	7	61	55	6	59	49	10
45–49	91	75	16	143	121	22	165	142	23
50–54	146	118	28	224	172	52	254	213	23
55–59	290	237	53	365	286	79	347	290	57
60–64	400	334	66	529	444	85	515	433	82
65–69	359	298	61	489	405	84	563	467	96
70–74	200	163	37	348	277	71	428	356	72
75–79	67	58	9	150	121	29	195	154	41
80–84	19	17	2	33	29	4	59	47	12
85–89	4	2	2	6	2	4	10	5	5
90–	1	1	0	0	0	0	0	0	0
Total	1,639	1,354	285	2,374	1,930	444	2,610	2,167	443

Pathologically proved lymph node metastasis (p-N) is shown in Table VI. The frequency of metastasis negative lymph node was 36.4–45.2% in 1969 to 1986, and there was no difference between these years. Table VII shows the distribution of M0 and M1. Distribution of histologic type is shown in Table VIII, and there was no remarkable change in any histologic type during the 18 years.

Survival Rates

Patients registered from 1969 to 1980 were followed up, their survival rate up to ten years was computed, and the results are shown in Table IX. There were 10,113 patients registered at 234 institutions in this period. To compute the survival rate necessitated following the patients accurately. Seventy-eight institutions were excluded, because their five-year follow up rate was below 80%. Thus, 8,948 patients were included for the computation of ten-year survival rate.

The survival rate of all registered cases, with or without surgery, is shown in Table IX. Five- and ten-year survival rates were 15.3% and 12.3%, respectively, with the female rate being significantly higher both times. Five thousand four hundred and eighty-one patients had undergone resection, among which 410 cases of operative death were excluded, thus 5,071 cases were the basis of computation of 10-year survival rate in patients receiving resection. Table X shows their five- and ten-year survival rates: 23.8% and 18.7%, respectively, the rate of females being significantly higher than males.

Survival rate was highest among those with abdominal esophageal cancer, followed by cervical cancer, and thoracic cancer (Table XI).

The highest survival was found in those where tumor length was less than 1 cm, followed by 1–2 cm and 2–3 cm (Table XII). In cases with tumor over 10 cm, survival rate dropped abruptly. Correlation between p-T classification and survival rate is shown in Table XIII. As T advanced survival rate dropped, with T4 showing the

by Sex and Year

1978–1980			1981–1983			1984–1986		
All	Male	Female	All	Male	Female	All	Male	Female
2	0	2	2	2	0	2	0	2
6	4	2	10	8	2	7	6	1
26	20	6	24	22	2	30	23	7
77	58	19	93	81	12	107	92	15
244	214	30	287	244	43	262	227	35
431	373	58	643	561	82	576	501	75
550	461	89	894	795	99	1,000	908	92
649	540	109	879	728	151	975	838	137
796	640	156	998	814	184	914	776	138
663	533	130	919	719	200	881	711	170
338	270	58	457	372	85	528	420	108
78	64	14	149	114	35	197	160	37
20	16	4	25	21	4	42	31	11
2	0	2	3	3	0	3	3	0
3,872	3,193	679	5,383	4,484	899	5,524	4,696	828

TABLE III. Double Primary Carcinoma of Other Organs by Year

	1969–1971	1972–1974	1975–1977	1978–1980	1981–1983	1984–1986
None	1,504	2,197	2,375	3,530	4,820	4,889
Synchronous	43	49	101	162	282	327
Metachronous	27	49	71	98	208	232

TABLE IV. Location of Tumor by Year

	1969–1971	1972–1974	1975–1977	1978–1980	1981–1983	1984–1986
Cervical	68	126	136	178	304	321
Upper	140	178	241	349	523	567
Middle	907	1,325	1,410	2,176	2,939	3,059
Lower	340	486	565	814	1,168	1,177
Abdominal	97	124	125	199	316	231
Others	87	135	133	156	133	169

Upper, Middle, and Lower indicate intrathoracic upper, middle, and lower esophagus.

TABLE V. p-T (TNM Classification) by Year

	1969–1971	1972–1974	1975–1977	1978–1980	1981–1983	1984–1986
p-T1	38	81	112	218	511	644
p-T2	156	263	284	488	708	704
p-T3	426	658	770	1,231	1,763	1,776
p-T4	147	238	270	409	571	735
Unknown	89	83	125	113	144	131
p-T1%	4.4	6.1	7.1	8.8	13.8	16.1

p-T1% indicates percent of T1 patients among all resected cases.

TABLE VI. p-N (TNM Classification) by Year

	1969–1971	1972–1974	1975–1977	1978–1980	1981–1983	1984–1986
p-N0	282	479	578	903	1,313	1,448
p-N1	455	673	798	1,384	2,172	2,316
Unknown	122	177	191	182	213	231
p-N0%	32.8	36.0	36.9	36.6	35.5	36.2

p-N0% indicates percent of N0 patients in all resected cases.

TABLE VII. M (TNM Classification) by Year

	1969–1971	1972–1974	1975–1977	1978–1980	1981–1983	1984–1986
M0	1,242	1,853	2,118	3,189	4,548	4,611
M1	183	278	255	438	549	545
Unknown	214	243	237	245	286	359

TABLE VIII. Histologic Type by Year

	1969–1971	1972–1974	1975–1977	1978–1980	1981–1983	1984–1986
Squamous	226	282	293	375	525	284
Well	217	368	427	684	1,021	1,133
Moderate	214	335	463	820	1,330	1,672
Poor	115	213	225	388	558	593
Adeno	37	66	64	74	89	89
Undifferentiated	7	10	12	23	40	53
Carcinosarcoma	6	3	13	12	16	20
Others	16	14	28	57	77	73
Unknown	21	38	42	36	42	61

Squamous: only squamous cell carcinoma is cited. Well: well differentiated squamous cell carcinoma. Moderate: moderately differentiated. Poor: poorly differentiated. Adeno: adenocarcinoma. Undifferentiated: undifferentiated carcinoma. Others: includes adenoacanthoma, basal cell carcinoma, adenoid cystic carcinoma, and mucoepidermoid carcinoma.

TABLE IX. Survival Rate of Registered Cases by Sex and Year

	No. patients	Survival rate (%)					
		1	2	3	4	5	10 years
All	8,948	40.9	24.6	19.2	16.7	15.3	12.3
Male	7,388	39.0	39.0	17.6	15.2	13.8*	10.8**
Female	1,560	49.9	32.5	26.4	23.4	22.4*	18.8**

*$p < 0.001$, **$p < 0.01$.

TABLE X. Survival Rate of Resected Cases by Sex and Year

	No. patients	Survival rate (%)					
		1	2	3	4	5	10 years
All	5,071	57.7	37.1	29.6	25.8	23.8	18.7
Male	4,133	56.0	35.1	27.7	23.9	21.7*	16.6**
Female	938	65.1	45.7	37.9	33.9	32.5*	27.3**

*$p < 0.005$, **$p < 0.025$.

TABLE XI. Survival Rate of Resected Cases According to Location of the Tumor

	No. patients	Survival rate (%)					
		1	2	3	4	5	10 years
All	5,071	57.7	37.1	29.6	25.8	23.8	18.7
Pharynx	21	58.1	39.5	30.2	24.6	25.2	—
Cervical	225	60.3	39.7	34.4	31.9	28.2	26.4
Upper	355	50.8	26.8	21.8	18.1	16.7	11.5
Middle	2,736	56.9	36.8	29.0	24.9	22.5	17.0
Lower	1,241	58.6	38.9	30.7	27.3	25.7	20.2
Abdominal	292	64.4	40.3	33.3	32.1	29.1	28.7
Esophagogastric	123	64.0	41.6	31.0	26.8	26.5	22.7
Cardia	76	59.8	40.2	39.6	33.8	33.0	20.2

TABLE XII. Survival Rate of Resected Cases According to Length of Filling Defect on X-ray Film

	No. patients	Survival rate (%)					
		1	2	3	4	5	10 years
All	5,071	57.7	37.1	29.6	25.8	23.8	18.7
No examination	6	51.0	34.7	17.7	18.1	18.6	
0–1 cm	19	86.0	77.0	78.8	80.8	82.9	45.3
1–2 cm	83	75.7	68.2	61.7	53.6	48.8	32.7
2–3 cm	250	74.7	53.8	42.9	42.1	37.6	32.6
3–5 cm	1,271	65.7	43.3	34.6	30.0	27.2	20.2
5–7 cm	1,636	57.1	35.1	27.4	24.0	21.9	17.9
7–10 cm	1,436	50.7	31.5	25.1	21.2	20.0	15.5
10–15 cm	338	41.5	24.6	19.1	16.4	14.9	12.1
15–18 cm	22	16.7	5.7	0.0			
Unknown	100	59.7	42.1	35.5	29.6	30.3	24.1

TABLE XIII. Survival Rate of Resected Cases According to p-T Classification

	No. patients	Survival rate (%)					
		1	2	3	4	5	10 years
All	5,071	57.7	37.1	29.6	25.8	23.7	18.6
p-T1	367	81.7	67.3	59.1	53.6	49.9	36.1
p-T2	954	67.4	47.6	38.8	35.2	31.0	24.8
p-T3	2,626	59.5	36.8	28.3	24.2	22.4	17.8
p-T4	865	33.4	14.6	11.0	8.9	8.2	5.9
Unknown	181	50.6	34.8	29.9	27.2	27.2	22.5

TABLE XIV. Survival Rate of Resected Cases According to p-N Classification

	No. patients	Survival rate (%)					
		1	2	3	4	5	10 years
All	5,071	57.7	37.1	29.6	25.8	23.7	18.6
N0	1,843	74.1	57.1	48.7	44.5	41.2	32.4
N1	1,736	57.0	32.3	23.7	19.7	17.9	14.1
Unknown	430	45.1	28.1	21.7	17.1	16.9	15.4
(M1 Lym)[a]	1,134	35.4	13.9	9.1	6.4	5.5	2.9

[a] Metastasis to lymph nodes beyond regional nodes.

TABLE XV. Survival Rate of Resected Cases According to M classification

	No. patients	Survival rate (%)					
		1	2	3	4	5	10 years
All	5,071	57.7	37.1	29.6	25.8	23.7	18.6
M0	3,885	64.8	44.2	35.9	31.7	29.3	23.9
M1	1,186	34.4	13.4	8.9	6.5	5.5	3.0

TABLE XVI. Survival Rate of Resected Cases According to Stage Classification

	No. patients	Survival rate (%)					
		1	2	3	4	5	10 years
All	5,071	57.7	37.1	29.6	25.8	23.7	18.6
Stage I	232	91.6	78.9	73.8	69.5	64.2	48.0
Stage IIA	1,306	75.6	58.2	49.1	44.3	40.9	32.2
Stage IIB	336	62.6	40.2	31.6	28.1	24.7	18.6
Stage III	1,484	56.4	31.1	22.5	18.5	17.2	13.8
Stage IV	1,105	35.5	13.6	9.0	6.5	5.4	2.9
Unknown	608	47.0	31.7	24.3	20.9	19.8	18.1

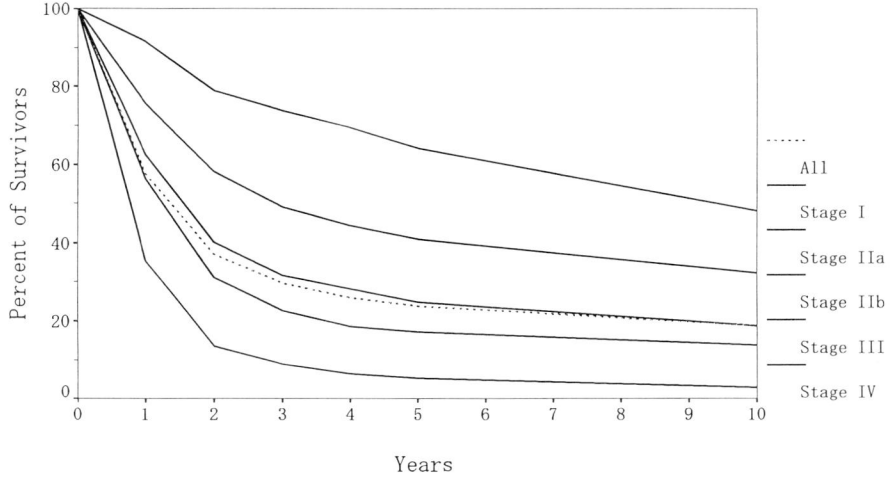

FIG. 1. Survival rate by stage

lowest survival. According to the p-N classification and survival rate, N0 had significantly higher rate than N1. In TNM classification, metastases to lymph nodes beyond the regional nodes were classified as M1 (LYM), and these had lower survival rate, but there was a reasonable number of patients who survived more than five years as shown in the bottom line of Table XIV. The M0 patients had a clearly higher survival rate than M1 cases as shown in Table XV.

Relationship between stage of TNM classification and survival is shown in Table XVI. Stage I had the best survival and there was a clear difference of survival in each stage classification (Fig. 1).

Comments and Conclusion

Number of esophageal cancer deaths in females has decreased by 50% during the last 20 years, but it remains relatively constant in males (7). Improved dietary conditions after World War II may have contributed to this reduction in females, but drinking and smoking habits of males may have counteracted the positive effect. The incidence rate of esophageal cancer itself showed a similar trend. The number of patients registered by JSDE has been about 2,000 over the past five years, and this is estimated to be one-fourth to one-fifth of all cases in Japan (S. Watanabe; personal communication). The age distribution of those recorded by JSDE, however, tended to be younger than that of the population based cancer registry.

It is noteworthy that multiple primary cancers increased to more than 10% in the past five years. Early diagnosis may contribute to finding small cancers, but the increase in metachronous cancer (more than one year from the initial cancer) suggests the necessity of careful follow-up for many years.

Location and histological type did not change markedly during the 18 years surveyed. Increase of adenocarcinoma of the esophagus, mostly from Barrett's esophagus was reported in the U.S.A. and European countries (1), but this trend was not observed by our registry in 1986. Frequency of Barrett's esophagus itself is very rare in Japan.

With early detection, the size of tumor and metastasis to the lymph nodes and other organs can be much improved. The survival rate reflected this improvement. An upgraded operation method, especially of lymph node dissection, also contributed to improved survival (3, 4, 6). Combination chemotherapy and radiotherapy for esophageal cancer improved survival rates a little, but complete resection and careful follow-up is still the best method of treatment.

Acknowledgments

We are grateful to 205 institutions for their registration of patients with esophageal carcinoma. This registration of patients was partly supported by research funds from the Ministry of Health and Welfare of Japan. We are grateful to Dr. S. Watanabe for editing this manuscript.

REFERENCES

1. Blot, W.J. and Fraumeni, J.F. Jr. Trends in esophageal cancer mortality among U.S. blacks and whites. *Am. J. Public Health*, **77**, 296–298 (1987).
2. Cutler, S.J. and Ederer, F. Maximum utilization of the life table method in analyzing survival. *J. Chron. Dis.*, **8**, 699–712 (1958).
3. Iizuka, T. and Kato, H. Statistics in esophageal cancer. *In* "Clinical Statistics in Japan," pp. 1281–1295 (1983) (in Japanese). Nihon Rinshosya, Tokyo.
4. Iizuka, T., Isono, K., Kakegawa, T., and Watanabe, H. Parameters linked to ten-year survival of resected esophageal carcinoma. *Chest*, **96**, 1005–1011 (1989).
5. Japanese Society for Esophageal Diseases, Guidelines for Clinical and Pathologic Studies on Carcinoma of the Esophagus, 8th ed. (1992) (in Japanese). Kanehara Shuppan, Tokyo.
6. Kato, H., Tachimori, Y., Watanabe, H., and Iizuka, T. Evaluation of the new TNM classification for thoracic esophageal tumors. *Int. J. Cancer*, **53**, 220–223 (1993).
7. Watanabe, S. Etiology and pathology of esophageal cancer. *Geriatric Med.*, **27**, 1425–1429 (1989).

TREATMENT RESULTS OF GASTRIC CANCER PATIENTS: AN ANALYSIS OF NATIONWIDE DATABASE

The Japanese Research Society for Gastric Cancer*

The results of treatment of gastric cancer between 1979 and 1982 in Japan were studied using the nationwide database collected by the Japanese Research Society for Gastric Cancer. A steady increase of early gastric cancer was observed and the result of treatment was excellent (5-year survival rate: 91.5%). The highest peak of age distribution was in the range between 60 and 69 years, which was 10 years younger than in Western countries. The 5-year survival rate after gastric resection in Japan was higher than in other countries. The proportions of proximal cancer and type 4 gastric cancer were smaller than in Western countries, and the proportion of total gastrectomy was also lower in Japan. The Japanese nationwide database showed that the outcome after D2 systematic lymph node dissection was superior to that of conventional dissection. Thus D2 dissection has become standard treatment for patients with gastric cancer in Japan.

The nationwide data collection of gastric cancer patients was started by the Japanese Research Society for Gastric Cancer and the National Cancer Center in 1963. The purpose was to promote the improvement of gastric cancer management by demonstrating the latest diagnostic and treatment methods as well as treatment results. In order to standardize the documentation of clinical, surgical, and pathological findings, the manual, "The General Rules for Gastric Cancer Study" was published by the Society in 1962. Since then approximately 10,000 new patients have been registered annually, which was estimated to cover approximately 15% of the primary gastric cancer patients in Japan. In this article, we show the status of registration and treatment results in Japan using the data between 1979 and 1982.

Data Collection and Analysis of Gastric Cancer Patients

The data were collected from approximately 180 leading institutions, mainly from the department of surgery. Each institution was requested to have surgical oncologists and a full-time pathologist and to report the detailed data of individual patients on a special registration form. An important requirement for member institutions was a high follow-up rate. When the 5-year follow-up rate in an institution was less than 80%, all data from that institution were abandoned. Survival rate was

---

* Manuscript was prepared by Hitoshi Katai, Keiichi Maruyama, Takeshi Sano, and Mitsuru Sasako, Department of Surgical Oncology, National Cancer Center Hospital, 5-1-1 Tsukiji, Chuo-ku, Tokyo 104, Japan; Kiyoshi Miwa, Miwa Registry Institute for Gastric Cancer, 2-2-22 Funabashi, Setagaya-ku, Tokyo 156, Japan

calculated by life table method. Thirty nine reports were published by the Society with the cooperation of the National Cancer Center since 1963 and, in addition, Miwa Registry Institute For Stomach Cancer since 1985.

Trends in Nationwide Registration

A total of 245,646 primary gastric cancer patients were registered in the 26 year period between 1963 and 1988 (Table I). Steady increase in resection rate and the proportion of early gastric cancers was observed (Fig. 1). The resection rate was 91.1% and proportion of early gastric cancer was as high as 44.1% in 1988.

Treatment Result

The latest 5-year survival rate available is that of those treated in 1982. To better interpret these results, we studied the database of primary gastric cancer patients treated in the 4 year period between 1979 and 1982. A total of 44,384 patients with primary cancer were registered in this period. The data from institutions with low follow-up rates were excluded. When we excluded non-resected cases, multiple cancers, and operative deaths, the number of patients analyzed was 18,189. The operative death rate was 1.7% and the loss to follow-up rate was 3.5%.

TABLE I. Nationwide Registration of Gastric Cancer Patients

Year	Hospitals	Total	Primary	Resected	Resection rate
1963	143	5,870	5,633	3,826	67.9%
1964	158	7,105	6,691	4,505	67.3
1965	143	6,837	6,546	4,682	71.5
1966	132	5,792	5,527	3,955	71.6
1967	129	6,006	5,753	4,192	72.8
1968	159	7,128	6,864	5,039	73.4
1969	187	8,040	7,752	5,497	70.9
1970	192	8,167	7,793	5,824	74.7
1971	154	7,456	7,080	5,352	75.6
1972	158	7,008	6,711	5,078	75.7
1973	155	7,526	7,269	5,602	77.1
1974	192	9,588	9,214	7,194	78.1
1975	174	8,710	8,504	6,785	79.8
1976	182	9,644	9,403	7,627	80.9
1977	168	8,600	8,389	6,881	82.0
1978	179	9,689	9,452	7,820	82.7
1979	184	10,726	10,468	8,731	83.4
1980	188	11,293	11,041	9,354	84.7
1981	192	11,832	11,565	9,938	85.9
1982	192	11,624	11,309	9,836	86.4
1983	238	12,399	12,130	10,565	87.1
1984	208	12,638	12,376	10,991	88.9
1985	237	13,985	13,632	12,213	89.6
1986	255	15,692	15,272	13,813	90.4
1987	241	15,808	15,427	14,006	90.8
1988	215	14,219	13,845	12,609	91.1
Total	4,758	253,382	245,646	201,915	82.2
Average	183	9,745	9,448	7,766	82.2

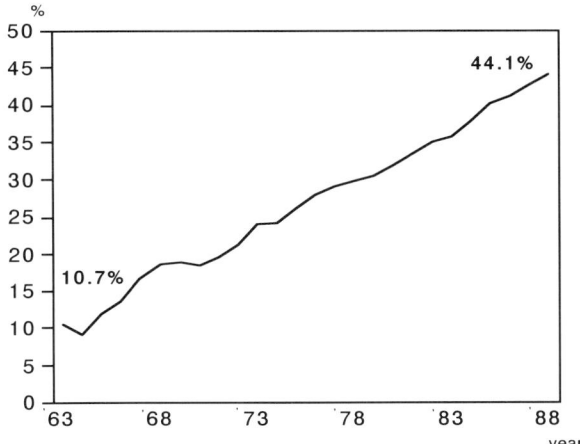

FIG. 1. Trends of proportion of early gastric cancer
(number of patients with early gastric cancer/resected cases)

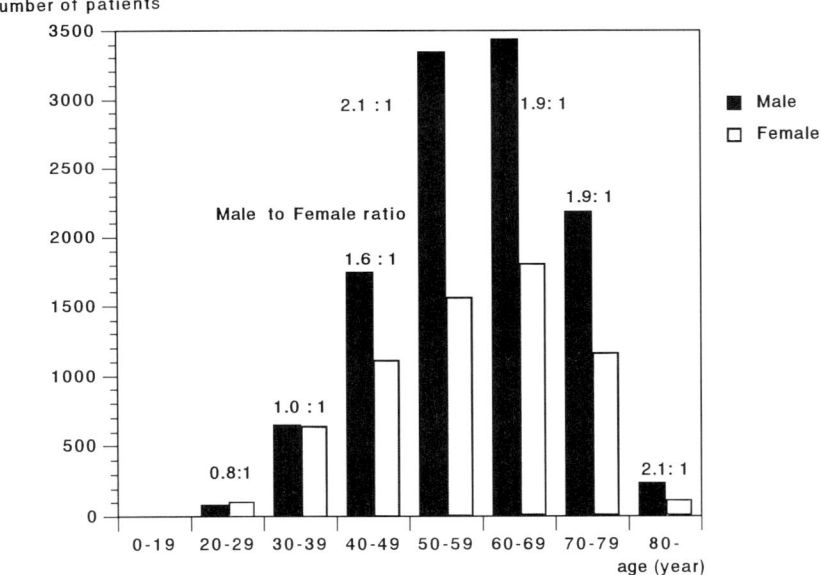

FIG. 2. Age distribution and sex ratio

The male to female ratio was almost 2:1 among those older than 50 years of age (Fig. 2). The peak incidence was between 60 and 69 years of age in both sexes.

The 5-year survival rate for all cases treated by gastric resection was 57.8% (Fig. 3). There was no difference in survival between male and female. The majority of tumors were located in the lower two thirds of the stomach and the proportion of proximal third cancer was only 15.3% (Fig. 4). The 5-year survival rate was 57.0%, 64.7%, and 45.0% in the distal, middle, and proximal third, respectively. Type 0 cancer (early gastric cancer) accounted for 32.0% with a 91.5% 5-year survival rate. In contrast, type 4 cancer (diffuse carcinoma) accounted for 10.6% with only a 13.5%

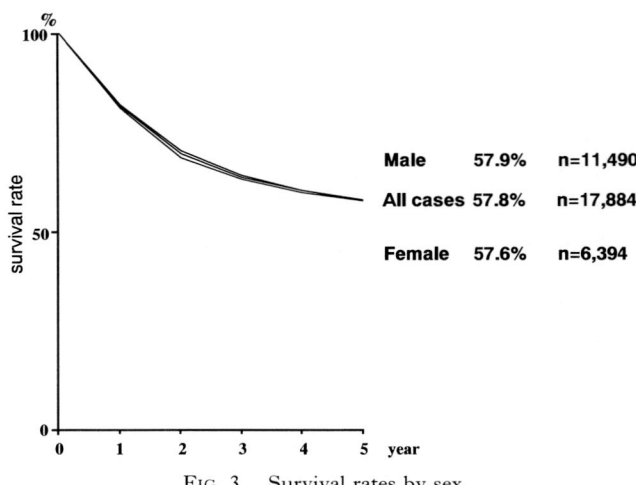

FIG. 3. Survival rates by sex

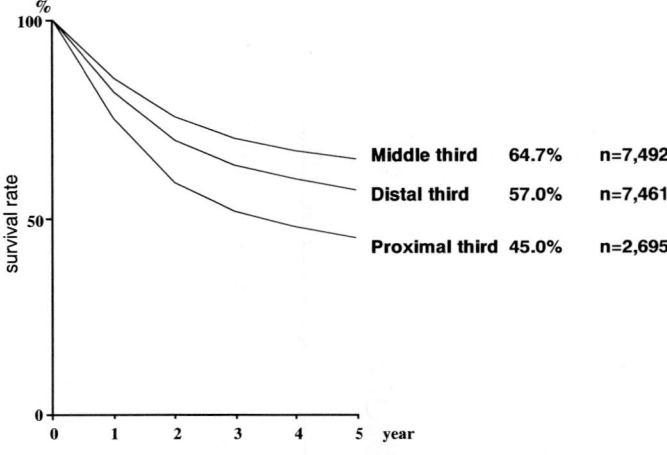

FIG. 4. Survival rates by location of tumor

5-year survival rate (Fig. 5). The Japanese histologic classification is similar to the WHO classification. Histological type seemed to have little impact on survival (Fig. 6), while the depth of invasion clearly correlated with survival (Fig. 7). When the tumor invasion was limited to the muscularis propria, the outcome of a patient was good and the 5-year survival rate was more than 75%. However, once the tumor invaded the subserosa, the outcome became poor and the 5-year survival rate was less than 50%. Lymph node metastasis was another important prognostic factor (Fig. 8). Survival correlated with extent of node involvement. The outcome of patients with peritoneal, liver or other distant metastasis was very poor. With peritoneal metastasis, the 5-year survival rate was only 7.6%; with liver metastasis, it was 5.2%. There were no 5-year survivors when the patient had multiple scattered metastases to both lobes of the liver. The 5-year survival rate was closely correlated with histological staging (Fig. 9).

With regard to resection method, distal gastrectomy predominated and 69.9% of

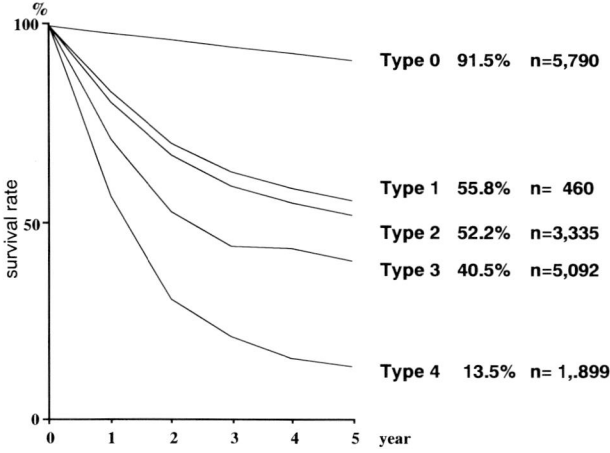

FIG. 5. Survival rates by macroscopic type of tumor

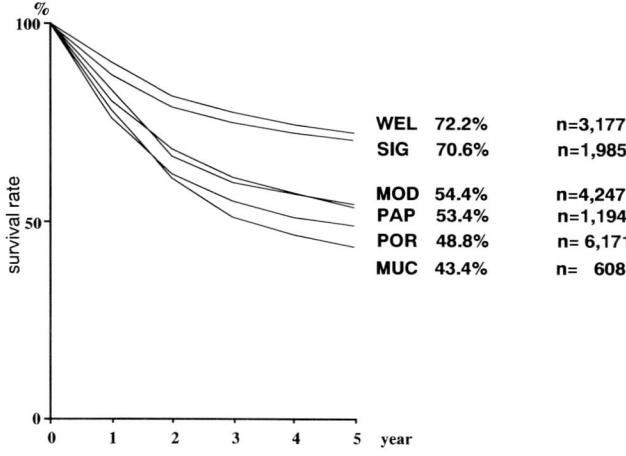

FIG. 6. Survival rates by histologic type of tumor
PAP: papillary adenocarcinoma. WEL: well-differentiated tubular adenocarcinoma. MOD: moderately differentiated tubular adenocarcinoma. POR: poorly differentiated adenocarcinoma. SIG: signet-ring cell carcinoma. MUC: mucinous adenocarcinoma.

the patients were treated by this procedure. Very few patients (3.6%) were treated by proximal gastrectomy. The 5-year survival rates after distal, proximal, and total gastrectomy was 65.6%, 54.8%, and 36.3%, respectively (Fig. 10). D2 lymph node dissection was standard procedure in Japan, accounting for 65.9%, and the 5-year survival rate following that was 65.8% (Fig. 11). A curative resection was performed in 74.4% of patients and their 5-year survival rate was 71.9% (Fig. 12).

Discussion

With regard to patient age, the highest peak was observed in the range between 60 and 69 years. This range was 10 years younger than that in Western countries (*3,*

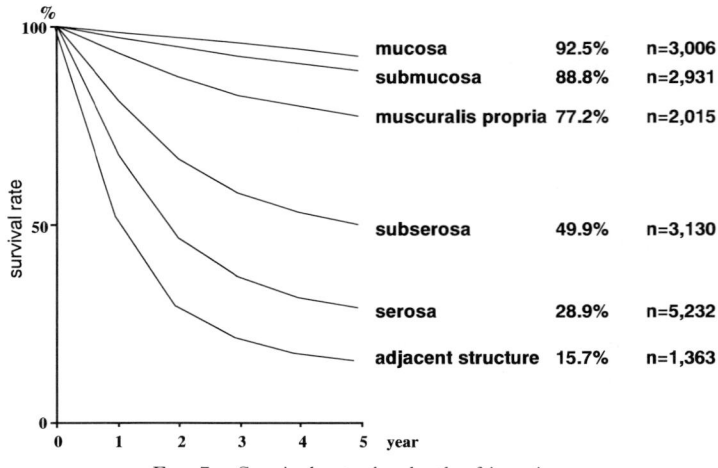

FIG. 7. Survival rates by depth of invasion

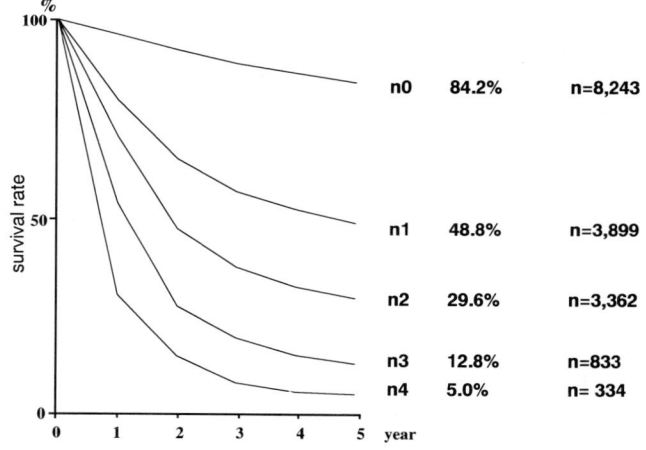

FIG. 8. Survival rates by lymph node metastasis

16, 21). The cure rate for gastric cancer in Japan was high with overall 5-year survival rate in our series being 57.8%. It was 10–24% in Germany (*16*) and was almost 5% in England (*2*). The proportion of proximal cancers in Japan was smaller than that in Western countries (*16, 21*), however, a steady increase of proximal cancer is being observed in Japan (*8*). The proportion of type 4 (diffuse) gastric cancer was almost 10% in Japan in this four year period and smaller than that in Western countries (*11*). The prognosis of this type of cancer was remarkably poor. The proportion of early gastric cancer was 44.1% in 1988 in Japan, while it was only 9.2% in Germany between 1982 and 1989 (*14*), and 7.4% in the U.S.A. between 1977 and 1979 (*3*). There was also an increase of early gastric cancer. Advancement of diagnostic imaging and a widespread mass-screening system seems to have contributed to the high rate of early detection.

Classification of lymph node metastasis differs between the Japanese and the TNM systems (*20*). Meticulous studies in Japan in the past revealed that the path-

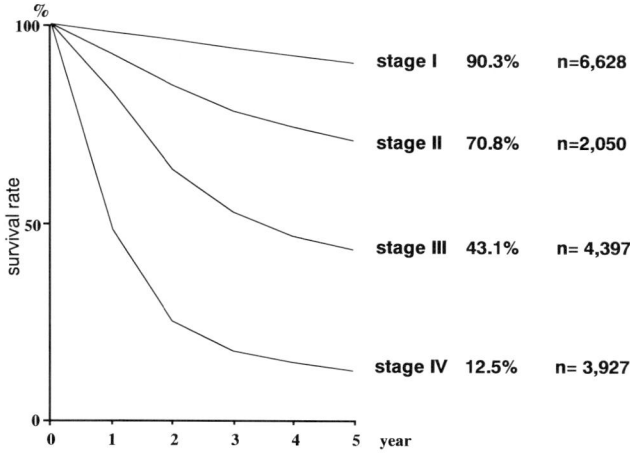

FIG. 9. Survival rates by stage

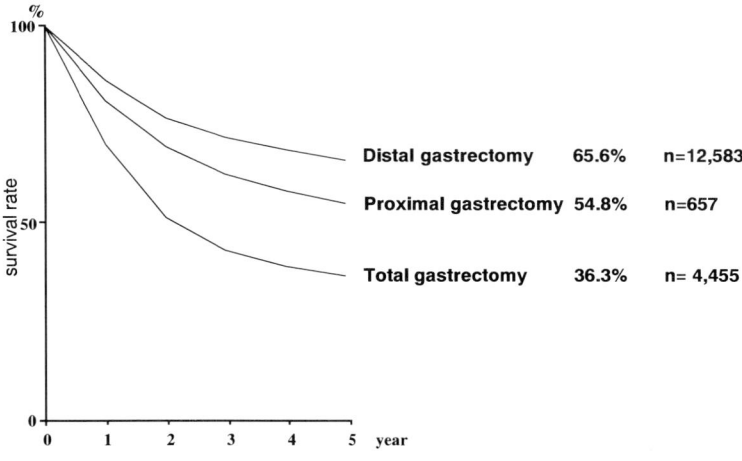

FIG. 10. Survival rates by method of resection

ways of lymph drainage were related to the location of tumors. From these studies, lymph node stations can be numbered from 1 to 16 and subsequently categorized into four groups designated N1 to N4 in the Japanese Rules (6). The grouping of stations depends on the tumor location. In the TNM classification, N1 and N2 are considered regional LN levels conventionally, while metastasis in N3 and N4 level nodes is regarded as distant metastasis due to low survival rate. The 5 year survival rate was 14.0% in N3, and only 5.5% in N4 even in this study.

The staging systems were also different between the Japanese Rules and the TNM classification. However, the prognosis was well correlated with staging in both systems.

With regard to surgical treatment, some special characters were noted in this database. The proportion of total gastrectomy was low in Japan, only 25.2%, while in Western countries it was much higher. In Germany, total gastrectomy was performed in 50.9% of patients with curative intention (15). This was apparently because

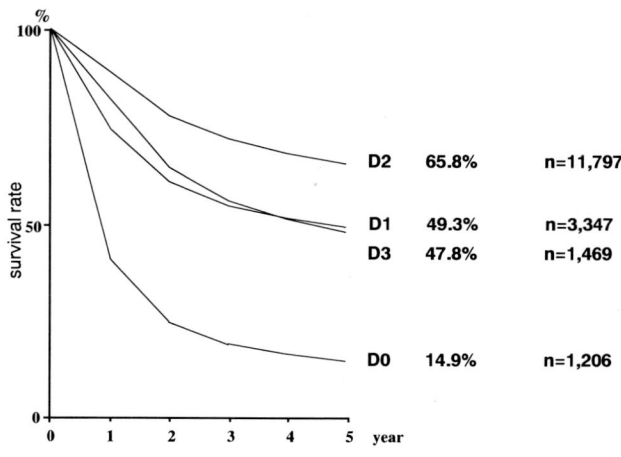

FIG. 11. Survival rates by lymph node dissection

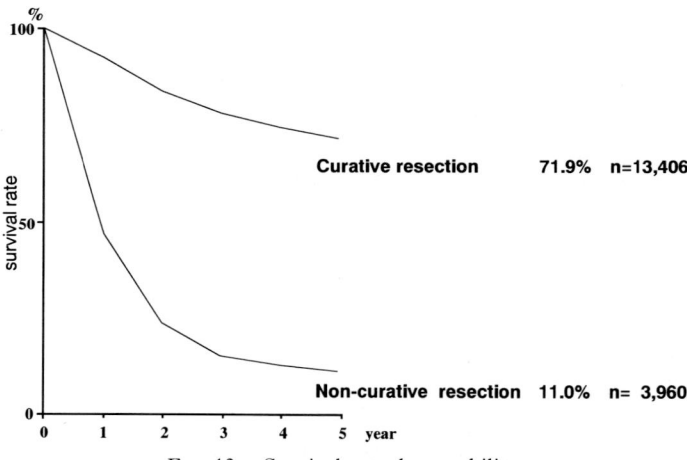

FIG. 12. Survival rates by curability

of high incidence of proximal, diffuse tumors, and advanced disease. Complete removal of the N1 lymph nodes was defined as "D1 dissection", and that of N1 and N2 was defined as "D2 dissection". The Japanese nationwide database showed that the prognosis after D2 systematic lymph node dissection was superior to that following conventional dissection. The D2 systematic lymph node dissection has now become standard treatment for patients with gastric cancer in Japan. The grounds to support thorough node dissection were that many long-term survivors after resection of stomach cancer had node metastasis (9, 10), that the procedure gave better survival rates than in historic control (12, 19), and that this decreased the incidence of local recurrence without added morbidity or mortality (10, 13). In most Western countries, however, lymph nodes were regarded as indicators rather than governors of disease and it was believed that radical lymphadenectomy only improved the accuracy of tumor staging (1). Furthermore, the absence of convincing evidence for beneficial effects and the reports of increased morbidity and mortality after D2 dissection had limited the indication for this procedure in Western countries (5). More recently, the effectiveness of D2 LN dissection has been recognized internationally and has been evaluated in some multi-center trials (4, 18).

Mode of recurrence is important to evaluate surgical treatment. Mode information was collected in the nationwide database but the accuracy was low due to difficulty of follow up study. To cover this, a study of 1,994 advanced cancers reported that peritoneal dissemination dominated the mode of recurrence (44.2%), followed by local (23.0%), liver (13.8%) and distant metastases other than peritoneal cavity and liver (10.6%) (7). Another study of 1,475 early gastric cancer patients reported that 1.4% died of recurrence and 6.6% of other causes. Hematogenous metastasis was the most common mode of recurrence (17).

The Japanese Research Society published a 12th edition of the General Rules in July 1993. The editorial board made great effort to harmonize the terminology and definition with the TNM classification in order to avoid confusion in international research activities. The major changes are: classification of depth of invasion was changed from "S" to "T" classification, as in the TNM manual. The new "Staging" is now almost the same as the TNM Staging System except that it includes N3, N4, and subdivision of stage IV. One of the major improvements is the change of character from "R" to "D" to document the grade of LN dissection. "R2 operation" was used to describe "complete removal of N1 and N2 lymph nodes" in the former Japanese manual, but the character "R" meant "residual tumor" in the TNM classification. To avoid confusion, the Japanese manual now uses "D2 operation" instead of "R2 operation". Based on this new manual, the Japanese Research Society started a new registration system using a personal computer in 1992 replacing the paper registration form.

REFERENCES

1. Cady, B. Lymph node metastases. Indicators, but not governors of survival. *Arch. Surg.*, **119**, 1067 (1984).
2. Craven, F.L. End results of surgical treatment: British experience. *In* "Gastric Cancer," ed. M. Nishi, H. Ichikawa, T. Nakajima, K. Maruyama, and E. Tahara, pp. 341–348 (1993). Springer-Verlag, Tokyo.
3. Curtis, R.E., Kennedy, B.J., Myers, M.H., and Hankey, B.F. Evaluation of AJC stomach cancer staging using the SEER population. *Semin. Onco.*, **12**, 21–31 (1983).
4. Cuschieri, A. Gastrectomy for gastric cancer: definitions and objectives. *Br. J. Surg.*, **73**, 513–514 (1986).
5. Dent, D.M., Madden, M.V., and Price, S.K. Randomized comparison of R1 and R2 gastrectomy for gastric carcinoma. *Br. J. Surg.*, **75**, 110–112 (1988).
6. Japanese Research Society for Gastric Cancer. The General Rules for the Gastric Cancer Study in Surgery and Pathology. *Jpn. J. Surg.*, **11**, 127–139 (1981).
7. Katai, H., Maruyama, K., Sasako, M., Sano, T., Okajima, K., Kinoshita, T., and Naparkov, A. Mode of recurrence after gastric cancer surgery. *Dig. Surg.*, **11**, 99–103 (1994).
8. Kinoshita, T., Maruyama, K., Sasako, M., and Okajima, K. Treatment results of gastric cancer patients: Japanese experience. *In* "Gastric Cancer," ed. M. Nishi, H. Ichikawa, T. Nakajima, K. Maruyama, and E. Tahara, pp. 293–305 (1993). Springer-Verlag, Tokyo.

9. Maruyama, K., Okabayashi, K., and Kinoshita, T. Progress in gastric cancer surgery in Japan and its limits of radicality. *World J. Surg.*, **11**, 418–425 (1987).
10. Maruyama, K., Sasako, M., Kinoshita, T., and Okajima, K. Effectiveness of systematic lymph node dissection in gastric cancer surgery. *In* "Gastric Cancer," ed. M. Nishi, H. Ichikawa, T. Nakajima, K. Maruyama, and E. Tahara, pp. 293–305 (1993). Springer-Verlag, Tokyo.
11. Meyer ,W.C., Damiano, R.J., Postlethwait, R.W., and Rotolo, F.S. Adenocarcinoma of the stomach, changing patterns over the last 4 decades. *Ann. Surg.*, **205**, 1–8 (1987).
12. Mine, M., Majima, S., Harada, M., and Etani, S. End results of gastrectomy for gastric cancer: effect of extensive lymph node dissection. *Surgery*, **68**, 753–758 (1970).
13. Papachristou, D.N. and Fortner, J.G. Local recurrence of gastric adenocarcinomas after gastrectomy. *J. Surg. Oncol.*, **18**, 47–53 (1981).
14. Rohde, H., Stutzer, H., Bauer, P., Heitmann, K., Gebbensleben, B., and the German Gastric Cancer TNM Study Group. Early gastric cancer in comparison to advanced gastric cancer. *Langenbeacks Arch. Chir.*, **376**, 16–22 (1991).
15. Rohde, H., Bauer, P., Stützer, H., Heitmann, K., Gebbensleben, B., and the German Gastric Cancer TNM Study Group. Proximal compared with distal adenocarcinoma of the stomach: difference and consequences. *Br. J. Surg.*, **78**, 1242–1248 (1991).
16. Rohde, H. and the German Gastric Cancer TNM Study Group. End results of surgical treatment: German experience. *In* "Gastric Cancer," ed. M. Nishi, H. Ichikawa, T. Nakajima, K. Maruyama, and E. Tahara, pp. 349–357 (1993). Springer-Verlag, Tokyo.
17. Sano, T., Sasako, M., Kinoshita, T., and Maruyama, K. Recurrence of early gastric cancer: Follow-up of 1475 patients and review of the Japanese literature. *Cancer*, **72**, 3174–3178 (1993).
18. Sasako, M., Maruyama, K., Kinoshita, T., Bonenkamp, J.J., van de Velde C.J.H., Hermans, J., and cooperating investigators. Quality control of surgical technique in a multicenter, prospective, randomized, controlled study on the surgical treatment of gastric cancer. *Jpn. J. Clin. Oncol.*, **22**, 41–48 (1992).
19. Shiu, M.H., Papachristou, D.N., Kosloff, C., and Eliopoulos, G. Selection of operative procedure for adenocarcinoma of the midstomach. Twenty years' experience with implications for future treatment strategy. *Ann. Surg.*, **192**, 730–737 (1980).
20. UICC TNM Classification of Malignant Tumours, 4th ed., pp. 43–46 (1987). Springer-Verlag, Tokyo.
21. Wanebo, H.J., Kennedy, B.J., Chmiel, J., Steele, G. Jr., Winchester, D., and Osteen, R. Cancer of the stomach — a patient care study by the American College of Surgeons. *Ann. Surg.*, **218**, 583–592 (1993).

A GENERAL VIEW OF LARGE BOWEL CANCER IN JAPAN

Registry Committee, Japanese Society for Cancer
of the Colon and Rectum[*1]

The large bowel cancer registry began in 1980 with the collection of detailed clinical and pathological information of colorectal and anal cancer patients going back to 1974. A total of 24,234 patients, 11,371 with colon cancer and 12,863 with rectum cancer, have been registered so far and analyzed for clinicopathological characteristics and survival rates. An increase over the years in the ratio of the number of colon cancer to rectum cancer patients and a shift to more aged patients has been observed. In 1982 and 1983, surgical operations were carried out in 8,310 (98.3%) out of 8,448 registered patients. Resection of the tumor was performed in 7,798 (92.3%) cases, of which 5,901 (69.9%) were assessed to be curative by postoperative histological evaluation. Operative mortality was 1.7% for the 8,310 surgically treated patients, and overall (TNM Stage I to IV) five year survival rates were 60.6% (95% confidence interval, 58.9–62.3) and 55.6% (95% confidence interval, 53.9–57.3) for colon and rectum cancer, respectively. The survival rates by stage did not change in the three periods of 1974–1977, 1978–1981, and 1982–1983.

The Japanese Society for Cancer of the Colon and Rectum (JSCCR), which was organized by the leading institutes treating large bowel cancer in Japan, began a registry of this cancer in 1980 to determine detailed clinical and histopathological aspects of cancer of the colon, rectum and anus in Japan. Patients with colorectal cancer treated at these member hospitals since 1974 were registered. The registration files consist of demographic data of the patients, detailed clinicopathological findings of the tumor and follow-up information. Clinicopathological findings were recorded and classified according to the "General Rules for Clinical and Pathological Studies on Cancer of the Colon, Rectum and Anus" originated and issued by JSCCR in 1977 and published in English in 1983 (3). The first report of the registry appeared in 1985 (Multi-Institutional Registry of Large Bowel Cancer in Japan Vol. 1 — Cases treated in 1974 and 1975 — Registry Committee of the JSCCR, 1985, Tokyo) containing data of 3,007 cases (1,300 colon and 1,707 rectum cancer). As of November 1993, seven reports[*2] had been published and the number of patients registered who were treated between 1974 and 1983 totalled 24,234. Contents of these reports are summarized here and compared with data of the regional registries in Japan.

[*1] Manuscript was prepared by Yasuo Koyama and Kenjiro Kotake, Tochigi Cancer Center, 4-9-13 Yohnan, Utsunomiya 320, Japan
[*2] The report has been published in English since 1992 (Vol. 7).

Collection of Data and Outline of Registered Cases

Reports of the JSCCR registry published up to 1993 (Volumes No.1 through No. 7) are summarized. Crude cumulative survival rates were calculated by the lifetable method and the statistical analysis was performed using the chi-square test, Greenwood method, and logrank test.

1. Number of registered cases by year, sex, and site

Table I shows number of the registered cases by sex and site in two-year increments. There was an increasing trend in total number of registered patients in each two-year interval, and this is especially noticeable in females with colon cancer. Also, the ratio of colon cancer to rectum cancer (C/R) patients has markedly increased in recent years and has exceeded 1.0 since 1980 in females (Table I and Fig. 1).

2. Age distribution

Patient age groups are shown in Table II and Fig. 2 by sex and site. There was

TABLE I. Number of Patients Registered by Year, Site, and Sex

Year	Colon			Rectum			C/R ratio			Grand total
	Male	Female	Subtotal	Male	Female	Subtotal	Male	Female	Subtotal	
1974–75	709	591	1,300	1,017	690	1,707	0.70	0.86	0.76	3,007
1976–77	862	737	1,599	1,191	827	2,018	0.72	0.89	0.79	3,617
1978–79	801	678	1,479	916	695	1,611	0.87	0.98	0.92	3,090
1980–81	1,487	1,333	2,820	1,838	1,271	3,109	0.81	1.05	0.91	5,929
1982–83	2,211	1,962	4,173	2,668	1,750	4,418	0.83	1.12	0.94	8,591
Total	6,070	5,301	11,371	7,630	5,233	12,863	0.80	1.01	0.88	24,234

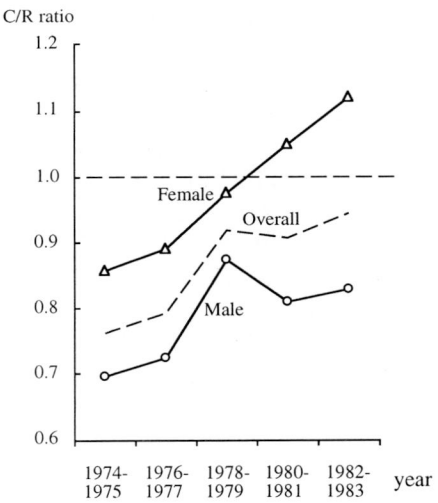

FIG. 1. Change in incidence of colon cancer and rectum cancer shown by change in C/R ratio (ratio of number of patients with colon cancer to those with rectum cancer)

TABLE II. Age Groups of Patients by Year, Site of Tumor, and Sex

Colon, male

Year	−29	−39	−49	−59	−69	−79	80−	Total
1974–75	17	53	125	135	227	139	13	709
1976–77	20	54	132	176	267	180	33	862
1978–79	11	42	103	201	214	188	42	801
1980–81	15	76	201	360	440	325	70	1,487
1982–83	19	95	268	598	604	520	107	2,211
Estimated 1984[a]	66	362	947	2,420	2,650	3,057	1,364	10,866

Colon, female

Year	−29	−39	−49	−59	−69	−79	80−	Total
1974–75	12	47	91	147	187	95	12	591
1976–77	14	47	113	198	213	130	22	737
1978–79	13	37	105	172	188	138	25	678
1980–81	18	68	179	318	378	320	52	1,333
1982–83	12	94	238	488	547	470	113	1,962
Estimated 1984[a]	59	255	807	1,630	2,541	2,789	1,517	9,598

Rectum, male

Year	−29	−39	−49	−59	−69	−79	80−	Total
1974–75	27	100	176	207	291	197	19	1,017
1976–77	17	78	211	257	360	232	36	1,191
1978–79	10	59	149	217	278	173	30	916
1980–81	18	114	261	496	525	364	60	1,838
1982–83	20	103	390	783	713	561	98	2,668
Estimated 1984[a]	28	197	956	1,919	2,267	2,036	917	8,320

Rectum, female

Year	−29	−39	−49	−59	−69	−79	80−	Total
1974–75	16	83	116	180	166	112	17	690
1976–77	13	50	170	207	222	138	27	827
1978–79	8	42	123	190	185	126	21	695
1980–81	14	77	235	310	361	223	51	1,271
1982–83	15	107	263	475	443	373	74	1,750
Estimated 1984[a]	8	127	753	1,228	1,623	1,651	921	6,311

[a] Estimated number of patients in Japan calculated from regional registry data.

a shifting to older years with time in both sexes, and this trend was similar in both colon and rectum cancer patients. The last line of each table and figure represents the estimated number of colon and rectum cancers by patient age, based on data of the population-based cancer registry in Japan. As shown clearly in Fig. 2, the proportion of older age patients is more remarkable in the data of regional registry than those of the JSCCR registry. This may suggest that hospitals belonging to the JSCCR treat more young patients than older among the overall colorectal cancer patients in Japan. Comparing the number of the JSCCR registry with that of the estimation, the rate of the former is about 20% of all colon cancer and about 30% of all rectum cancer.

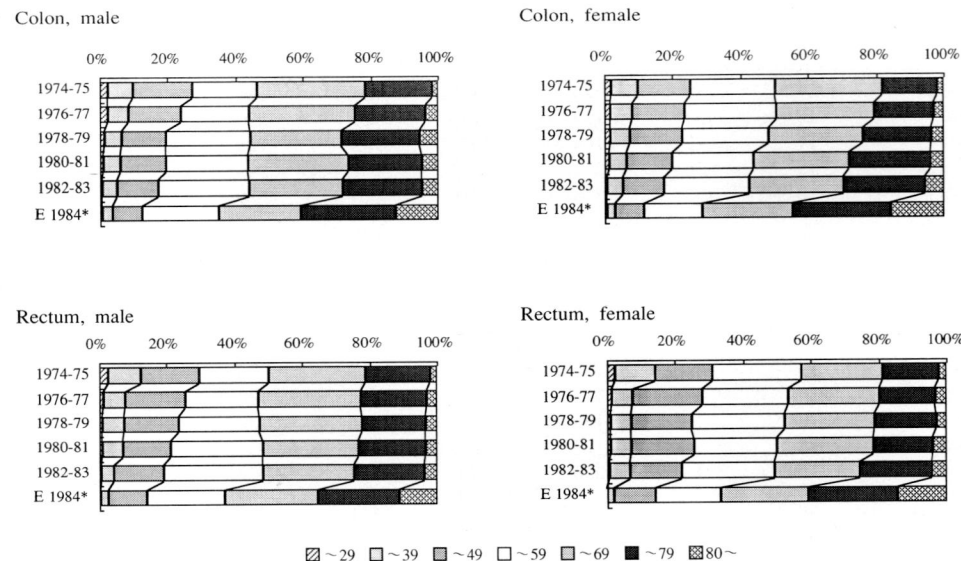

FIG. 2. Age distribution of patients by site and year
*: Estimated incidence in Japan from regional registry data.

3. Histological type and subtype of the tumor

Almost all of the registered tumors were adenocarcinoma. Histological type, subtype, and their frequency did not essentially change during the 10 year period from 1974–1983. Table III shows histological type of tumors treated in 1983. Adenocarcinomas were divided into five subtypes corresponding to the grade of differentiation and character of mucin production, *i.e.*, well, moderately and poorly differentiated adenocarcinoma, mucinous carcinoma, and signet-ring cell carcinoma. Proportion of well differentiated adenocarcinoma of the colon and rectum was 54.9% and 54.6%, respectively, followed by moderately differentiated (29.2%, 32.1%), poorly differentiated (5.2%, 3.4%) adenocarcinoma, mucinous carcinoma (4.4%, 3.1%), and signet-ring cell carcinoma (0.3%, 0.6%).

Malignant tumors other than adenocarcinoma accounted for only 1.6% of all tumors: 21 squamous cell carcinoma, 14 malignant carcinoid, 9 undifferentiated carcinoma, 6 adenosquamous carcinoma, 6 malignant lymphoma, and others. Because the number of cases with malignant tumors other than adenocarcinoma was very small, these were eliminated from the subsequent analysis.

4. Resectability and operative mortality

Table IV shows modality of treatment, mode of surgery, resectability and operative mortality of patients treated in 1982 and 1983. Surgical operation was carried out in 98.1% of those with colon cancer (4,038/4,113) and 98.5% of those with rectum cancer (4,272/4,335). Surgical resection of the tumor was performed in 3,808 patients with colon cancer and in 3,990 with rectum cancer. All told, this was done in 7,798 out of the 8,448 registered patients (resection rate was 92.3%). The surgical opera-

TABLE III. Histological Type and Subtype of Malignant Neoplasm Registered by JSCCR

	Colon		Rectum		Anal canal		Total	
	No.	%	No.	%	No.	%	No.	%
Adenocarcinoma:								
well-differentiated	1,115	54.9	1,135	54.6	30	34.1	2,280	54.3
moderately differentiated	594	29.2	668	32.1	14	15.9	1,276	30.4
poorly differentiated	105	5.2	71	3.4	5	5.7	181	4.3
mucinous carcinoma	89	4.4	65	3.1	17	19.3	171	4.1
signet-ring cell carcinoma	7	0.3	12	0.6	0		19	0.5
adenocarcinoma NOS[a]	103	5.1	99	4.8	1	1.1	203	4.8
Subtotal	2,013	99.1	2,050	98.7	67	76.1	4,130	98.4
Other malignancies:								
squamous cell carcinoma	1	0.05	5	0.24	15	17.05	21	0.50
adenosquamous carcinoma	1	0.05	4	0.19	1	1.14	6	0.14
undifferentiated carcinoma	6	0.30	3	0.14	0		9	0.21
basaloid cell carcinoma	0		0		3	3.41	3	0.07
carcinoid	1	0.05	13	0.63	0		14	0.33
malignant melanoma	0		0		2	2.27	2	0.05
leiomyoblastoma	0		1	0.05	0		1	0.02
leiomyosarcoma	1	0.05	1	0.05	0		2	0.05
malignant lymphoma	6	0.30	0		0		6	0.14
others	3	0.15	1	0.05	0		4	0.10
Subtotal	19	0.9	28	1.3	21	23.9	68	1.6
Grand total	2,032	100	2,078	100	88	100	4,198	100

[a] NOS: not otherwise specified.

TABLE IV. Modality of Treatment, Mode of Surgery, and Operative Mortality by Site of Tumor

	Surgical										Non-surgical		Grand total
	Resected				Not resected		Surgery NOS[a]		Total				
	Curative		Not-curative										
	No.	%	No.	%	No.	%	No.	%	No.	%	No.	%	
Colon	2,750	66.9	1,058	25.7	101	2.5	129	3.1	4,038	98.1	75	1.8	4,113
operative mortality	20	0.7	30	2.8	18	17.8	9	7.0	77	1.9			
Rectum	3,151	72.7	839	19.4	157	3.6	125	2.9	4,272	98.5	63	1.5	4,335
operative mortality	2.8	0.9	11	1.3	16	10.2	6	4.8	61	1.4			
Grand total	5,901	69.9	1,897	22.4	258	3.1	254	3.0	8,310	98.4	138	1.6	8,448
operative mortality	48	0.8	41	2.2	34	13.2	15	5.9	138	1.7			

[a] NOS: not otherwise specified.

tions were assessed to be curative in 5,901 cases (69.9% of all cases) and non-curative in 1,897 cases (22.4%) by post-operative histological evaluation. Overall operative mortality was 1.7% of the 8,310 surgically treated patients. It was the lowest (0.8%) in curative resection and highest (13.2%) in non-resected surgery.

Stage and Survival

1. Clinical and pathological stage

Distribution of patients in each pathological TNM stage is shown in Table V and Fig. 3. Except for the significant decrease of stage IV in both colon and rectum cancer since 1976 ($p < 0.01$), distribution of patients in each stage was essentially unaltered during the decade, and approximately half of them were classified as stage III or IV (*i.e.*, advanced cancer with metastasis).

2. Survival rate

Figure 4 shows survival rate of all patients treated from 1974 to 1983 in terms of site and pTNM stage. Five year survival rate of stage III colon cancer was 59.3%, while that of rectum cancer was 45.1%. To know whether the survival rates had changed during the ten years from 1974 to 1983, we divided the ten years into three periods, the first and the second four years and the last two years. As shown in Table VI and Fig. 5, however, the survival rates in these three periods were essentially unchanged not only overall (stage 0 was excluded) but in any subset of the stage.

Figure 6 shows survival rates according to the mode of surgery. When patients

TABLE V. pTNM Stage of Tumor by Site and Year

Colon

Year	Stage 0	Stage I	Stage II	Stage III	Stage IV	Total
1974–75	24	85	399	254	300	1,062
	2.3	*8.0*	*37.6*	*23.9*	*28.2*	*100*
1976–77	26	105	506	339	216	1,192
	2.2	*8.8*	*42.4*	*28.4*	*18.1*	*100*
1978–79	36	67	488	332	249	1,172
	3.1	*5.7*	*41.6*	*28.3*	*21.2*	*100*
1980–81	36	137	861	677	501	2,212
	1.6	*6.2*	*38.9*	*30.6*	*22.6*	*100*
1982–83	62	296	1,376	968	694	3,396
	1.8	*8.7*	*40.5*	*28.5*	*20.4*	*100*

Rectum

Year	Stage 0	Stage I	Stage II	Stage III	Stage IV	Total
1974–75	27	227	393	446	226	1,319
	2.0	*17.2*	*29.8*	*33.8*	*17.1*	*100*
1976–77	15	175	590	527	150	1,457
	1.0	*12.0*	*40.5*	*36.2*	*10.3*	*100*
1978–79	20	183	432	434	157	1,226
	1.6	*14.9*	*35.2*	*35.4*	*12.8*	*100*
1980–81	49	311	879	864	346	2,449
	2.0	*12.7*	*35.9*	*35.3*	*14.1*	*100*
1982–83	89	563	1,202	1,314	493	3,661
	2.4	*15.4*	*32.8*	*35.9*	*13.5*	*100*

Italicized figures in each column show percentage.

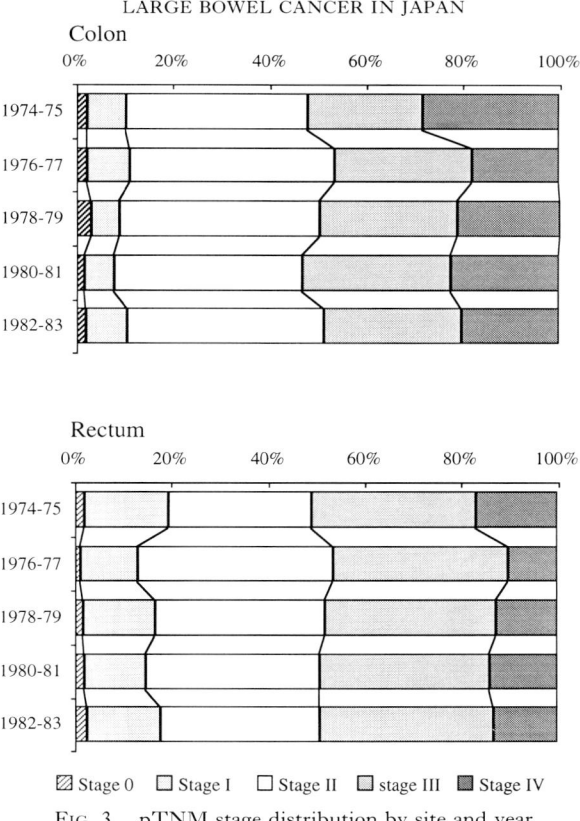

FIG. 3. pTNM stage distribution by site and year

with colon and rectum cancer underwent curative resection, more than 75% of the former and 66% of the latter survived for more than five years, while the five year survival rate of those who had non-curative resection was only 15%.

Comparison of Survival with Population-based Cancer Registry

Numerous basic analyses on the clinical and histopathological data of large bowel cancer in Japan, other than that of the JSCCR registry, have been reported by researchers based on various sources of data. Hanai *et al.* (2) reported the relative five year survival rate of patients with cancer of the colon and rectum in Osaka Prefecture, based on data of the regional cancer registry at a workshop held in September 1988 in Tokyo. These rates had improved from 30.3% to 35.9% in colon cancer and from 26.3% to 37.0% in rectum cancer over the period 1970 to 1980. They (1) reported more recently that the survival rates of both colon and rectum cancer rose to 40% in the 1984–1986 period. The report of the JSCCR registry using crude cumulative survival rates for the same period showed a reasonably better survival rate of both cancers. One possible reason for the discrepancy in the rates of these registries could be the difference in objects. As stated above, the age structure inclined toward younger age groups in the JSCCR registry; in that registry for 1980 and 1981, patients with localized disease of the colon and rectum were 47% and 49%, respectively.

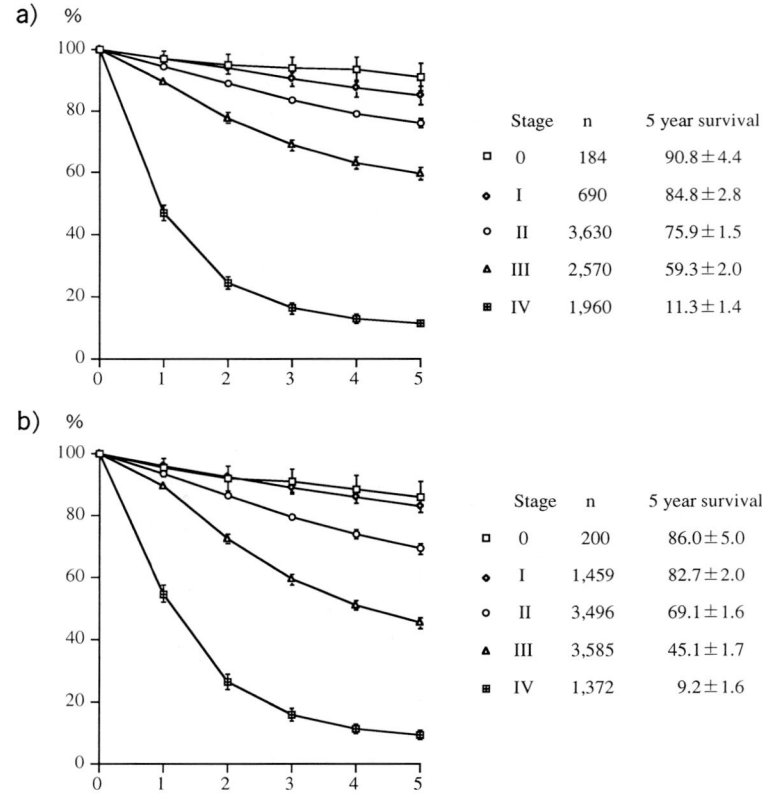

FIG. 4. Five year survival rates by pTNM stage (total patients from 1974 to 1983)
a. Colon cancer.   b. Rectum cancer.

In the regional registry of Osaka, in contrast, patients with localized disease accounted for 28% and 35%, respectively, in 1978–1980 (*1*). This suggests that the regional registry contained more records of patients with advanced cancer than did the JSCCR registry. Furthermore, a multivariate analysis of prognostic factors for large bowel cancer using the JSCCR registry data (*6*) showed that, apart from the factors directly related to the tumor, factors such as age, sex, mode of surgery, and grade of lymph node dissection were also independently and significantly prognostic. Although the treatment modality and types of surgery were not given in the reports from the regional registry, it is assumed that the JSCCR registry systems mainly covered patients who had a chance to receive more sound and radical mode of treatment at a high level hospital such as a university hospital, large-scale general hospital, or cancer center hospital in their district. This population bias may also reflect the aforementioned differences in survival rates.

Different Survival Rates Depending on Hospital Size

Murakami *et al.* (*5*) reported that the morbidity of cancers in any site of the colon is drastically increasing, especially in the sigmoid colon of the female. Similarly, the JSCCR registry showed a steeper increase in colon cancer in the female than in the

TABLE VI. Patient Lifetables by pTNM Stage, Site, and Year

Colon
1794–77

Stage	No.	1	2	3	4	5
0	50	100±0	97.9±4.2	97.9±4.2	95.7±5.9	93.4±7.3
I	190	99.5±1.1	96.8±2.6	94.0±3.5	90.1±4.4	88.9±4.7
II	905	94.4±1.5	89.1±2.1	83.6±2.5	78.8±2.8	75.7±2.9
III	593	89.7±2.5	78.1±3.4	69.7±3.8	63.7±4.1	58.9±4.2
IV	516	52.5±4.4	28.7±4.1	20.3±3.6	18.0±3.5	17.2±3.4

1978–81

Stage	No.	1	2	3	4	5
0	72	93.0±6.1	91.5±6.6	91.5±6.6	91.5±6.6	90.0±7.2
I	204	95.5±2.9	90.9±4.1	87.8±4.7	83.6±5.3	80.3±5.8
II	1,394	93.0±1.4	86.6±1.9	81.0±2.2	76.2±2.4	73.0±2.5
III	1,009	88.6±2.0	77.6±2.6	68.4±3.0	62.5±3.1	59.1±3.2
IV	750	50.2±3.7	28.6±3.3	19.9±3.0	15.6±2.7	13.6±2.6

1982–83

Stage	No.	1	2	3	4	5
0	62	98.4±3.2	96.7±4.6	93.4±6.4	93.4±6.4	89.7±8.0
I	296	96.3±2.2	93.8±2.8	89.3±3.6	87.8±3.9	85.4±4.2
II	1,376	95.8±1.1	90.6±1.6	85.6±1.9	82.2±2.1	79.2±2.3
III	968	89.8±1.9	77.8±2.7	69.7±3.0	64.7±3.1	61.1±3.2
IV	694	53.4±3.8	29.6±3.5	18.7±3.0	13.7±2.7	11.8±2.5

Rectum
1974–77

Stage	No.	1	2	3	4	5
0	42	95.2±6.6	90.5±9.1	88.1±10.0	83.1±11.6	83.1±11.6
I	402	93.2±2.5	89.9±3.0	86.2± 3.5	81.7± 3.9	76.3± 4.4
II	983	93.3±1.6	84.5±2.3	76.4± 2.8	71.2± 2.9	66.6± 3.1
III	973	88.0±2.1	69.9±3.0	56.2± 3.2	48.1± 3.3	42.6± 3.3
IV	376	53.1±5.2	25.2±4.6	15.2± 3.8	12.6± 3.5	9.7± 3.2

1978–81

Stage	No.	1	2	3	4	5
0	69	98.5±2.9	91.1±6.9	89.6± 7.4	88.1± 7.9	86.5± 8.4
I	494	97.1±1.5	93.2±2.3	90.1± 2.7	88.4± 2.9	85.7± 3.2
II	1,311	92.8±1.4	86.6±1.9	79.9± 2.2	73.8± 2.5	70.1± 2.6
III	1,298	88.1±1.8	71.4±2.5	58.7± 2.8	50.1± 2.8	44.1± 2.8
IV	503	53.2±4.5	26.3±3.9	16.0± 3.3	10.7± 2.8	9.6± 2.7

1982–83

Stage	No.	1	2	3	4	5
0	89	93.2±5.3	93.2±5.3	93.2± 5.3	90.8± 6.2	87.0± 7.3
I	563	96.8±1.5	93.7±2.1	90.1± 2.5	86.7± 2.9	84.5± 3.1
II	1,202	94.1±1.4	87.1±1.9	81.0± 2.3	75.4± 2.5	70.0± 2.7
III	1,314	91.6±1.5	74.9±2.4	61.8± 2.7	53.5± 2.8	47.9± 2.8
IV	493	57.0±4.5	26.7±4.0	15.9± 3.4	11.0± 2.9	8.3± 2.6

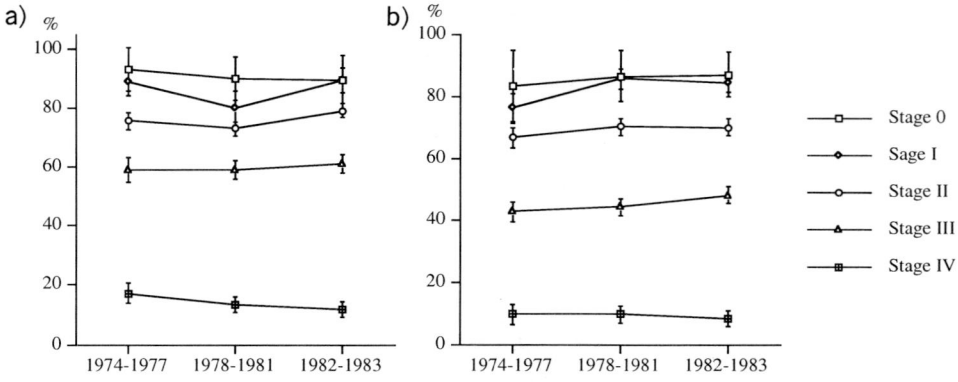

FIG. 5. Change of five year survival rate by year and pTNM stage
a. Colon cancer. b. Rectum cancer.

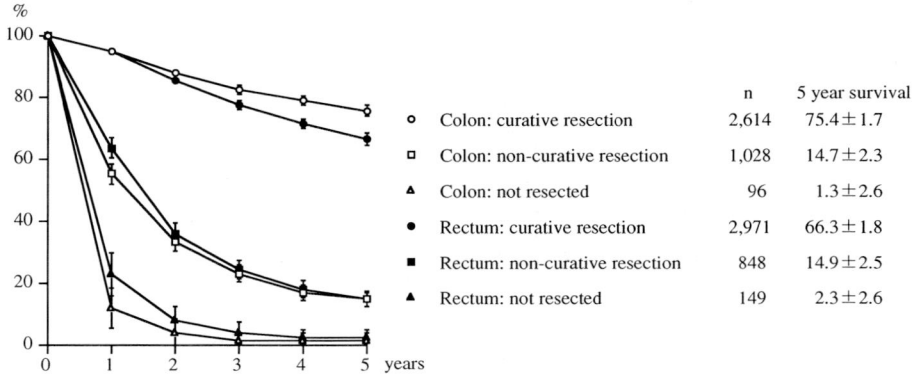

	n	5 year survival
Colon: curative resection	2,614	75.4±1.7
Colon: non-curative resection	1,028	14.7±2.3
Colon: not resected	96	1.3±2.6
Rectum: curative resection	2,971	66.3±1.8
Rectum: non-curative resection	848	14.9±2.5
Rectum: not resected	149	2.3±2.6

FIG. 6. Five year survival rate by mode of surgery and site of tumor

male. "The Fifth Report of Research on the Actual Condition of Malignant Neoplasms" (4) conducted by the Ministry of Health and Welfare in 1989 is the latest nationwide information on cancer in Japan. Cancers of stomach, colon and rectum, liver, bronchus, breast, and uterus that were treated from May 1 to July 31, 1985 at 18 regions where regional cancer registration had been made were investigated. According to this report, curative resection was carried out in 65.0% of 906 colon cancers and in 68.7% of 696 rectum cancers. These figures are slightly but significantly ($p < 0.01$) lower than those of the JSCCR registry. Another interesting result of the research was that three year survival rates were apparently different in terms of hospital type. The highest rate (69.8 ± 5.8% of colon cancer, 78.9 ± 6.4% of rectum cancer) was found in cancer center hospitals, followed by university hospitals (58.2 ± 4.0%, 61.8 ± 4.2%), so-called general hospitals* (51.9 ± 1.7%, 56.2 ± 2.0%), and small-scale clinics (46.9 ± 8.6%, 30.6 ± 11.7%). Seventy-two percent of the patients with large bowel cancer were treated at general hospitals. These facts may account for differences in the rate of curative resection and survival rates between the JSCCR

---

* Hospitals with more than 20 beds other than cancer center or university hospitals.

registry and the regional registry. Results attained by the cancer center hospitals may reflect the state of the art today, while the accumulated data of the JSCCR registry includes high-quality clinical and pathological information and represents standardized treatment of large bowel cancer in Japan.

Acknowledgments

A part of this work was supported by a Grant-in-Aid for Cancer Research from the Ministry of Health and Welfare of Japan. The registration committee appreciates Dr. Masayuki Yasutomi, President of the Japanese Society for Cancer of the Colon and Rectum, and the member doctors who contribute to this registry. Member hospitals are listed at the end of this book.

REFERENCES

1. Hanai, A., Kitagawa, T., Tsukuma, H., and Fujimoto, I. Trend of cancer incidence and survival in Japan. *CRC*, **2**, 823–834 (1993) (in Japanese).
2. Hanai, A., Sakata, S., Kitagawa, T., and Fujimoto, I. Change of survival rate of cancer patients in Osaka Prefecture, 1996–1980. *In* "Databook of Workshop on the Evaluation of Change of Survival Rate in Cancer Patients," pp. 106–122 (1988) (in Japanese).
3. Japanese Research Society for Cancer of the Colon and Rectum. General rules for clinical and pathological studies on cancer of the colon, rectum and anus. *Jpn. J. Surg.*, **13**, 557–573 (1983).
4. Ministry of Health and Welfare. *In* "Cancer Shown by Figures '90 — Report of the 5th Research for Actual Condition of Malignant Neoplasm in Japan," ed. K. Suemasu, Ministry of Health and Welfare and Foundation for Promotion of Cancer Research. Part I. Research on Patients. pp. 36–58 (1991) (in Japanese). Sogo-Igaku-shya, Tokyo.
5. Murakami, R., Kitagawa, T., Tsukuma, H., and Hanai, A. Descriptive epidemiology of colon cancer in Osaka, Japan. *CRC*, **2**, 854–863 (1993) (in Japanese).
6. Registry Committee, Japanese Research Society for Cancer of Colon and Rectum. A multivariate analysis of prognostic factors of colorectal cancer. *KARKINOS*, **6**, 515–526 (1993) (in Japanese).

REGISTRY OF FAMILIAL ADENOMATOUS POLYPOSIS

The Polyposis Committee of the Japanese Research Society for
Cancer of the Colon and Rectum*

The Polyposis Center of Japan had registered 1,104 (male 616, female 488) cases of familial adenomatous polyposis (FAP) and 722 families as of January, 1993. A family survey revealed 11,054 family members which included 2,136 affected cases. There were at least 5,146 persons who were at risk of being FAP gene carriers. Epidemiological and clinical data were presented. Frequency of FAP at birth in Japan was estimated as 1/17,400. Cumulative prevalence of colorectal cancer exceeded 50% in the age category of 40 to 44 years for both men and women, and exceeded 90% at around 60 years. Out of 414 deaths among FAP patients, 81% were from colorectal cancer. The importance of family examinations in preventing death from colorectal cancer was stressed. Total colectomy with ileo-rectal anastomosis was the most frequent surgery. Desmoid tumor and periampullary cancer was the most important target to watch next to colorectal cancer. Function-preserving surgery and minimal intervention for FAP patients should be sought by early detection of FAP and by periodic follow up. Registry of FAP patients combined with molecular diagnosis will be helpful for this purpose.

In 1972 Dr. J. Utsunomiya treated a patient with familial adenomatous polyposis (FAP) whose relatives had previously been reported twice in the literature as independent families, in 1930 and 1958 (*33*). This demonstrated the necessity of a central registry system for FAP families throughout the nation and maintenance of this record over generations to collect information on FAP and prevent colorectal cancer. The Center for Analyzing Familial Polyposis was established at Tokyo Medical and Dental University in 1975 through the great efforts of Dr. Utsunomiya (*37*). The registry was later expanded to include other types of gastrointestinal polyposis and hereditary colorectal cancer: Peutz-Jeghers syndrome, juvenile polyposis, and hereditary non-polyposis colorectal cancer (HNPCC). In 1982, the registry system went under the management of Drs. T. Iwama and Y. Mishima at the Research Center for Polyposis and Intestinal Diseases (the Polyposis Center). This Center was a national institute for a 10-year-period. Since April 1993 the registry and its related activities have been maintained at the Research Center for Genes and Genetic Diseases, Tokyo Medical and Dental University.

To promote nationwide registration of FAP, the Polyposis Center was recognized in 1982 as the registry office of the Polyposis Committee of the Japanese Re-

---

* Manuscript was prepared by Takeo Iwama and Yoshio Mishima, The Research Center for Polyposis and Intestinal Diseases, The 2nd Department of Surgery, Tokyo Medical and Dental University, 1-5-45 Yushima, Bunkyo-ku, Tokyo 113, Japan

search Society for Cancer of the Colon and Rectum. Since that time, the Center has reported annually on the number of registered patients and families with FAP, age- and sex-specific distribution of colorectal cancer, and prefecture- and institute-specific registered number of FAP cases. The purposes of the registry of hereditary colorectal cancer at the Polyposis Center include: 1) epidemiological study, 2) genetic study including molecular biology, and 3) clinical study on the natural history of these diseases, diagnosis, early treatment of cancer, preventive treatment of the disease, reasonable follow-up care of patients and their family members, and improving and developing surgical treatment for these diseases.

Data Collection

FAP is clinically defined as a condition in which more than 100 adenomas are distributed throughout the colon and rectum (*6*). Gardner's syndrome has been proven to be a variation of FAP (*18, 24*). Our material has been collected according to clinical definition. Information regarding the proband of FAP as well as other types of polyposis and hereditary colorectal cancer has been gathered through five different sources: 1) inquiries to hospitals throughout the nation, 2) autopsy records, 3) published literature, 4) voluntary visits by patients, and 5) the Japanese Research Society for Cancer of the Colon and Rectum. The most constant and important source of registration has been inquiries to doctors who published literature related to this disease and voluntary registration. The Polyposis Center serves as an information center for doctors who want to know about the epidemiological and genetic details of FAP or recent developments in FAP studies and other polyposis conditions. At the Department of Cytogenetics, Tokyo Medical and Dental University, fibroblasts, lymphocytes, and cancer cells are stored for cytogenetic studies. For each family, an exact pedigree map, a "working pedigree", has been constructed using the national family register system (Koseki) which has been legally maintained for more than 90 years. In order to identify family members, a permanent coding system was devised (*35*). The affected members are identified through hospital records, death certificates, and information from patients and their family members. The Polyposis Center sends a list of these high risk people to the regional physician who registered the case and the doctor encourages family members of the patient to have health examinations (Fig. 1). By this means, an increased number of cases linking two or more pedigrees which were registered independently has been discovered. Recently, the importance of a national or regional registry of polyposis patients has been recognized in many countries. National and regional registers all over the world are represented in the "Leeds Castle Polyposis Group", which was established in 1985 and holds plenum meetings every second year (*5*). In Europe, "Euro FAP" has been organized.

Basic Data on Registered Patients

The number of registered cases among gastrointestinal polyposis cases and hereditary colorectal cancer is shown in Table I. There were 1,104 cases (616 males, 488 females) of FAP and 722 families registered as of January 1993. Among them, 112 families (15.5%) were composed of two or more fused families. A family survey revealed 11,054 family members which included 2,136 affected cases. There are at

TABLE I. Registered Cases as of January 1993

	FAP	P-J	HNPCC	Juvenile polyposis
Registered cases	1,104	183	142	12
No. of families	722	173	120	12
Completed pedigree maps	676	158	103	5

FAP: familial adenomatous polyposis. P-J: Peutz-Jeghers syndrome.
HNPCC: hereditary nonpolyposis colorectal cancer (does not necessarily fulfill the definition of HNPCC).

TABLE II. Results of a Family Survey from Proband Cases as of January 1993

Cases	1,104
Families	722
Fused families (15.5% of 722)	112
Completed working pedigree maps	676
Members	11,054
Affected cases (alive 924, dead 1,212)	2,136
Persons at risk of FAP	5,146

TABLE III. Age and Sex Specific FAP Cases, and Cases with Colorectal Cancer among the Registered 1,091 FAP Cases[a]

Age	Male			Female		
	Colorectal cancer		Total	Colorectal cancer		Total
	+ (m, sm)	−		+ (m, sm)	−	
0–9	0	9	9	2(2)	5	7
10–13	1(1)	12	13	2(1)	14	16
15–19	6(3)	28	34	6(4)	29	35
20–24	22(11)	48	70	30(9)	40	70
25–29	43(13)	46	89	46(9)	28	74
30–34	44(8)	50	94	43(7)	28	71
35–39	74(14)	34	108	46(7)	25	71
40–44	49(3)	20	69	47(5)	11	58
45–49	35(5)	3	38	22(2)	6	28
50–54	29(3)	9	38	20(2)	3	23
55–59	20	1	21	10	1	11
60–	19(2)	5	24	15(1)	5	20
Total	342(63)	265	607	289(49)	195	484

m, sm: carcinoma *in situ* or cancer restricted to submucosa.
[a] Cases with insufficient clinical information were excluded.

least 5,146 persons who are at risk of being FAP gene carriers (Table II). There is no particular geographic cluster of FAP cases in Japan. Based on these data in 1981, Murata *et al.* (*22*) estimated the frequency of FAP at birth as 5.74/100,000 or 1/17,400. Comparable data were 1/23,790 in England, 1/7,437 in the U.S.A (*6*), 1/7,646 in Sweden (*1*), 1/10,000 in Denmark with the point prevalence rate of 26 per million inhabitants at the end of 1982 (*3*), and between 1/24,840 and 1/14,740 in Finland (*17*). Sex ratio (male/female) of the registered FAP cases was 1.24 (Table III), but it was 1.19 among cases that were found by family examination (Table IV).

TABLE IV. Age and Sex Specific Number of FAP cases and Cases with Colorectal Cancer Found by Examination of FAP Families or by Extracolonic Manifestations of FAP

Age	Male	Female	Total	% of colorectal cancer
0–9	9 (0)	3 (0)	12 (0)	0
10–13	12 (0)	9 (0)	21 (0)	0
15–19	11 (1)	16 (0)	27 (1)	3.7
20–24	24 (2)	23 (3)	47 (5)	10.6
25–29	19 (1)	19 (5)	38 (6)	15.8
30–34	25 (5)	15 (3)	40 (8)	20.0
35–39	26 (12)	17 (4)	43 (16)	37.2
40–44	18 (8)	12 (6)	30 (14)	46.7
45–49	2 (1)	7 (4)	9 (5)	55.6
50–54	5 (2)	4 (2)	9 (4)	44.4
55–59	1 (1)	2 (1)	3 (2)	66.7
60–	2 (0)	2 (0)	4 (0)	0
Total	154 (33)	129 (28)	283 (61)	21.6

( ): number of patients with colorectal cancer.

TABLE V. Initial Symptoms of Primary Cases

	Number	%
No symptom	145	11.9
Feces with blood	377	30.9
Diarrhea	328	26.9
Abdominal pain	187	15.3
Anemia	51	4.2
Others	131	10.7

Clinical Details

Three dominant initial symptoms were feces with blood, 31%; diarrhea, 27%; and abdominal pain, 15% (Table V). Age at diagnosis of FAP and the number of cancer cases among them are shown in Table IV. Cumulative prevalence of colorectal cancer (except early cancer) exceeded 50% in the age category of 40 to 44 years for both men and women, and exceeded 90% at around 60 years (13) (Fig 2). Prevalence of colorectal cancer among patients who were diagnosed predominantly by family examination or partly by extra-colonic checkup for a clinical symptom is shown in Table IV. The overall morbidity rate from colorectal cancer was 21.6% in this group, substantially lower than the morbidity of 47.6% among background cases (Table IV). This demonstrates the importance of family examinations in preventing death from colorectal cancer (17). There was a notable improvement in prognosis in patients who had surveillance and surgery (25). Because of rapid recent developments in molecular biological studies on FAP (29) and hereditary nonpolyposis colorectal cancer (2, 8), molecular diagnosis may soon be clinically applicable for these conditions. Colonic carcinoma in FAP occurs frequently in multiple form. In the general population, multiple carcinoma was only found in 4.5% of colorectal carcinoma cases, but multiple lesions were found in 38% of 497 FAP carcinoma cases (Table VI).

Although the site of carcinoma in FAP was similar to that in the general popula-

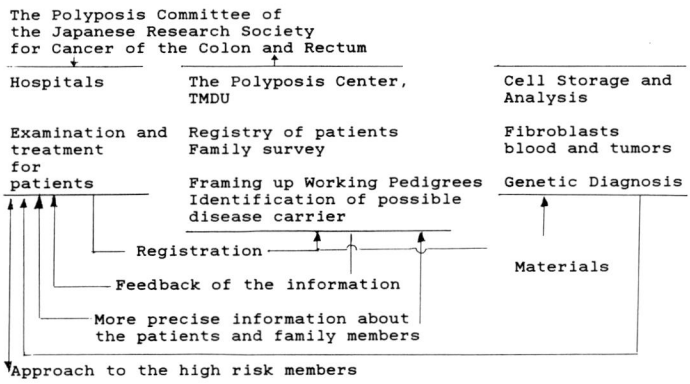

FIG. 1. Working system of the Polyposis Center of Japan for familial adenomatous polyposis

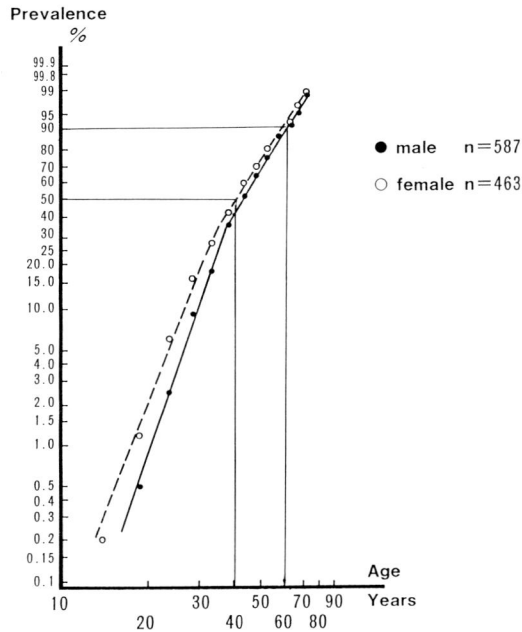

FIG. 2. Cumulative prevalence of colorectal cancer in 1,050 patients with FAP

tion, the actual occurrence of carcinoma at each location was greater than this distribution figure because of the multiplicity of carcinomas (Table VII). For example, 274 cases with rectal cancer actually represented 55.1% of 497 FAP cases. The incidence of extra-colonic tumors is shown in Table VIII (*13*). Mean age at diagnosis was higher than that of colorectal cancer except for desmoid tumor and thyroid cancer.

1. *Cause of death*

Three hundred and thirty five (81%) of 414 deaths among FAP patients were due to colorectal cancer. Gastric cancer (*34*), periampullary cancer (including duodenal

TABLE VI. Multiplicity in Colorectal Cancer Patients

Number of cancers	FAP[a]		General population	
	497 cases		24,616 cases[b]	
Single	308	62.0%	23,504	95.5%
2	113	22.7	895	3.6
3	34	6.8	148	0.6
4	10	2.0	39	0.2
5–	31	6.2	30	0.1

[a] Advanced cancer.
[b] The 16th meeting of Jpn. Soc. Large Bowel Cancer Res.

TABLE VII. Location of Colorectal Cancer

Location	497 FAP cases		General population Jpn. Soc. Large Bowel Cancer Res. (%)
	Number of patients[a]	Proportion of tumors (%)	
Cecum	31	4.2	5.7
Ascending	65	8.9	7.6
Transverse	91	12.4	7.2
Descending	61	8.3	4.5
Sigmoid	210	28.7	24.5
Rectum	274	37.4[b]	45.1

[a] Multiple cancers in one location were counted as one in that location.
[b] Rectal cancer occurred in 274 (55.1%) out of 497 cancer cases.

TABLE VIII. Extra Colonic Tumors among FAP Patients

	Cases		Mean age at diagnosis (mean ± SD)
	Male	Female	
Thyroid cancer	2	9	32.5 ± 11.8
Cancer of the duodenum and small intestine	13	10	43.7 ± 11.8
Gastric cancer	17	10	49.2 ± 12.7
Desmoid tumor	26	45	32.2 ± 9.4

TABLE IX. Cause-specific Observed/Expected Mortality Ratios or Standardized Mortality Ratios

Cause of death	Standardized mortality ratios (95% confidence interval)			p
	Male	Female	Total	
Duodenal or small intestinal carcinoma[a]	177 (65–386)	493 (160–1,148)	250 (112–447)	<0.001
Gastric carcinoma	2.77 (1.11–5.69)	5.18 (1.68–12.1)	3.43 (1.77–6.0)	<0.002
Colorectal carcinoma	175 (152–202)	286 (241–338)	210 (183–241)	<0.001
All deaths	6.26 (5.5–7.12)	14.8 (12.7–17.1)	8.3 (7.53–9.15)	<0.001

p values refer to total cases. (Iwama, T. Ann. Surg., **217**, 101 (1993))
[a] Including periampullary carcinoma.

TABLE X. Rectal Cancer Risk after Rectum Preserving Operation in FAP Patients

Institute	Postoperative years			
	5	10	15	20
St Mark's Hosp. (1)	1.5%	3.6	3.6	3.6
Scandinavia[a]	3.1	4.5	5.7	9.4
Mayo Clinic[b]	5	13	25	42
Polyposis Center[c]	4.0	12.8 (11.1–14.5)[d]	24.2 (17.2–31.2)[d]	—

[a] De Cosse, J.J. et al. Br. J. Surg., **79**, 1372–1375 (1992).
[b] Moertel, C.G. Cancer, **28**, 160–164 (1971).
[c] Iwama, T. Dis. Colon Rectum, **37**, 1024–1026 (1994).
[d] 5% confidence interval.

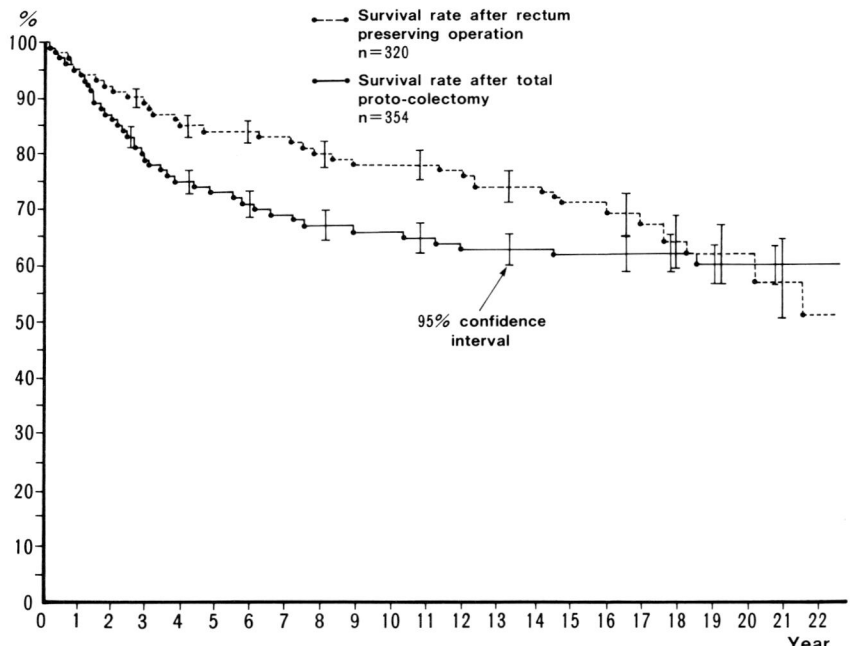

FIG. 3. Procedure specific survival rate after colorectal surgery performed in Japan

and small intestinal cancer) (*12*), desmoid tumor (*20*), and other malignant tumors caused 2 to 3% of deaths (*13*). The periampullary carcinoma was most important, because its standardized mortality rate is as high as that of colorectal cancer (Table IX), and no follow-up system of treatment has yet been established (*12, 13, 26*).

2. Surgical treatment of colorectal polyposis and its prognosis

Among registered cases, initial surgery included total procto-colectomy with ileostomy (197 cases), total procto-colectomy with ileo anal anastomosis (*36*) (143 cases), and total colectomy with ileo rectal anastomosis (*19*) (272 cases). Of all surgeries performed, 320 cases underwent rectum-preserving surgery and 354 underwent total colorectal resection. Survival curves for these two groups are shown in Fig. 3.

TABLE XI. Overall Relative Mortality in FAP Family Members Less Than 20 Years of Age

Sex	Exposed persons (person-yr)	Observed deaths	Expected deaths	Relative mortality rate (95% CI)	z	p
Male	13,400	36	23.04	1.56 (1.09–2.17)	2.4	0.016
Female	11,508	22	16.03	1.37 (0.86–2.07)	1.4	0.16
Total	24,908	58	39.07	1.48 (1.13–1.92)	2.7	0.007

CI: confidence interval. z: z score of normal distribution. (Iwama, T. *Cancer*, **73**, 2065 (1994))

TABLE XII. Relative Risk of Cancer Death in FAP Family Members

Age	Sex	Exposed persons (person-yr)	Observed deaths	Expected deaths	Relative mortality rate (95% CI)	z	p
0	Male	925	0	0.055	—	0.47	>0.5
	Female	839	0	0.045	—	0.42	>0.5
1–4	Male	3,469	4	0.26	15.4 (4.19–39.4)	3.0	0.003
	Female	3,178	3	0.20	15 (3.09–43.8)	2.57	0.01
5–9	Male	3,836	2	0.21	9.25 (1.15–21.8)	1.91	0.06
	Female	3,541.5	0	0.14	—	0.75	>0.4
10–14	Male	3,077.5	0	0.14	—	0.75	>0.4
	Female	2,852.5	0	0.1	—	0.63	>0.5
15–19	Male	2,092.5	2	0.13	15.4 (1.86–55.6)	2.11	0.035
	Female	1,097	1	0.08	12.5 (0.31–69.6)	1.43	>0.1
20–25	Male	1,036	2	0.06	33.3 (4.02–120)	2.34	0.02
	Female	1,031.5	6	0.04	150 (55.1–327)	4.50	0.001

(Iwama, T. *Cancer*, **73**, 2065 (1994))

Initially, the survival curve of the total colorectal resection group decreased rapidly because of the poor prognosis of already present rectal cancer. This was later followed by a faster decrease in the survival of the rectum-preserving group because of the development of rectal cancer. Postoperative risk of cancer in the preserved rectum in Japan was 4% at 5 years, 13% at 10 years, and 24% at 15 years (Table X). Main contributing factors to these figures are the length of preserved rectum, age or follow-up period, density of polyps, and method of follow-up observation (*16*). A randomized, double blind and controlled trial showed the effectiveness of the nonsteroidal anti-inflammatory drug Sulindac in reducing colonic polyps, but failed to show that it can replace colectomy as primary therapy (*10*).

3. Treatment of other tumors

There is no proven effective treatment for desmoid tumor except complete removal. Although a long-term nonsteroidal anti-inflammatory drug seems effective, spontaneous regression sometimes occurs (*32*). Following colorectal cancer, periampullary carcinoma is the most important tumor because at least 70% of cancer in the duodenum develops in the ampullary portion (*28*). Indications for local excision of the ampulla of Vater were proposed for the early stage of this tumor (*15*). This proposal may justify periodic observation of the duodenum, because this kind of treatment is far more beneficial than pancreatico-duodenectomy for FAP patients; the latter procedure is a very severe operation for patients with FAP who have already had total colectomy. The incidence of gastric cancer among FAP patients in Japan is 4.5 to 13.6 % (*13, 38*), 3.1 times higher than that in the general population (*13*), but outside Japan, gastric carcinoma is a rare complication (*26*). The incidence of thyroid cancer is 19 to 100 times higher than that in the general population (*4, 13*). However, regular thyroid examination is not indicated, as thyroid cancer is uncommon and the prognosis is excellent (*4*).

There is limited data about the risk of cancer or mortality among very young first-degree family members of FAP patients (*9*). In Japan, overall relative mortality rate in these young members (<20 years) of FAP patients was 1.48 (Table XI). Relative cancer mortality in the age group between 1 and 4 years was significantly higher (Table XII), because the relative mortality from hepatoblastoma in this group was 176 (*14*).

Discussion

These registered cases were collected from several sources as described previously. There may be some bias or deviation due to the length of time required to obtain these data, the main source of registration being our requests to doctors who published findings, and because of our having to depend on their willingness. We do not view this as serious, however, because our registry was complementary with the Cancer Registry of Colorectal Cancer. Recently, more cases have been diagnosed by examination of family members; this tendency will be accelerated by the use of molecular diagnosis (*7, 21, 23, 29*).

The site of FAP gene mutation seems related to the expressed manifestation of FAP. A less severe form of FAP is caused by mutated sites which are located very close to the 5' end of the APC gene (*31*). Germline mutations between codon 1250 and 1464 were observed in profuse type polyposis, whereas in patients with fewer polyps no mutation was observed in that region. Congenital hypertrophy of retinal pigment epithelium (CHRPE) lesions are almost always absent if the mutation occurs before exon 9, which is a rather early part of the gene, but are systematically present if the mutation occurs after this exon (*27*). However, a recent paper found a substantial phenotypic variability of FAP in 11 unrelated families with identical APC gene mutation (*11*). It is very interesting that inactivation of the APC gene by two mutations (germinal and somatic) is necessary in the development of adenoma in FAP (*21*). The protein product of APC gene is a 2,844 amino acid polypeptide, but its function has not yet been identified. The APC protein was recently found to be associated with beta-catenin (*30*), and it is speculated that reduced affinity of the mutant APC protein with beta-catenin may contribute to the APC phenotype. Beta-catenin associates with the cytoplasmic tail of the cell adhesion molecule E-cadherin and is thought to be essential for the normal function of E-cadherin in maintaining the adhesion junction of epithelial cells. These studies suggest that the APC protein with catenin is closely related to the differentiation of the gastrointestinal mucosa.

The molecular diagnosis of FAP is now very expensive. The cost should be reduced so that the method can be accepted as a routine medical test. Greater merit from early diagnosis will be achieved by developing more effective and diminished therapeutic interventions for FAP patients. In the future, this registry system and molecular diagnosis should be expanded to include HNPCC (*2, 8*). HNPCC patients will be more effectively treated than FAP patients by periodic follow-up with endoscopy since the number of colonic lesions of HNPCC is limited. Consequently, endoscopic polypectomy or laparoscopic colectomy may replace traditional colectomy in the stage of early cancer or at least during the adenoma stage in HNPCC patients. As a matter of course, the Polyposis Center has been very careful to safeguard the privacy of registered patients. The Center will continue to function to improve the welfare of patients with FAP and other hereditary gastrointestinal tumors.

Acknowledgments

Quotations have been used from "Pathological and Genetic Aspects of Adenomatosis Coli in Japan" by J. Utsunomiya appearing in Gann Monograph on Cancer Research No. 35; "Genetics of Human Tumors in Japan", Japan Scientific Societies Press, 1988; and "Current Status of the Registration of Familial Adenomatous Polyposis at the Polyposis Center in Japan" by T. Iwama, Y. Mishima *et al.*, in "Hereditary Colorectal Cancer", Springer-Verlag, Tokyo, 1990.

A part of this work was supported by the Cancer Research Fund of the Ministry of Health and Welfare, and the Ministry of Education, Science and Culture of Japan.

REFERENCES

1. Alm, T. and Licznerski, G. The intestinal polyposis. *Clin. Gastroenterol.*, **2**, 577–602 (1973).
2. Bronner, C.E., Baker, S.M., Morrison, P.T. *et al.* Mutation in the DNA mismatch repair gene homologue hMLH1 is associated with hereditary non-polyposis colon cancer. *Nature*, **368**, 258–261 (1994).
3. Bulow, S., Holms, N.V., and Hauge, M. The incidence and prevalence of familial polyposis coli. *Scand. J. Soc. Med.*, **14**, 67–74 (1986).
4. Bülow, S., Holm, N.V., and Mellemgaard, A. Papillary thyroid carcinoma in Danish patients with familial adenomatous polyposis. *Int. J. Colorect. Dis.*, **3**, 29–31 (1988).
5. Bülow, S., Burn, J., Neal, K., Northover, J., and Vasen, H. The establishment of a polyposis register. *Int. J. Colorect. Dis.*, **8**, 34–38 (1993).
6. Bussey, H.J.R. *In* "Familial Polyposis Coli," pp. 1–93 (1975). The Johns Hopkins University Press, Baltimore.
7. Cottrell, S., Bicknel, D., Kalamanis, L., and Bodmer, W.F. Molecular analysis of APC mutations in familial adenomatous polyposis and sporadic colon carcinomas. *Lancet*, **340**, 626–630 (1992).
8. Fisher, R, Lescoe, M.K., Rao, M.R.S., Copeland, N.G., Jenkins, N.A., Garber, J., Kane, M., and Kolodner, R. The human mutator gene homolog MSH2 and its association with hereditary nonpolyposis colon cancer. *Cell*, **75**, 1027–1038 (1993).
9. Giardiello, F.M., Johan, G., Offerhaus, J.A., Krush, A., and Booker, S.V. Risk of hepatoblastoma in familial adenomatous polyposis. *J. Pediat.*, **119**, 766–768 (1991).
10. Giardiello, F.M., Hamilton, S.R., Krush, A.J., Piantadosi, S., Hylind, L.M., Celano, P., Booker, S.V., Robinson, C.R., and Offerhaus, G.J. Treatment of colonic and rectal adenomas with Sulindac in familial adenomatous polyposis. *N. Engl. J. Med.*, **328**, 1313–1316 (1993).
11. Giardiello, F.M., Krush, A.J., Petersen, G.M., Brooker, S.V., Kerr, M., Tong, L.L., and Hamilton, S.R. *Gastroenterology*, **106**, 1542–1547 (1994).
12. Iida, M., Yao, T., Itoh, H. *et al.* Natural history of duodenal lesions in Japanese patients with familial adenomatous coli. *J. Surg. Oncol.*, **38**, 19–21 (1988).
13. Iwama, T., Mishima, Y., and Utsunomiya, J. The impact of familial adenomatous polyposis on the tumorigenesis and mortality at the several organs. *Ann. Surg.*, **217**, 101–108 (1993).

14. Iwama, T. and Mishima, Y. Mortality in young first-degree relatives of patients with familial adenomatous polyposis. *Cancer,* **73**, 2065–2068 (1994).
15. Iwama, T., Tomita, H., Kawachi, Y., Yoshinaga, K., Kume, S., Maruyama, H., and Mishima, Y. Indication of local excision for ampullary lesion associated with familial adenomatous polyposis. *J. Am. Coll. Surgeons,* **179**, 462–464 (1994).
16. Iwama, T. and Mishima, Y. Analysis of factors which may affect the risk of rectal cancer after rectum preserving operation in patients with familial adenomatous polyposis. *Dis. Colon Rectum,* **37**, 1024–1026 (1994).
17. Jarvinen, H.J. Epidemiology of familial adenomatous polyposis in Finland: impact of family screening on the colorectal cancer rate and survival. *Gut,* **33**, 357–360 (1992).
18. Kinzler, K.W., Nilbert, M.C., Su, L. *et al.* Identification of FAP locus genes from chromosome 5q21. *Science,* **253**, 661–665 (1991).
19. Lockhart-Mummery, H.E., Dukes, C.E., and Bussey, H.J.R. The surgical treatment of familial polyposis of the colon. *Br. J. Surg.,* **43**, 476–481 (1956).
20. McAdam, W.A.F. and Goligher, J.C. The occurrence of desmoid tumor in patients with familial polyposis coli. *Br. J. Surg.,* **57**, 618–631 (1970).
21. Miyaki, M., Konishi, M., Yanosita, R.K. *et al.* Characteristic of somatic mutation of adenomatous polyposis coli gene in colorectal tumors. *Cancer Res.,* **54**, 3011–3020 (1994).
22. Murata, M., Utsunomiya, T., Iwama, T., and Tanimura, M. Frequency of adenomatosis coli in Japan. *Jpn. J. Human Genet.,* **26**, 19–30 (1981).
23. Nagase, H., Miyoshi, Y., Nakamura, Y. *et al.* Correlation between the location of germ-line mutation in the APC gene and the number of colorectal polyposis in familial adenomatous patients. *Cancer Res.,* **52**, 4055–4057 (1992).
24. Nishisho, I., Nakamura, Y., Miyoshi, Y. et al. Mutation of chromosome 5q21 gene in FAP and colorectal cancer patients. *Science,* **253**, 665–669 (1991).
25. Nugent, K.P., Spigelman, A. D., and Phillip, R.K.S. Life expectancy after colectomy and ileorectal anastomosis for familial adenomatous polyposis. *Dis. Colon Rectum,* **36**, 1059–1062 (1993).
26. Offerhaus, G.J.A., Giardiello, F.M., Krush, A.J., Brooker, S.V., Tersmette, A.C., Kelley, K., and Hamilton, S.R. The risk of upper gastrointestinal cancer in familial adenomatous polyposis. *Gastroenterology,* **102**, 1980–1982 (1992).
27. Olshwang, S., Tiret, A., Laurent-Puig, P., Muleris, M., Parc, R., Thomas, G., and Thomas, G. Restriction of ocular fundus lesions to a specific subgroup of APC mutations in adenomatous polyposis coli patients. *Cell,* **75**, 959–968 (1993).
28. Ono, C., Iwama, T., and Mishima, Y. A case of familial adenomatous polyposis complicated by thyroid carcinoma, carcinoma of the ampulla of Vater and adrenocortical adenoma. *Jpn. J. Surg.,* **21**, 234–240 (1991).
29. Powell, S.M., Petersen, G.M., Krush, A.J., Brooker, S., Giardiello, F.M., Hamilton, S.R., Vogelstein, B., and Kinzler, K.W. Molecular diagnosis of familial adenomatous polyposis. *N. Engl. J. Med.,* **329**, 1982–1987 (1993).
30. Rubinfeld, B., Polakis, P., Albert, I., Muller, O., Chamberlain, S.H., Masiaz, F.R., Munemitsu, S., and Polakis, P. Association of the APC gene product with beta-catenin. *Science,* **262**, 1731–1734 (1993).
31. Spiro, L., Olschwang, S., Groden, J. *et al.* Alleles of the APC gene: an attenuated form of familial polyposis. *Cell,* **75**, 951–957 (1993).
32. Tsukada, K., Church, J., Jagelman, D.G., Fazio, W.V., McGannon, E., George, C.R., Schroder, T., Lavery, I., and Oakley, J. Noncytotoxic drug therapy for intra-abdominal desmoid tumor in patients with familial adenomatous polyposis. *Dis. Colon Rectum,* **35**, 29–33 (1992).

33. Utsunomiya, J., Iwama, T., Suzuki, H., and Komatsu, I. Long-time follow-up of a family of familial polyposis of the colon. *Igaku no Ayumi,* **81**, 493–498 (1972) (in Japanese).
34. Utsunomiya, J., Maki, T., Iwama, T., Matsunaga, Y., Ichikawa, T., Shimomura, T., Hamaguchi, E., and Aoki, N. Gastric lesion of familial adenomatous polyposis coli. *Cancer,* **34**, 745–754 (1974).
35. Utsunomiya, J. and Iwama, T. Adenomatosis coli in Japan. *In* "Colorectal Cancer: Prevention, Epidemiology, and Screening," ed. S. Winawer and S.D. Sherlock, pp. 83–94 (1980). Raven Press, New York.
36. Utsunomiya, J., Iwama, T., Imajo, M., Matsuo, S., Sawai, S., Yaegashi, K., and Hirayama, R. Total colectomy, mucosal proctectomy, and ileoanal anastomosis. *Dis. Colon Rectum,* **23**, 2459–2464 (1980).
37. Utsunomiya, J. Pathology and genetic aspects of adenomatosis coli in Japan. *In* "Genetics of Human Tumors in Japan," ed. H. Takebe and J. Utsunomiya, pp. 45–59 (1988). Japan Sci. Soc. Press, Tokyo.
38. Watanabe, H., Enjoji, M., Yao, T., and Ohsato, K. Gastric lesions in familial adenomatosis coli. *Hum. Pathol.,* **9**, 269–283 (1978).

PRIMARY LIVER CANCER IN JAPAN

The Liver Cancer Study Group of Japan*

Primary liver cancer is common in Japan as in other Asian countries. Over 90% of liver cancers are hepatocellular carcinoma, and many patients have a past history of hepatitis and frequently have hepatic cirrhosis. HBs antigen was detected in 40% of hepatocellular carcinoma cases in 1970, but incidence of the antigen had gradually but clearly decreased to 20% by 1990. HCV virus hepatitis now plays an important role as an etiological factor in hepatocellular carcinoma.

Recent advances in diagnostic techniques, especially imaging diagnosis, has made it possible to detect small liver cancer (less than 2 cm in diameter) in approximately 10% of all cases. Survival rate after surgical treatment, such as segmental resection, is improving and postoperative death is decreasing.

Factors allowing prediction of survival rate or those governing risk of recurrence have been more clearly identified.

Primary liver cancer is common in Japan, as in other Asian countries, but it is not as common in Western countries. In Japan, its incidence now ranks next to that of stomach cancer, and the number of patients with liver cancer is showing a gradual and definite increase.

The Liver Cancer Study Group of Japan has been conducting follow-up studies since 1965 with the cooperation of institutions throughout the country. Records of patients have been collected and analyzed by computer. The pathogenesis of primary liver cancer was unknown in 1970, and its diagnosis was difficult. Patients who could be treated in the early stage were scarce. The records of these patients show that primary liver cancer in Japan has the following characteristics:

1) Over 90% of liver cancers are hepatocellular carcinomas.
2) The incidence of primary liver cancer is highest in the sixth decade of life.
3) Primary liver cancer is more common in men than in women.
4) Many patients have a past history of hepatitis and frequently have hepatic cirrhosis; however, the number of HBs antigen carriers has definitely been decreasing.

On the basis of these characteristics, examinations of high risk patients and greater use of ultrasonography and computed tomography imaging have made it possible to detect primary liver cancer in the early stage. The 9th report by the Liver Cancer Study Group of Japan showed that small liver cancers (less than 2 cm in diameter) were detected in 10% of the patients.

---

* Manuscript was prepared by Shigeki Arii and Takayoshi Tobe, Hamamatsu Rosai Hospital, 25 Shogencho, Hamamatsu 430, Japan

TABLE I. Number of Patients

Report	Duration	Histologic diagnosis proven			Total	Clinical diagnosis	Total
		Male	Female	Unknown			
3rd	1960–1974	2,153	563	—			2,716
4th	1968–1977	2,299	530	—	2,829	1,202	4,031
5th	1978–1979	934	231	33	1,198	1,198	2,396
6th	1980–1981	1,824	421	41	2,286	2,372	4,658
7th	1982–1983	1,811	425	15	2,251	3,316	5,567
8th	1984–1985	2,021	484	9	2,514	4,806	7,320
9th	1986–1987	2,621	636	6	3,263	6,301	9,564
10th	1988–1989	2,924	666	48	3,638	7,062	10,700
11th	1990–1991	Now being collected					

The first and second reports were omitted because the classification and method of analysis were completely different. (Liver Cancer Study Group of Japan)

The number of operable cases has also shown a gradual but definite increase. Safe surgical procedures for liver cancer associated with severe hepatic cirrhosis are now well established in Japan; recent reports indicate that postoperative complications after hepatectomy occur in only 3–4% of cases, with none being recorded in a few institutes. Further advances have been made through the identification of various backgrounds and factors that influence the survival rate after hepatic resection, and the determination of important risk factors for recurrence.

Data Collection: Criteria, Hospital, Data Check, Data Processing

From 1965 to 1977, the Liver Cancer Study Group of Japan reported every 3 years an analysis of primary liver cancer in the country. In the fourth survey in 1980, a statistical analysis was done of 4,031 cases of primary liver cancer diagnosed in 155 institutions from January 1, 1968 to December 31, 1977.

In 1978 a new questionnaire designed for computerized analysis was introduced, and since then surveys have been performed every 2 years. The number of patients is shown in Table I. The current survey comprises the cases of primary liver cancer diagnosed and treated from January 1, 1988 to December 31, 1989. In addition, the survival curves of patients treated with hepatic resection from 1978 to 1989 were correlated with factors indicating the tumor stage.

The study was based on the answers to 258 questions from 562 institutes throughout the country. The survey and analysis, using mainly histologically proven cases, included gross anatomic and histologic features of the tumors, pathology of the noncancerous portion, distant metastases, past medical history, frequency of positive Hepatitis B surface antigen and Hepatitis B surface antibody, age distribution, various diagnostic procedures, surgical procedures, and survival rate in relation to operative curability and tumor stage.

Subjects and Methods

The participants in this survey were patients with primary liver cancer diagnosed and treated from January 1, 1988 to December 31, 1989. A questionnaire that covered 258 items including age, history, gross anatomic and histologic features of the tumors, noncancerous portions of the liver, grade of anaplasia, growth pattern, distant metastasis, diagnostic procedures, surgical treatment, and so on was sent to 562 hospitals and institutions throughout the country. The data were coded, fed into a computer, and analyzed in this article.

The calculation of the survival rates of the hepatocellular carcinoma patients receiving hepatic resections is based on a follow-up from January 1, 1978 to December 31, 1989, when a prototype of the present questionnaire, designed for computerized analysis, was introduced. Survival rates were also correlated with the factors indicating the histologic features and the developmental stages of the tumor. The calculation used the traditional lifetime table method of Cutler-Ederer (1). The date of admission, rather than the data of diagnosis or initial treatment, is the starting point in the calculation of survival time. The statistical significance of the difference in the survival pattern between the earlier and the later surveyed groups was analyzed by the log-rank test.

Basic Data on the Registered Patients: Number of Patients by Year, Age Distribution by Sex, Year, Histology, etc.

The registered patients from each report are listed in Table I. The first and second reports were omitted because the classification and method of analysis were completely different.

From the current 10th Report (January 1, 1988–December 31, 1989) of the 10,700 cases of primary liver cancer on file, 3,345 were diagnosed histologically: 963 at autopsy and 2,382 at operation or biopsy. The remaining cases were diagnosed as primary liver cancer by clinical findings, laboratory findings, computed tomography, hepatic angiography, ultrasonography, or laparoscopy. The survey presented here is based on the 3,638 histologically proven cases.

Number, Sex, and Age of Patients

Table II shows the number of patients classified by histology: 3,345 had hepatocellular carcinoma with a male/female ratio of 4.7 to 1; 173 had cholangiocarcinoma with a male/female ratio of 1.6 to 1; 26 had mixed carcinoma, 11 had hepatoblastoma,

TABLE II. Number of Patients: Histologic and Clinical Diagnosis

	Male $n=8,301$	Female $n=2,134$	Sex unknown $n=163$	Total
Hepatocellular carcinoma	7,955	1,975	152	10,082
Cholangiocellular carcinoma	222	114	9	345
Mixed type	23	8	0	31
Hepatoblastoma	19	11	0	30
Sarcoma	4	2	1	7
Cystoadenocarcinoma	3	6	0	9
Other primary liver cancer	75	18	1	94
Unknown (histologically)				102

n: number of patients.   (Liver Cancer Study Group of Japan (1988,1989))

TABLE III. Age Distribution

Age	HC M n=7,692	HC F n=1,921	HC Total n=9,613	CC M n=205	CC F n=110	CC Total n=315	MX M n=22	MX F n=7	MX Total n=29	HB M n=19	HB F n=10	HB Total n=29	SA M n=3	SA F n=2	SA Total n=5	CA M n=3	CA F n=6	CA Total n=9
0–4	0	1	4	0	0	0	0	0	0	7	5	12	0	0	0	0	0	0
5–9	2	1	3	0	0	0	0	0	0	2	0	2	0	0	0	0	0	0
10–14	8	0	8	0	0	0	0	0	0	0	0	0	0	0	0	0	0	0
15–19	0	4	4	0	0	0	1	0	1	0	0	0	0	0	0	0	0	0
20–24	5	3	8	0	0	0	0	0	0	0	0	0	0	0	0	0	0	0
25–29	9	2	11	1	1	2	0	1	1	0	0	0	0	0	0	0	0	0
30–34	24	3	27	0	0	0	0	0	0	0	0	0	0	0	0	0	0	0
35–39	110	15	125	5	2	7	0	1	1	0	0	0	0	0	0	0	0	0
40–44	217	23	240	12	2	14	0	1	1	0	0	0	0	0	0	1	0	1
45–49	406	72	478	9	6	15	3	1	4	0	0	0	1	1	2	1	1	2
50–54	1,113	132	1,245	21	7	28	3	0	3	1	0	1	0	0	0	0	2	2
55–59	1,933	319	2,252	36	19	55	2	0	2	5	0	5	1	0	1	0	1	1
61–64	1,675	434	2,109	41	17	58	6	1	7	1	0	1	0	0	0	0	1	1
65–69	1,008	404	1,412	24	16	40	3	1	4	0	4	4	0	1	1	1	0	1
70–74	676	275	951	34	21	55	4	1	5	1	1	2	1	1	2	0	1	1
75–79	367	177	544	16	11	27	0	0	0	1	0	1	0	0	0	0	0	0
80–84	106	38	144	5	6	11	0	0	0	1	0	1	0	0	0	0	0	0
85–89	30	16	46	1	2	3	0	0	0	0	0	0	0	0	0	0	0	0
90–	3	2	5	0	0	0	0	0	0	0	0	0	0	0	0	0	0	0
Mean	60.5	64.1		62.0	64.7		59.3	51.4		34.4	35.4		58.8	70.6		52.3	57.5	

HC, hepatocellular carcinoma; CC, cholangiocellular carcinoma; MX, mixed carcinoma; HB, hepatoblastoma; SA, sarcoma; CA, cystoadenocarcinoma.   (Liver Cancer Study Group of Japan (1988, 1989))

TABLE IV. Diagnostic Procedure

	HC n=9,607	CC n=317	MX n=29	HB n=29	SA n=5	CA n=9
US	3,465 (36.1%)	96 (30.3%)	10 (34.5%)	11 (38.0%)	0	3 (33.3%)
CT	2,017 (21.0%)	76 (24.0%)	5 (17.2%)	11 (38.0%)	2 (40.0%)	3 (33.3%)
Angiography	3,265 (34.0%)	60 (18.9%)	8 (27.6%)	2 (6.9%)	0	1 (11.1%)
Laparoscopy	26 (0.3%)	2 (0.6%)	0	0	1 (20.0%)	0
cytological	113 (1.2%)	18 (5.7%)	1 (3.4%)	0	0	0
Biopsy incisional	484 (5.0%)	22 (6.9%)	2 (6.9%)	3 (10.3%)	1 (20.0%)	0
Operation	178 (1.9%)	25 (7.9%)	2 (6.9%)	1 (3.4%)	0	2 (22.2%)
Others	59 (0.6%)	18 (5.7%)	1 (3.4%)	1 (3.4%)	1 (20.0%)	0

6 had sarcoma, and 70 had other malignancies, which were recorded as malignant liver tumor histologically but not classified as hepatocellular carcinoma, cholangiocellular carcinoma, mixed carcinoma, hepatoblastoma, or sarcoma. Hilar cholangiocarcinoma was regarded as primary liver cancer when the tumor was noted macroscopically to originate in an intrahepatic bile duct.

Because not all questionnaire items were answered, the numbers in some of the items reported here do not equal the total number of cases.

The age of the patients with each histologic type of tumor is listed in Table III.

The peak incidence of hepatocellular carcinoma was in patients who were in their 50s, while that of cholangiocellular carcinoma was in patients in their 60s. The mean ages were 60.5 years in men and 64.1 years in women with hepatocellular carcinoma, and 59.7 years in men and 62.2 years in women with cholangiocellular carcinoma.

Method of Diagnosis

Table IV lists a variety of diagnostic procedures and their effectiveness in clinical diagnosis. Hepatic angiography, computed tomography, and ultrasonography were performed in approximately 90% of the hepatocellular carcinoma patients and demonstrated positive findings in 90% of these individuals. In 51.5% of the hepatocellular carcinoma patients and in 9.0% of the cholangiocellular carcinoma patients, the serum alphafetoprotein (AFP) level was higher than 200ng/ml. Clinical stage of these patients is shown in Table V.

TABLE V. Clinical Stage of HCC

Stage	Male	Female	Total
I	3,203	735	3,938
II	2,297	629	2,926
III	1,553	369	1,922
Unknown	707	189	896

TABLE VI. Procedure for Hepatic Resection

	HC $n=2,639$	CC $n=118$	MX $n=19$	HB $n=12$	SA $n=2$	CA $n=5$	Total $n=2,795$
Extended lobectomy	123	27	1	3	0	1	155 (5.5%)
Lobectomy	440	60	4	6	0	4	514 (18.4%)
Segmentectomy	517	16	7	0	1	0	541 (19.4%)
Subsegmentectomy	623	6	3	1	1	0	634 (22.7%)
Partial resection	888	9	3	2	0	0	902 (32.3%)
Hepatectomy with additional surgical treatment	48	0	1	0	0	0	49 (1.8%)
	2,639/2,951 (89.4%)	118/169 (69.8%)	19/20 (95.0%)	12/15 (80.0%)	2/2 (100%)	5/5 (100%)	

TABLE VII. Survival Rate of HCC Patients Treated with Hepatic Resection

	n	1 year	2 years	3 years	5 years
Overall	4,152	71.9%	56.6%	45.6%	30.9%
Patients with curative resection	2,289	77.4%	64.8%	55.0%	36.6%
Tumor size smaller than 2 cm	347	79.3%	67.1%	57.4%	39.3%
Portal vein invasion					
V_{p0}	1,852	80.4%	69.1%	59.8%	39.0%
V_{p1}	124	70.4%	52.6%	42.9%	36.8%
Growth pattern					
expansive	1,663	81.1%	69.1%	59.7%	41.1%
infiltrative	120	65.4%	54.9%	47.8%	27.9%

(Liver Cancer Study Group of Japan (January 1, 1978–December 31, 1987))

Method of Treatment

1. *Surgical treatment*

As shown in Table VI, of the 2,795 resections, 155 were extended lobectomies, 514 were lobectomies, 541 were segmentectomies, and 1,536 were partial resections, including subsegmentectomies.

2. *Other treatment*

Lipiodolization-transhepatic arterial embolization (TAE) and percutaneous ethanol infusion therapy (PEIT) were established as the common treatment for hepatocellular carcinoma in Japan. Lipiodolization was performed in 5,858 patients including 213 for operative adjuvant therapy.

Survival

This article reports the survival rates of patients with hepatocellular carcinoma and with cholangiocellular carcinoma treated by partial hepatic resection, on the basis of responses received from January 1, 1978, when a prototype of the present questionnaire was introduced, to December 31, 1987. As stated earlier, the survival rates of those with primary liver cancer (hepatocellular carcinoma and cholangiocellular carcinoma) were calculated by the traditional lifetime table method of Cutler-Ederer (*1*). The date of admission, not the date of diagnosis or initial treatment, is the starting point in the calculation of survival time. The statistical significance of differences in the survival pattern was analyzed by the log-rank test.

The abbreviations used here are based on the General Rules for the Clinical and Pathological Study of Primary Liver Cancer. Special attention is paid to the survival rates in relation to clinicopathological factors, which provide significant information for estimating the prognosis in patients with primary liver cancer.

1. *Survival rate of hepatocellular carcinoma (HCC) patients treated with curative or non-curative partial hepatic resection*

The overall 1-, 2-, 3-, and 5-year survival rates were 71.9%, 56.6%, 45.6%, and 30.9%, respectively (Table VII, Fig. 1). The survival rates of patients with curative resection were 77.4% at 1 year, 64.8% at 2 years, 55.0% at 3 years, and 36.6% at 5 years (Fig. 2), while those of the non-curative group were 66.6%, 47.8%, 34.7%, and 23.3%, respectively (Fig. 3).

The difference between the curative and non-curative surgery groups is statistically significant. Curability of surgery was defined by the General Rules for the Clinical and Pathological Study of Primary Liver Cancer (*9*).

The survival rates of patients with curative resection in relation to clinical and histopathological factors are listed below:

1) Tumor size (Fig. 4). In patients with tumors smaller than 2cm in diameter, the 1-, 2-, 3-, and 5-year survival rates were 86.9%, 81.5%, 74.5%, and 60.5%, respectively. Patients with tumors larger than 2cm in diameter had a poorer prognosis (2.1–5.0cm: 1 year, 79.3%; 2 years, 67.1%; 3 years, 57.4%; and 5 years, 39.3%; 5.1–10.0cm: 1 year, 74.3%; 2 years, 57.7%; 3 years, 48.0%; and 5 years, 26.8%). The differences among these 3 groups were significant.

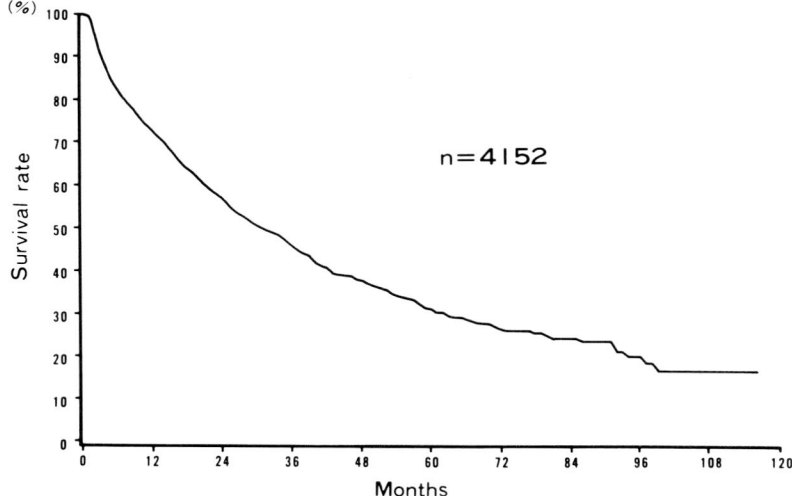

FIG. 1. Cumulative survival rate of HCC patients with partial hepatectomy

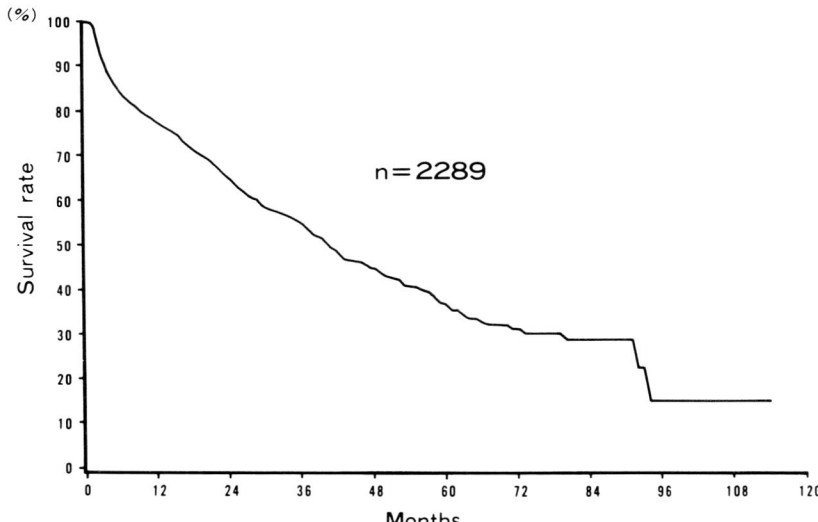

FIG. 2. Cumulative survival rate of HCC patients with curative hepatic resection

2) Tumor number (Fig. 5). The survival rates of patients with solitary tumors were 80.0% at 1 year, 67.8% at 2, 57.2% at 3, and 38.2% at 5 years, whereas those of patients with two tumors were 66.8% at 1 year, 48.8% at 2, 39.9% at 3, and 29.9% at 5 years. There was a significant difference between patients with single tumors and those with two or more tumors, but no significant difference between those with two tumors and those with three.

3) Fibrous tumor capsule (Fc) and infiltration of cancer cells into tumor capsule (Fc-inf) (Fig. 6). Capsular formation surrounding the tumor did not significantly influence the survival rate, possibly because a relatively large proportion of non-

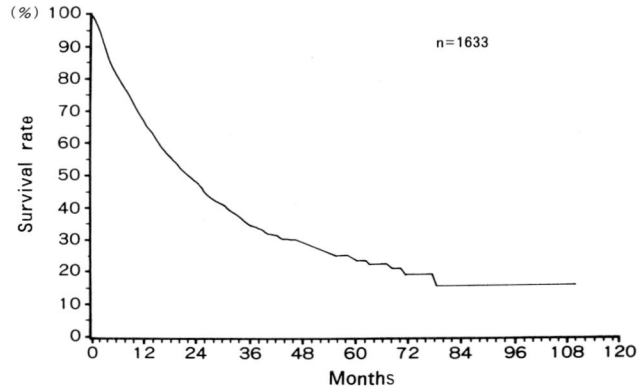

FIG. 3. Cumulative survival rate of HCC patients with non-curative hepatic resection

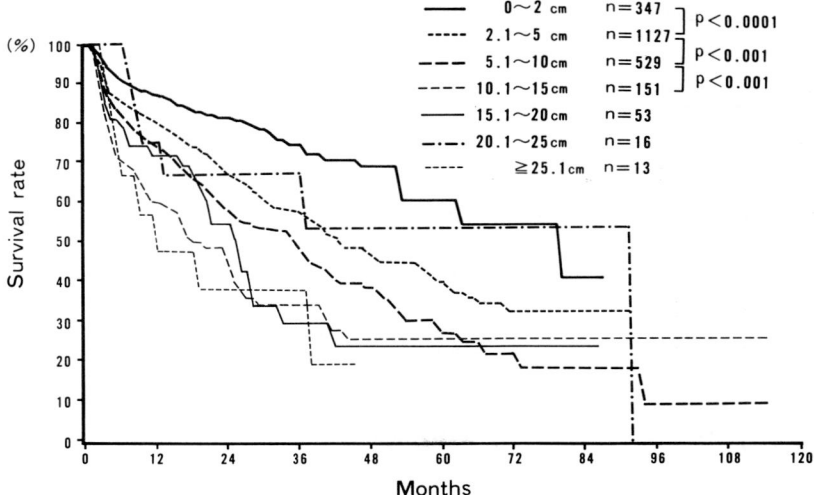

FIG. 4. Cumulative survival rates of HCC patients with curative resection in relation to tumor diameter

encapsulated tumors were small. However, the infiltration of cancer cells into the fibrous capsule of the tumor led to a low survival rate: in patients without capsular infiltration, 1-, 2-, 3-, and 5 year survival rates were 81.3%, 71.0%, 61.8%, and 40.1%, respectively, while in those with infiltration, they were 76.6%, 61.2%, 50.3%, and 34.6%.

4) Portal vein invasion of the tumor (V_p) (Fig. 7). There was a significant difference between V_{p0} and V_{p1}, and between V_{p0} and V_{p2}, but no significant difference between V_{p1} and V_{p2} (V_{p0}: 80.4% at 1 year, 69.1% at 2, 59.8% at 3, 39.0% at 5 years; V_{p1}: 70.4% at 1 year, 52.6% at 2, 42.9% at 3, 36.8% at 5 years).

5) Growth pattern of tumor (Fig. 8). Growth patterns were classified as expansive growth (Eg), in which the tumor had macroscopically clear margins, and infiltrative growth (Ig) with unclear margins. The Eg-group had better survival rates than

the Ig-group (Eg: 81.1% at 1 year, 69.1% at 2, 59.7% at 3, and 41.1% at 5; Ig: 65.4% at 1 year, 54.9% at 2, 47.8% at 3, and 27.9% at 5).

6) Grade of anaplasia of cancer cells (Edmondson-Steiner classification) (Fig. 9). There was no significant correlation between survival rates and the Edmondson-Steiner classification.

7) Tumor extent (Fig. 10). The extent of the tumor affected the survival rate significantly. In the H_s group (tumor localized to one Couinaud's segment), the 1-, 2-, 3-, and 5-year survival rates were 85.4%, 78.7%, 69.3%, and 53.3%, respectively.

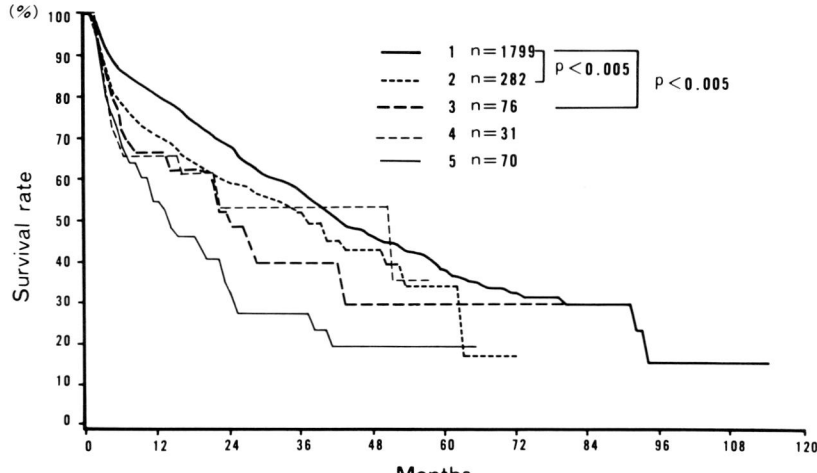

FIG. 5. Cumulative survival rates of HCC patients with curative resection in relation to number of tumors

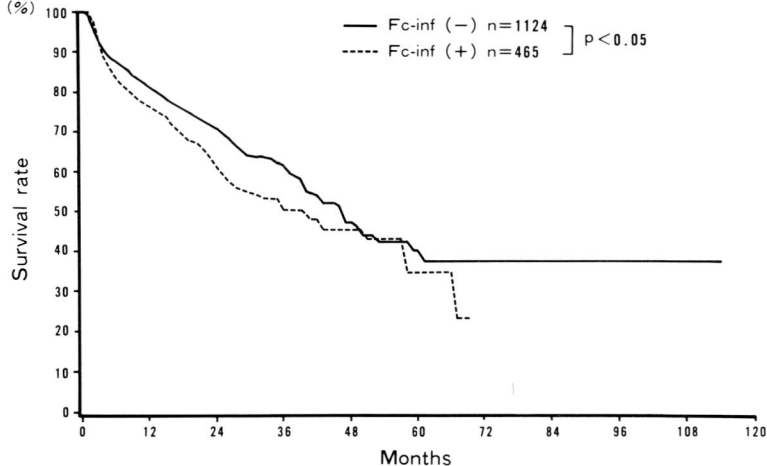

FIG. 6. Cumulative survival rates of HCC patients with curative resection in relation to macroscopic infiltration of tumor capsule
Fc-inf (−) and Fc-inf (+) represent the absence and presence of macroscopic infiltration, respectively.

There were statistically significant differences between H_s and H_1, and between H_s and H_2, but not between H_1 and H_2.

2. *Survival rates of cholangiocarcinoma (CCC) patients treated with curative or non-curative partial hepatic resection*

The overall 1-, 2-, 3-, and 5-year survival rates were 54.6%, 38.8%, 31.5%, and 29.8%, respectively (Fig. 11). Patients treated with curative surgery (Fig. 12) had better survival rates than those treated with non-curative surgery (Fig. 13) (curative surgery group: 69.4% at 1 year, 65.5% at 2, 43.5% at 3, and 43.5% at 5; non-curative surgery group: 45.5% at 1 year, 22.4% at 2, 22.4% at 3, and 19.6% at 5 years).

Survival rates in relation to clinical and histopathological factors are listed below:

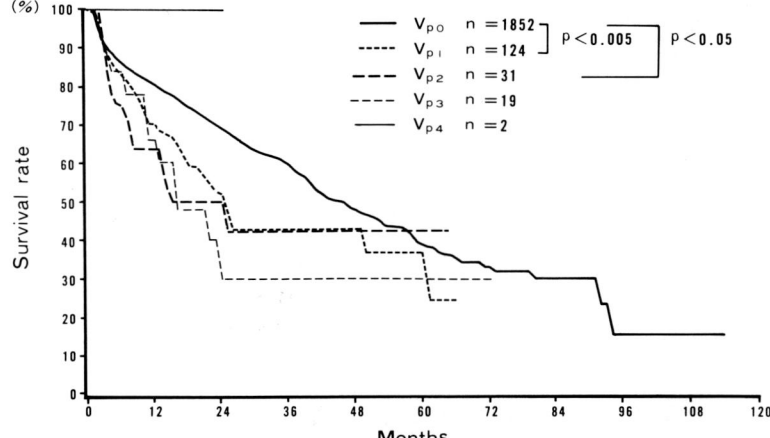

FIG. 7. Cumulative survival rates of HCC patients with curative resection in relation to the degree of macroscopic portal involvement
V_{p0}, no portal involvement; V_{p1}, involvement to more than the 3rd branch of the peripheral tract; V_{p2}, V_{p3}, V_{p4}, involvement to the 2nd branch, 1st branch, and portal trunk, respectively.

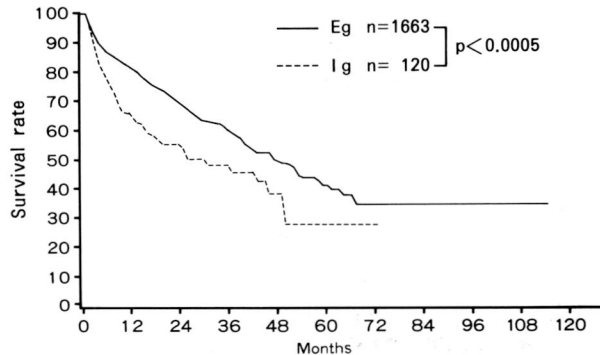

FIG. 8. Cumulative survival rates of HCC patients with curative resection in relation to growth pattern of the tumor. Eg and Ig represent expansive and infiltrative growth, respectively

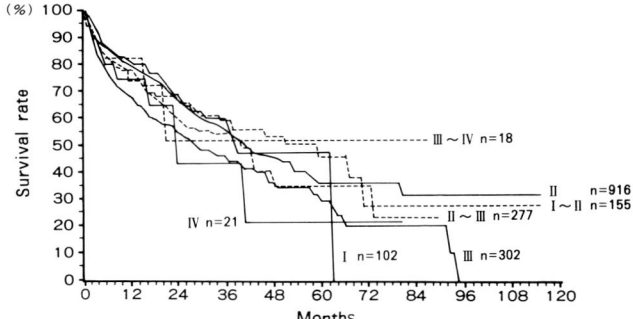

FIG. 9. Cumulative survival rates of HCC patients with curative resection in relation to grade of Edmondson-Steiner classification

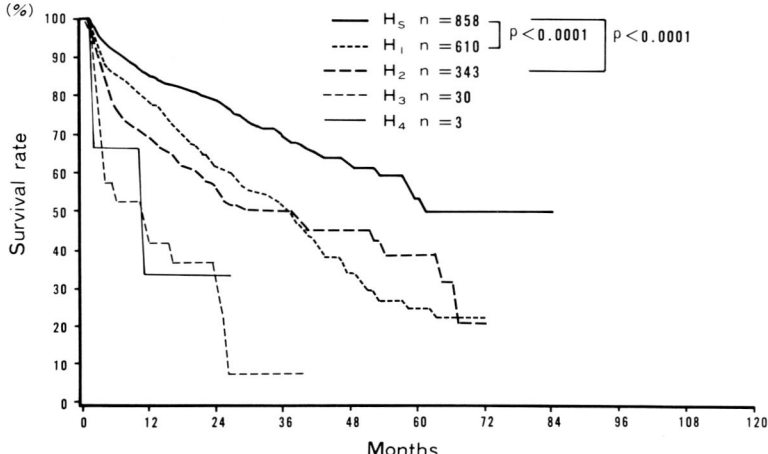

FIG. 10. Cumulative survival rates of HCC patients with curative resection in relation to extent of the tumor
Hs, located in one subsegment (Couinaud's segment); H1, located in one segment; H2, located in two segments; H3, located in three segments; H4, located in four segments.

1) Tumor size (Fig. 14). All patients with tumors smaller than 2 cm in diameter are alive, but the number of cases (9 patients) is too small to evaluate the significance as a prognostic indicator. In the group with tumors 2.1–5.0 cm in diameter, the survival rates were 62.3% at 1 year, 43.3% at 2, 37.9% at 3, and 31.6% at 5.

2) Lymph node metastasis (Fig. 15). In the N_0 group, 1-, 2-, 3-, and 5-year survival rates were 64.2%, 51.4%, 41.9%, and 38.4%, respectively, while in the N_1 group they were 39.7% at 1 year and 29.8% at 2 years, a great difference.

3) Type of histology (Fig. 16). Patients with cystopapillary cholangiocellular carcinoma have a relatively better survival rate: (microtubular: 51.6% at 1 year, 46.3% at 2, and 18.4% at 3; macrotubular: 56.6% at 1 year, 46.3% at 2, and 44.7% at 3; cystopapillary: 67.9% at 1 year, 58.4% at 2, and 44.7% at 3).

4) Tumor extent (Fig. 17). There were no significant differences among the groups, although the H_s group tended to survive longer than the others.

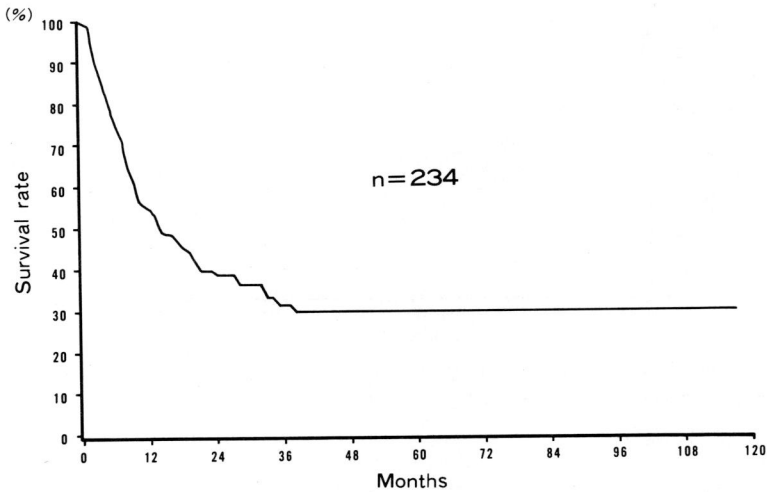

Fig. 11. Cumulative survival rate of CCC patients with partial hepatic resection

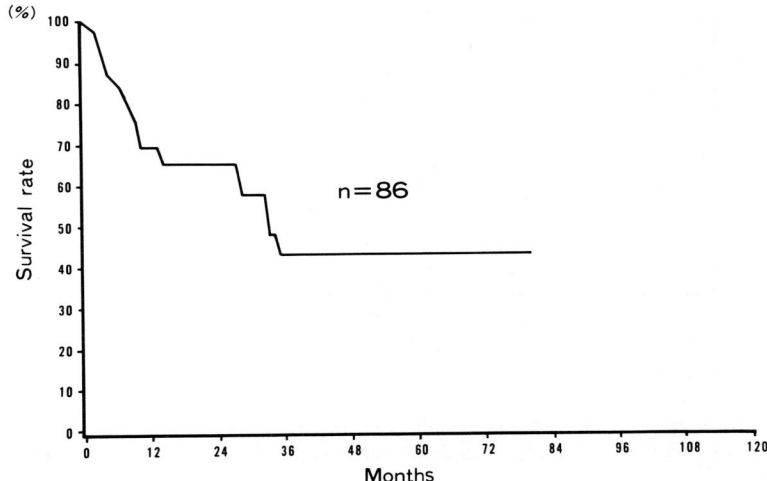

Fig. 12. Cumulative survival rate of CCC patients with curative resection

Comments and Discussion

The number of patients with HCC has increased in Japan during the past 10 years, and HCC is now the third cause of cancer death in males. In the 1970s, there were very few resectable cases because the tumor was far advanced by the time it was diagnosed and concomitant severe liver cirrhosis was often present. However, the recent development of noninvasive and precise diagnostic modalities such as computed tomography (CT) and ultrasonography (US) has made it possible to diagnose HCC at an earlier stage, thereby increasing the number of resectable tumors. The current report showed 10% of liver cancer in Japan can be detected as small liver

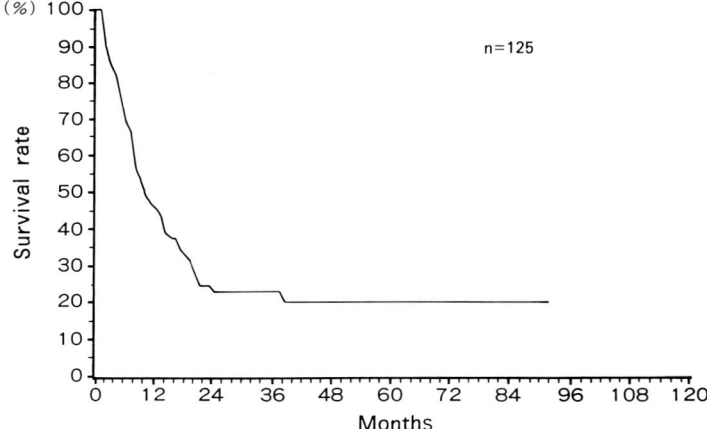

FIG. 13. Cumulative survival rate of CCC patients with non-curative resection

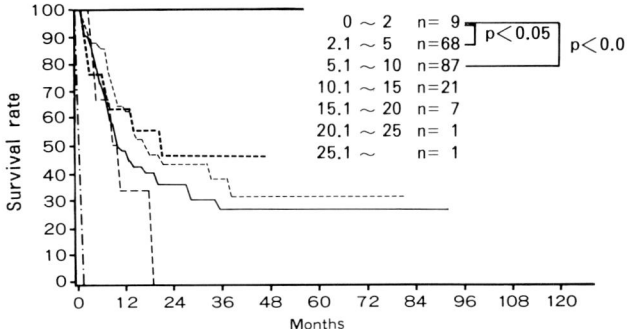

FIG. 14. Cumulative survival rates of CCC patients with partial hepatectomy in relation to tumor diameter (cm)

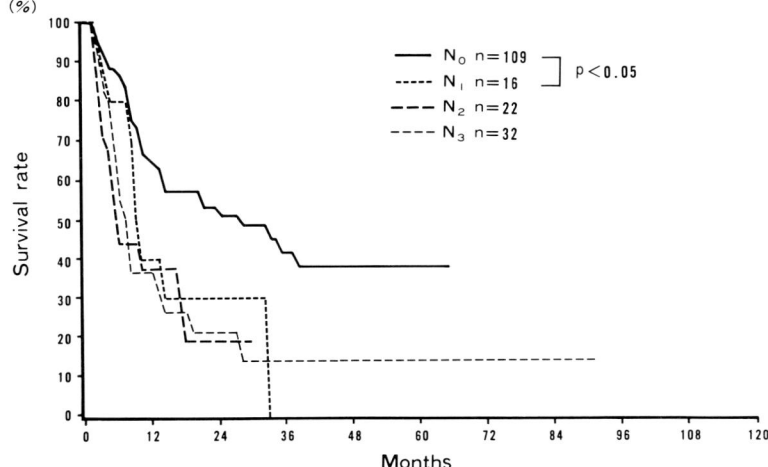

FIG. 15. Cumulative survival rates of CCC patients with partial hepatectomy in relation to the grade of lymph node metastasis
N_0–N_3 are defined by the General Rules for the Clinical and Pathological Study of Primary Liver Cancer.

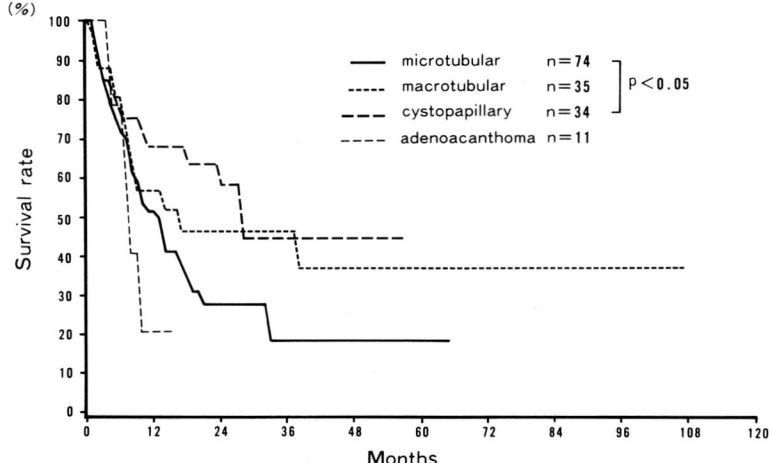

Fig. 16. Cumulative survival rates of CCC patients with partial hepatectomy in relation to the type of histology

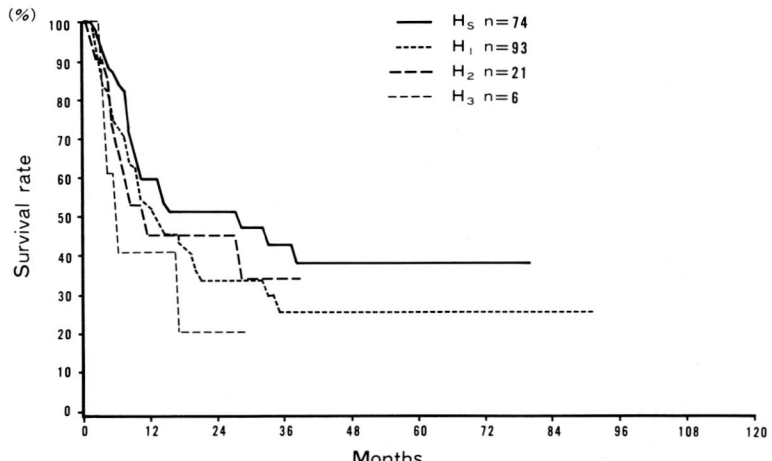

Fig. 17. Cumulative survival rates of CCC patients with partial hepatectomy in relation to extent of the tumor
Hs, located in one subsegment (Couinaud's segment); H1, located in one segment; H2, located in two segments; H3, located in three segments.

cancer (less than 2 cm in diameter). Furthermore, the operative mortality rate is now lower, because of better pre- and postoperative management, development of surgical techniques and improved preoperative evaluation of hepatic functional reserve for preoperative liver failure.

The Follow-up Studies of the Liver Cancer Study Group of Japan (2–8) have played an important role as a guide in the diagnosis of and treatment for primary liver cancer.

The most important and greatest changes during the period of registration are the incidence of HB antigen carriers. The number of HBs antigen showed a gradual but definite decrease from 40% in 1970 to 22.5% in 1987. On the other hand, based on the clinical characteristics of primary liver cancer studied by the Liver Cancer Group in Japan, the high risk group was men in the sixth decade of life with a past history of blood transfusion or hepatitis, patients with hepatic cirrhosis caused by blood transfusion or hepatitis and HB antigen carriers or HCV antigen carriers; all of these are carefully followed up.

Serum AFP is screened regularly and US and CT are frequently used for lesions suspected of being malignant. The operability of primary liver cancer especially for hepatocellular carcinoma is gradually but definitely increasing, however, the extent of resection has gradually become smaller. In the earlier 10 year-period, the Japanese surgeons used large resections in an attempt to remove the cancer, and trisegmentectomy and lobectomy were commonly performed. However, limited but anatomically precise hepatectomies are now the rule. The way in which survival rates after hepatic resection are affected by various backgrounds and other factors is being studied.

Thus the factors in primary liver cancer, especially in hepatocellular carcinoma patients, which are indicative of good survival rates following surgery are being determined, as are the most important risk factors portending recurrence after hepatic resection.

REFERENCES

1. Cutler, S.J. and Ederer, F. Maximum utilization of the life table method in analyzing survival. *J. Chronic Dis.*, **8**, 699–712 (1958).
2. Ishikawa, K. and Kosaka, K. Results of hepatic resection for primary liver cancer. *Acta Hepatol. Jpn.*, **14**, 409–410 (1973).
3. Ishikawa, K. Follow-up study of patients with primary liver cancer: Report 3. *Acta Hepatol. Jpn.*, **17**, 460–465 (1976).
4. Murakami, F. Okamura, T., Ohta M. *et al.* Liver disease and surgical treatment, particularly hepatic resection and transplantation. *Shinryo*, **23**, 265–277 (1970) (in Japanese).
5. Okuda, K. and The Liver Cancer Study Group of Japan. Primary liver cancer. *Cancer*, **45**, 2663–2669 (1980).
6. The Liver Cancer Study Group of Japan. Primary liver cancer in Japan. *Cancer*, **54**, 1747–1755 (1984).
7. The Liver Cancer Study Group of Japan. Primary liver cancer in Japan. *Cancer*, **60**, 1400–1411 (1987).
8. The Liver Cancer Study Group of Japan. The general rules for the clinical and pathological study of primary liver cancer. *Jpn. J. Surg.*, **19**, 98–129 (1989).
9. The Liver Cancer Study Group of Japan. Primary liver cancer in Japan: Clinicopathologic features and results of surgical treatment. *Ann. Surg.*, **211**, 277–287 (1990).

STATISTICS REGISTRY OF BILIARY TRACT CANCER

Japanese Society of Biliary Surgery*

Cancer incidence statistics for 1988–1992 were compiled and edited based on the data collected by the research group for the Statistics Registry of Biliary Tract Cancer in Japan. Data were obtained from 144 medical institutions.

A total of 5,293 patients were registered during the five year period. This chapter includes the following statistical analysis of biliary cancer: 1) background of cancer registrants; 2) number of patients by year and age distribution by sex; 3) incidence of pre-existing disease (cholelithiasis); 4) methods of diagnosis and treatment; 5) clinical stage and survival.

Biliary tract cancer has a poorer prognosis than any other gastrointestinal cancer. Its incidence is lower than those of stomach and colon cancers. To improve therapeutic results of biliary tract cancer, the Japanese Society of Biliary Surgery prepared General Rules for Surgical and Pathological Studies on Cancer of the Biliary Tract in 1981 so that the same criteria would be used to evaluate results obtained at various institutions. The third edition of this publication (3) was issued in January 1993. To effectively keep track of the patients with biliary tract cancer, the Japanese Society of Biliary Surgery undertook national registration in 1987. In keeping with the General Rules, a questionnaire was prepared for patients, and the data obtained for the five years from 1988 to 1992 were compiled in 1994. This report deals with the background factors, results of examination, methods of treatment, and prognosis in cases of biliary tract cancer registered for that five year period.

Data Collection

Criteria, hospital, data check, and data processing

Data were obtained from 144 medical institutions in Japan (the testing facilities are listed at the end of this report). There were no special criteria for testing facilities and patients could be registered from any facility wishing to participate in this survey. Questionnaires for collecting data on bile duct, gallbladder, and ampullary cancers (carcinoma of the papilla of Vater) according to the above-mentioned General Rules were delivered to each testing facility. After they were returned to the registration office, the data were checked for entry error and input into a personal computer (NEC 9,800 series). Statistical analysis was performed according to the analytical system developed by the registration committee.

---

* Manuscript was prepared by Takukazu Nagakawa and Masato Kayahara, Second Department of Surgery, School of Medicine, Kanazawa University, 13-1 Takaramachi, Kanazawa 920, Japan

Basic Data on the Registered Patients

1. Number of patients by year

Table I shows the number of patients registered with bile duct, gallbladder, and ampullary carcinomas by year; about 500, 450, and 120 cancer patients, respectively, were registered each year. There was no year-related difference in the number of those registered. A total of 5,293 patients were registered for the five years from 1988 to 1992: 2,312, 2,352, and 629 with bile duct, gallbladder, and ampullary cancer, respectively. Since the National Cancer Center estimated the number of gallbladder cancer patients in Japan in 1988 to be 13,167 (5,692 males and 7,475 females), those with that disease entered in this national registration of biliary tract cancer accounted for just 3.6%.

2. Age distribution by sex

Figures 1–3 show the sex and age distribution in the three cancer groups. In the bile duct group, 1,494 were males and 818 were females and the male to female ratio was 1.83:1. The peak incidence occurred among patients in their 60s. In the gallbladder cancer group, 814 were males and 1,538 were females with a male to female ratio of 1:1.89. The proportion of patients in their 60s to 70s was high as in the bile duct and gallbladder groups. In the ampullary cancer group, 339 were males and 290 were females with a male to female ratio of 1.17:1. In this group, the greatest number of patients were in their 50s to 70s.

TABLE I. Number of Patients by Year

	Bile duct cancer (n = 2,312)			Gallbladder cancer (n = 2,352)			Ampullary cancer (n = 629)		
	Male	Female	Total	Male	Female	Total	Male	Female	Total
1988	343	171	514	172	342	514	63	55	118
1989	279	136	415	158	296	454	65	63	128
1990	265	149	414	171	312	483	68	61	129
1991	277	183	460	170	282	452	71	55	126
1992	330	179	509	143	306	449	72	56	128

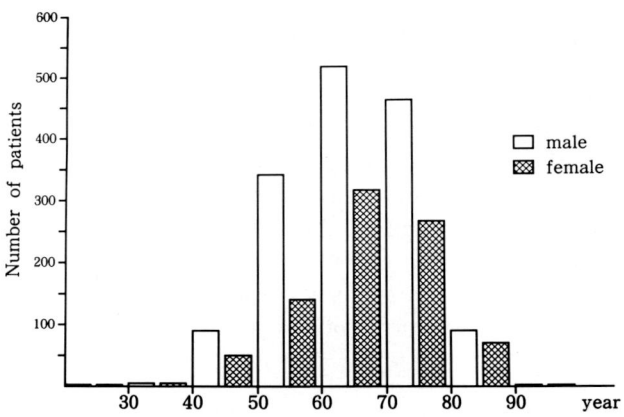

FIG. 1. Age and sex distribution for bile duct cancer

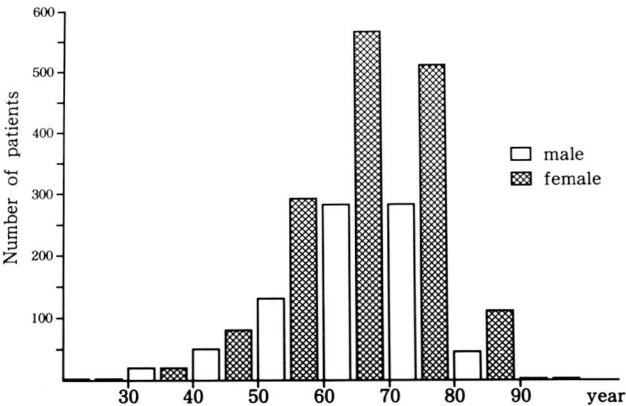
FIG. 2. Age and sex distribution for gallbladder cancer

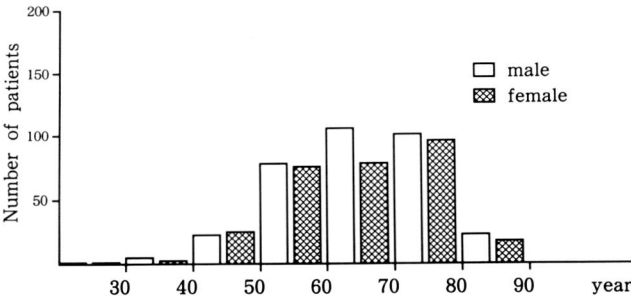
FIG. 3. Age and sex distribution for ampullary cancer

TABLE II. Pre-existing Disease

	n	Cholelithiasis
Bile duct cancer	2,312	305 (13.2%)
Gallbladder cancer	2,352	1,090 (46.3%)
Ampullary cancer	629	51 (8.1%)

3. Pre-existing disease

Cholelithiasis is the most frequent pre-existing disease. It was noted in 13.2%, 46.3%, and 8.1% of the patients in the bile duct, gallbladder, and ampullary cancer groups, respectively, thus being notably higher in the gallbladder group (Table II).

4. Methods of diagnosis

Table III shows the methods for first detection of each disease. The detection rate by ultrasonography (US) was high in the gallbladder and bile duct cancer groups with 75% of gallbladder being detected by this means. Understandably, the detection rate by endoscopic retrograde cholangiopancreatography (ERCP) was highest in the ampullary cancer group. Computed tomography (CT) was able to first detect the biliary lesion in less than 10% of the patients.

TABLE III. Methods for First Detection of Cancer

Procedure \ Site	Bile duct cancer n = 2,312	Gallbladder cancer n = 2,352	Ampullary cancer n = 629
US	50.0%	74.2%	32.4%
PTC	26.6%	3.8%	12.7%
ERCP	13.7%	2.8%	42.9%
CT	6.9%	8.6%	4.8%
Miscellaneous	2.8%	10.6%	7.2%

US; ultrasonography, PTC; percutaneous transhepatic cholangiography, ERCP; endoscopic retrograde cholangiography, CT; computed tomography.

TABLE IV. Methods of Treatment

Procedure \ Site	Bile duct n = 2,312	Gallbladder n = 2,352	Ampullary n = 629
Surgical resection	1,509	1,611	566
Palliative operation	216	92	30
Probe laparotomy	100	171	5
Others	46	132	1
No operation	441	346	27

TABLE V. Clinical Stage of Bile Duct Cancer (Surgical Cases 1,871)

	1988	1989	1990	1991	1992	Total
Stage I	53	42	43	38	48	224 (12.6%)
Stage II	65	53	54	61	60	293 (16.5%)
Stage III	87	86	93	83	94	443 (24.9%)
Stage IV	185	128	121	160	170	764 (43.0%)
Not judged	17	9	11	8	9	54 (3.0%)
Unknown	28	21	11	20	13	93

TABLE VI. Clinical Stage of Gallbladder Cancer (Surgical Cases 1,642)

	1988	1989	1990	1991	1992	Total
Stage I	116	89	99	101	119	524 (26.0%)
Stage II	24	46	36	38	29	173 (9.1%)
Stage III	51	38	32	50	36	207 (11.0%)
Stage IV	220	194	222	178	183	997 (52.4%)
Not judged	5	6	9	3	4	27 (1.6%)
Unknown	23	15	8	15	15	76

5. Methods of treatment

Table IV shows the methods of treatment for biliary tract cancer. Surgical resection was performed in 1,509 (65.3%), 1,611 (68.5%), and 566 (90.0%) patients from the bile duct, gallbladder, and ampullary groups, respectively. The proportion of patients with surgical resection was higher in the ampullary cancer group than in the other two groups. Palliative operation including bilioenterostomy (e.g., choledochojejunostomy) was performed in 216 (9.3%), 92 (3.9%), and 30 (4.8%) patients from the bile duct, gallbladder, and ampullary cancer groups, respectively, while no surgical operation was performed in 441 (19.1%), 346 (14.7%), and 27 (4.3%) of patients from these groups.

6. *Clinical stage by year in patients with surgical procedure*

In the classification of the clinical stage of patients with surgical procedure, 68% from the bile duct cancer group presented in Stage III or IV and 63% from the gallbladder cancer group presented in Stage III or IV. On the other hand, 61.5% of those from the ampullary cancer group presented in Stage I or II. Patient clinical stage showed no year-related difference in any group (Tables V to VII).

7. *Survival*
1) *Survival rate of patients according to the method of treatment*

Table VIII shows the survival rates by treatment method and disease. The prognosis of patients with surgical resection was more favorable than any other method of treatment in each type of biliary tract cancer, the 3-year survival rates for resection in the bile duct, gallbladder, and ampullary cancer groups being 36%, 46%, and 59%, respectively. The 5-year survival rates for these patients were 27%, 40%, and 52%, respectively. On the other hand, almost none of the patients without surgical resection lived as long as 3 years (Figs. 4 to 6).

2) *Survival rates of patients according to clinical stage*

Table IX shows the survival rates by degree of clinical stage. These rates were analyzed in those undergoing a surgical procedure. In clinical Stage I group, the 3-year survival rates for bile duct, gallbladder, and ampullary cancer individuals were 69%, 83%, and 78%, respectively; the 5-year rates were 59%, 76%, and 75%. In Stage II group, 3-year survival rates were 50%, 64%, and 63%, respectively, while 5-year were 37%, 56%, and 53%. In contrast, only 9% of the patients with bile duct cancer in

TABLE VII. Clinical Stage of Ampullary Cancer (Surgical Cases 486)

	1988	1989	1990	1991	1992	Total
Stage I	26	30	35	33	35	159 (26.2%)
Stage II	42	43	42	40	32	199 (35.3%)
Stage III	33	37	34	31	27	162 (28.5%)
Stage IV	11	9	13	10	19	62 (9.1%)
Not judged	0	1	0	3	0	4 (0.9%)
Unknown	3	4	0	4	5	16

TABLE VIII. Survival Rates of Patients According to Method of Treatment

	Bile duct cancer					Gallbladder cancer					Ampullary cancer				
	n	1 y	2 y	3 y	5 y	n	1 y	2 y	3 y	5 y	n	1 y	2 y	3 y	5 y
Surgical resection	(1,501)	67	46	36	27	(1,595)	67	51	46	40	(560)	86	69	59	52
Palliative operation	(212)	32	12	5		(91)	14	4	3		(29)	41	33	20	
Probe laparotomy	(98)	20	6			(170)	13	1			(5)	40			
Others	(45)	24	9	0		(131)	15	3			(1)	0			
No operation	(433)	21	7	2		(339)	7	1			(26)	40	7		

y: year.

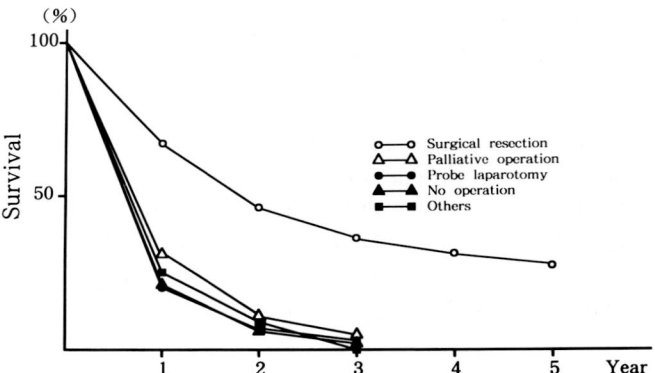

FIG. 4. Survival rates of patients with bile duct cancer by method of treatment

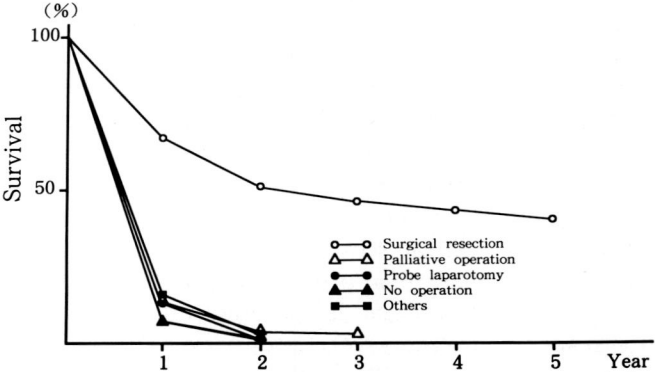

FIG. 5. Survival rates of patients with gallbladder cancer by method of treatment

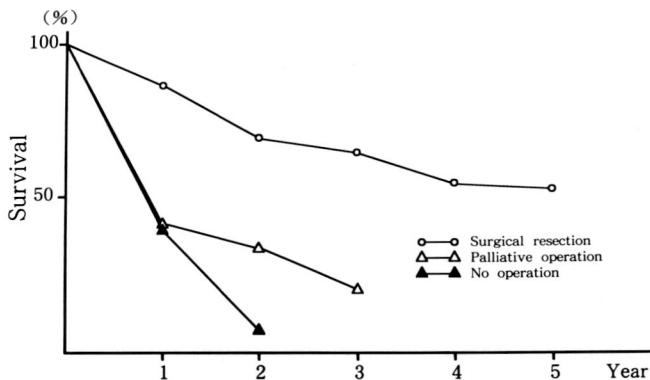

FIG. 6. Survival rates of patients with ampullary cancer by method of treatment

Stage IV group survived 5 years. None of those with ampullary cancer presenting in Stage IV survived even 5 years. There was a correlation between clinical stage and prognosis in every biliary cancer group (Figs. 7 to 9).

TABLE IX. Survival Rates (%) of Patients According to Clinical Stage

	Bile duct cancer					Gallbladder cancer					Ampullary cancer				
	n	1 y	2 y	3 y	5 y	n	1 y	2 y	3 y	5 y	n	1 y	2 y	3 y	5 y
Stage I	(221)	88	77	69	59	(518)	94	87	83	76	(159)	92	84	78	75
Stage II	(292)	79	58	50	37	(172)	86	72	64	56	(195)	88	72	63	53
Stage III	(441)	67	43	32	22	(206)	70	50	43	33	(160)	82	57	44	38
Stage IV	(757)	44	21	13	9	(986)	30	12	10	8	(62)	53	30	6	

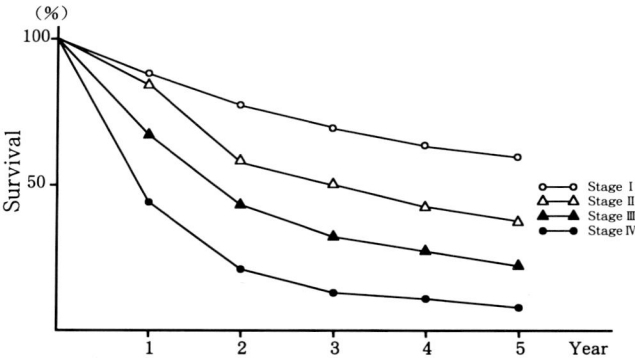

FIG. 7. Survival rates of patients with bile duct cancer by clinical stage

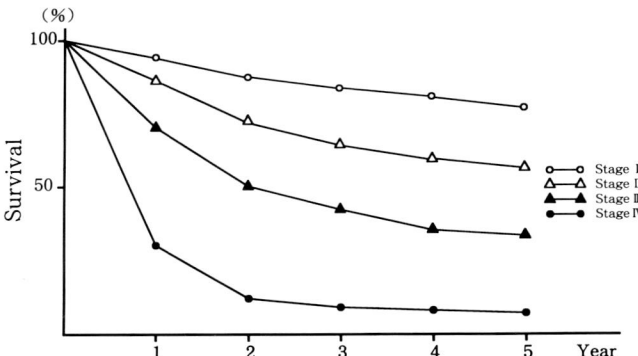

FIG. 8. Survival rates of patients with gallbladder cancer by clinical stage

Comments and Discussion

Since this registration survey was undertaken by the biliary tract cancer registration committee of the Japanese Society of Biliary Surgery, the testing facilities for the most part were those for surgical operation. Therefore, it seems probable that surgical procedures were slightly more common than other methods of treatment. With regard to the sex ratio of bile duct cancer, a review of the literature showed a slight overall predominance of the male sex (5, 10). The results of the French Surgical Association Survey (8) showed that 289 (52%) of 552 patients with bile duct cancer were male. Langer et al. (4) reported the same results. The male to female ratio for

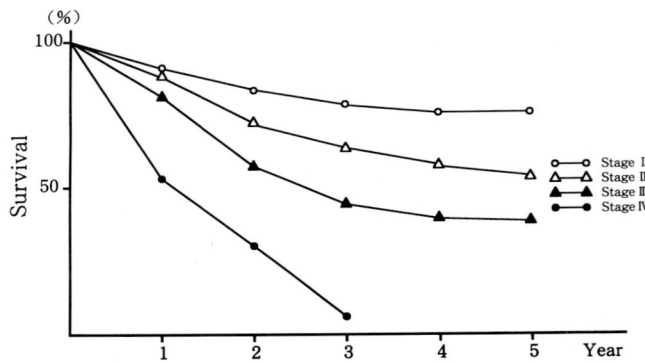

FIG. 9. Survival rates of patients with ampullary cancer by clinical stage

gallbladder cancer was reported to be between 1:1.76 and 1:3.5 (1, 2, 5, 7). Monson et al. (6) reported that the sex ratio for ampullary cancer was 1.3:1. Our registration study showed almost the same results as mentioned earlier.

The recent development of radiographic examinations has contributed to the detection of biliary tract malignancy. US is one of the most useful, non-invasive, and easily used methods for primary diagnosis; therefore, it has been the means first used for diagnosis if hepato-biliary-pancreatic disease is suspected. Our study shows, however, that it is difficult to detect ampullary cancer with US because of the anatomical site involved. The French Surgical Association Survey (8) reported that preoperative diagnostic investigations consisted of abdominal echography in 386 patients (70%), as well as transhepatic or endoscopic retrograde cholangiography in, respectively, 166 (30%) and 176 patients (32%).

Morrow et al. (7) reported that 103 (92%) of 112 patients with gallbladder cancer had cholelithiasis, while in our study cholelithiasis was observed in 46% of these patients. Although association with cholelithiasis is high among malignant tumors of the gallbladder, the data in primary extrahepatic bile duct cancer vary between 62% and 13% (average =36%) (10). One hundred forty-four (26%) of 552 patients in the French Surgical Association Survey were noted to have associated gallstones (8). Langer et al. (4) reported that the frequency of gallstones was 24% in patients with bile duct cancer. In our study, stones were found in only 13% of this group.

As to the clinical stage of biliary tract cancer, Mizumoto et al. (5) reported that 77% of patients with gallbladder cancer had Stage III or IV. They also reported that 79% of patients with bile duct cancer had Stage III or IV. In our study, 63% of the patients with gallbladder cancer and 68% of those with bile duct cancer presented Stage III or IV. In spite of the development of radiographic examination, more than 60% of the patients with biliary cancer other than ampullary cancer had an advanced stage of the disease.

Donohue et al. (1) reported that the resectability rate for gallbladder cancer was 65%. The overall resectability rate of bile duct cancer in the French Surgical Association Survey series (8) was reported to be 34%. Shyr et al. (9) reported the resectability for patients with ampullary cancer was 86%. These rates for patients with gallbladder, bile duct, and ampullary cancer in our series were 69%, 68%, and 90%, respectively.

The prognosis for patients with biliary tract cancer is low compared with that of patients with other gastrointestinal malignancy. The cooperative survey analysis by Mizumoto et al. (5) indicated that overall 3- and 5-year survival rates for patients with surgical resection in the gallbladder cancer group were 51% and 39%. That same report stated that survival rates in the bile duct cancer group were 61% and 37%, respectively. Langer et al. (4) reported that the predicted 5-year survival rate was 27% for patients with bile duct cancer. Our results showed that 3- and 5-year survival rates in the gallbladder cancer group were 46% and 40%, while rates in the bile duct cancer group were 36% and 27%, respectively. Ampullary cancer has the best prognosis among the biliary tract cancers. Monson et al. (6) reported that the 3- and 5-year survival rates were 48% and 34%, respectively, while Shyr et al. (9) reported this rate to be 37%. These data did not differ from our results.

With regard to the relationship between clinical stage and prognosis, Mizumoto et al. (5) stated that 5-year survival rates of patients with bile duct cancer in Stage I, II, III, and IV were 64.5%, 50.4%, 30.7%, and 9.4%, respectively; those in our study were 59%, 37%, 22%, and 9%. The rates in the gallbladder cancer group were reported to be 83.2%, 49.3%, 29.3%, and 7.0% (5), while in our study they were 76%, 56%, 33%, and 8%.

Acknowledgment

The authors appreciate contribution of members to this registry and Dr. Shaw Watanabe, Chief of Epidemiology Division, National Cancer Center for his constructive discussion.

This work was supported in part by Grants-in-Aid for Cancer Research from the Ministry of Health and Welfare of Japan.

REFERENCES

1. Donohue, J.H., Nagorney, D.M., Grant, C.S., Tsushima, K., Ilstrup, D.M., and Adson, M.A. Carcinoma of the gallbladder: Does radical resection improve outcome? *Arch. Surg.*, **125**, 237–241 (1990).
2. Hamrick, R.E. Jr., Liner, F.J., Hastings, P.R., and Cohn, I. Jr., Primary carcinoma of the gallbladder. *Ann. Surg.*, **195**, 270–273 (1982).
3. Japanese Society of Biliary Surgery. General Rules for Surgical and Pathological Studies of Cancer of Biliary Tract. 3rd ed. (1993) (in Japanese). Kanehara Shuppan, Tokyo.
4. Langer, J.C., Langer, B., Taylor, B.R., Zeldin, R., and Cummings, B. Carcinoma of the extrahepatic bile duct: Results of an aggressive surgical approach. *Surgery*, **98**, 752–759 (1985).
5. Mizumoto, R., Ogura, T., Matsuda, S., Kusuda, T., Taoka, T., Kaneda, M., Yajima, Y., and Tabata, M. Cooperative survey of surgical treatment for carcinoma of the biliary tract in Japan. *Biliary Tract and Pancreas*, **11**, 869–882 (1990) (in Japanese).
6. Monson, J.R.T., Donohue, J.H., McEntee, G.P., McIlrath, D., van Heerden, J.A., Shorter, R.G., Nagorney, D.M., and Ilstrup, D.M. Radical resection for carcinoma of the ampulla of vater. *Arch. Surg.*, **126**, 353–357 (1991).
7. Morrow, C.E., Sutherland, D.E.R., Florack, G., Eisenberg, M.M., and Grage, T.B. Primary gallbladder carcinoma: Significance of subserosal lesions and results of aggressive surgical treatment and adjuvant chemotherapy. *Surgery*, **94**, 709–714 (1983).
8. Reding, R., Buard, J.L., Lebeau, G., and Launois, B. Surgical management of 552 carcinomas of the extrahepatic bile duct (gallbladder and periampullary tumors excluded). Results of the French Surgical Association Survey. *Ann. Surg.*, **213**, 236–241 (1991).

9. Shyr, Y.M., Su, C.H., Wang, H.C., Lo, S.S., and Lui, W.Y. Comparison of resectable and unresectable periampullary carcinomas. *J. Am. Coll. Surg.*, **178**, 369–378 (1994).
10. Sons, H.U. and Borchard, F. Carcinoma of the extrahepatic bile ducts: A postmortem study of 65 cases and review of the literature. *J. Surg. Oncol.*, **34**, 6–12 (1987).

THE PRESENT STATUS OF PANCREATIC CANCER REGISTRATION

The Pancreatic Cancer Registration Committee of
the Japan Pancreas Society*

A total of 13,498 pancreatic cancer patients was registered by the Pancreatic Cancer Registration Committee of the Japan Pancreas Society from 345 major hospitals in Japan for the period 1981 through 1992. Past history, present symptoms, methods of diagnosis, treatment methods and survival were analyzed. Diagnosis with ultrasound and computed tomography have become more common, used in about 50% and 25% of the cases, respectively. Although one-fourth of the cases are still inoperable, tumor resection was performed in 40% of the total. More than half received intra- and/or post-operative chemotherapy, but the rate of success was less than 10%. Five year survival rates were 17.5% by resectional surgery, 1.6% by bypass operation, 0.4% by exploratory laparotomy, and 1.2% without operation. Among resected cases, islet cell carcinoma (65.3%), cystadenocarcinoma (54.3%), and papillary adenocarcinoma (32.6%) showed relatively good five-year survival rates.

The annual number of deaths from pancreatic cancer, along with lung cancer and colorectal cancer, has shown an annual increase in Japan and now exceeds 13,000. In the dynamic population statistics published by the Statistical Information Division of the Secretariat of the Ministry of Health and Welfare, the mortality rate in a population of 100,000 was 5.0 for men and 3.5 for women in 1970, 7.8 and 5.7 in 1980, and 12.1 and 9.6 in 1990 (3). Thus, during this 20-year period, the rate showed a marked increase of 2.4- to 2.7-fold. With regard to recent changes in the number of deaths from pancreatic cancer according to sex and age, the male-to-female ratio was 1.25 to 1.28:1, showing a tendency for a greater number of men than women, while the age of those dying was 60–65 years and 70–80 years for men, and 75–80 years for women. The increase in the death rate of males 60 to 65 years of age is noticeable in that it is earlier, but the increase in elderly patients as a whole seems to reflect an overall increase in this form of cancer.

The recent development of diagnostic and therapeutic measures for pancreatic diseases has been remarkable. With regard to pancreatic cancer, however, as known from circumstances in which the cancer has been regarded as synonymous with incurable disease, and since most cases upon detection are advanced, this cancer carries a very poor prognosis in comparison with other gastrointestinal cancers.

To improve therapeutic results for pancreatic cancer, and as a means of assessing

---

* Manuscript was prepared by Yoichi Saitoh, Masahiro Yamamoto, and Osamu Ohashi, First Department of Surgery, Kobe University School of Medicine, 7-5-2, Kusunoki-cho, Chuo-ku, Kobe 650, Japan

data on the basis of common criteria, the General Rules for the Study of Pancreatic Cancer were established by the Japan Pancreas Society in 1980 (2). On the basis of these rules, a nationwide pancreatic cancer registration has been undertaken by the Pancreatic Cancer Registration Committee of the Society every year since 1981 (1). With the cooperation of 345 major institutions throughout Japan, a total of 13,498 cases of pancreatic cancer to date had been documented through 1992.

This study describes the results of the nationwide survey and the totalization of data carried out by the Pancreatic Cancer Registration Committee of the Japan Pancreas Society.

Background of the Registered Patients

The total number of patients with pancreatic cancer registered in Japan during the 12-year period was 13,498 (Table I). Their background as well as the recent status of diagnosis and treatment for the disease in Japan were ascertained.

TABLE I. Annual Number of Patients Registered by the Pancreatic Cancer Registry in Japan

Year	Male	Female	Total
1981	751	440	1,191
1982	513	301	814
1983	656	419	1,075
1984	655	412	1,067
1985	661	409	1,070
1986	734	436	1,170
1987	781	519	1,300
1988	620	403	1,023
1989	716	481	1,197
1990	902	517	1,419
1991	612	358	970
1992	736	475	1,211
Total	8,337	5,170	13,507

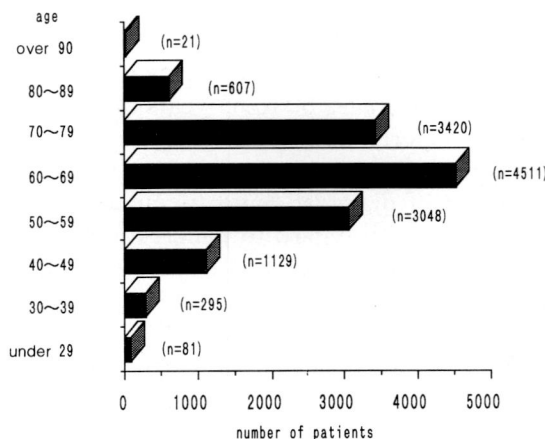

FIG. 1. Age distribution (1981–1992)

The male-to-female ratio of these patients was 1.6 to 1, the largest proportion being in their 60s, probably because many of these had undergone limited treatment (Fig. 1).

With regard to family history, 2.2% and 25.9% of the patients had family histories of pancreatic and other cancers, respectively. Whether or not hereditary and constitutional factors are involved in the occurrence of pancreatic cancer should be investigated in the future.

With regard to past history, 16.2%, 7.9%, 6.0%, 3.0%, 1.8%, 1.3%, 1.2%, 0.8%, 0.6%, and 0.6% of the registered patients had histories of diabetes mellitus, peptic ulcer, cholelithiasis, chronic pancreatitis, acute pancreatitis, chronic diarrhea, chronic alcoholism, (tumorous) pancreatic cyst, (non-tumorous) pancreatic cyst, and pancreatolithiasis, respectively (Table II). The incidence of diabetes mellitus associated with cancer other than pancreatic cancer is generally believed to be about 1%, and the incidence of pancreatic cancer in patients with diabetes mellitus has been reported to be three times as high as that in non-diabetic patients. These findings suggest a relationship between these two conditions. Since this type of survey includes diabetes mellitus secondarily to pancreatic cancer, however, it is impossible to conclude that diabetes mellitus is a risk factor for the disease.

With regard to diagnostic clues in patients presenting to hospitals, 86.9% had some symptoms, and only 3.1% made their visit for a medical checkup or a mass screening examination. The initial symptoms were mainly abdominal pain and jaun-

TABLE II. Past Histories

	No. of patients	% of patients
Diabetes mellitus	2,192	16.2
Peptic ulcer	1,072	7.9
Cholelithiasis	807	6.0
Chronic pancreatitis	410	3.0
Acute pancreatitis	245	1.8
Chronic diarrhea	170	1.3
Chronic alcoholism	156	1.2
Pancreatic cyst (tumorous)	103	0.8
(non-tumorous)	86	0.6
Pancreatolithiasis	78	0.6

TABLE III. Symptoms

Symptom	No. of patients	% of patients
Abdominal pain	4,142	30.7
Jaundice	2,087	15.5
Anorexia	1,059	7.8
Back pain	923	6.8
Malaise	684	5.1
Weight loss	522	3.9
Nausea	269	2.0
Abdominal mass	165	1.2
None	517	3.8
Others	3,130	23.2

TABLE IV. Annual Changes in Diagnostic Methods for First Detecting a Lesion of the Pancreas (%)

Year	US	CT	ERCP	PTC	UGI	EGD	DIC	SCINTI	ANGIO
1981	24.5	11.4	16.0	21.7	5.9	0.6	0.5	0.8	3.1
1982	31.7	13.5	14.8	19.2	4.8	0.9	0.6	0.6	0.9
1983	33.9	16.6	11.5	15.3	4.0	0.9	0.2	0.5	0.9
1984	35.5	17.9	11.2	12.5	3.7	0.7	0.3	2.5	1.9
1985	30.6	14.1	9.3	10.0	3.0	0.5	0.1	0.3	1.2
1986	36.8	16.5	10.8	9.1	3.0	0.7	0.1	0.1	0.9
1987	41.6	23.2	9.5	7.2	3.1	0.9	0.1	0.5	0.8
1988	42.9	21.1	8.1	8.0	2.2	1.0	0.2	0.0	0.7
1989	42.8	27.0	7.5	6.9	1.6	0.6	0.0	0.2	0.7
1990	43.9	22.9	6.8	7.0	1.3	0.5	0.1	0.1	0.4
1991	44.9	25.3	5.7	6.6	1.4	0.7	0.1	0.4	0.3
1992	49.7	25.8	5.8	4.3	1.1	0.7	0.1	0.0	0.2

US: ultrasound. CT: computed tomography. ERCP: endoscopic retrograde cholangiopancreatography. PTC: percutaneous transhepatic cholangiography. UGI: upper gastrointestinal series. EGD: esophagogastroduodenoscopy. DIC: drip infusion cholangiography. SCINTI: scintigram. ANGIO: angiography.

TABLE V. Annual Changes of Tumor Size (TS) (%)

Year	$TS_1 \leq 2.0$ cm	2.0 cm$<TS_2 \leq 4.0$ cm	4.0 cm$<TS_3 \leq 6.0$ cm	6.0 cm$<TS_4$
1981	2.9	14.9	19.1	33.8
1982	3.7	14.3	21.3	28.9
1983	2.6	17.0	16.5	32.1
1984	2.6	19.2	25.2	33.2
1985	4.3	17.2	17.2	28.4
1986	3.8	18.1	20.3	26.5
1987	3.7	15.8	19.5	26.1
1988	5.8	20.4	21.1	23.2
1989	4.1	19.0	19.9	22.0
1990	3.8	17.3	19.5	27.4
1991	1.4	6.7	3.8	2.9
1992	5.7	20.7	16.4	16.4

dice, the incidences of which accounted for 30.7% and 15.5%, respectively (Table III). Characteristically, the incidence of jaundice as the initial symptom increased with age, probably because complaints due to pain diminish in the elderly. This point should be kept in mind in routine examination.

The affected period was relatively short in the majority of patients and the proportion who had suffered from the cancer for at most three months accounted for 62.3%.

Among the various diagnostic measures, ultrasonography (US), and computed tomography (CT) have become increasingly important as methods for first detecting a lesion of the pancreas. The frequency of US, in particular, has recently reached 49.7%, although it was 24.5% at the beginning of the survey (Table IV).

The rates of positivity for abnormal levels on biochemical tests were 31.9% and 40.5% for amylase and lipase, respectively, in terms of blood pancreatic enzyme levels, and 48.9% and 79.1% for carcinoembryonic antigen (CEA) and CA19-9, respectively, in terms of tumor markers. The incidence of exocrine and endocrine dysfunction at the time of diagnosis was 62.3% by pancreatic function tests and 67.4% by oral glucose tolerance test.

Although small pancreatic cancers with tumors of 2 cm or less are not necessarily early ones, the rates of resection and prognosis are better than those of pancreatic cancers larger than this. Owing to the recent development of techniques such as diagnostic imaging, detection of small pancreatic cancers has increased slightly. The incidence of small pancreatic cancer among the registered patients in 1981, 2.9%, had increased to 5.7% by 1992 (Table V).

Treatment Tendencies in Pancreatic Cancer

By treatment method, the 13,498 registered cases were composed of 4,597 (34.1%) patients who underwent resection, 4,699 (34.8%) who underwent palliative operation, 921 (6.8%) who underwent exploratory laparotomy, 2,940 (21.8%) who had no operation, and 341 (2.5%) without operation who were autopsied (Fig. 2). In connection with this, 24.5% of all patients underwent resection in 1981 when nationwide registration was initiated, but this number had increased to 37.6% by 1992 (Table VI). This improvement in resection rate can be attributed mainly to the

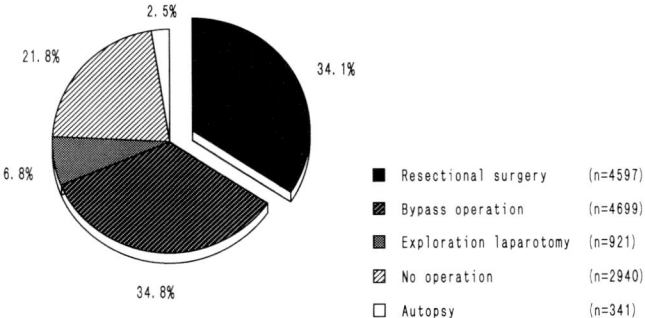

FIG. 2. Recent treatment status

TABLE VI. Annual Changes in Treatments and Proportion Found at Autopsy

Year	Resectional surgery		Bypass operation		Exploratory laparotomy		No operation		Autopsy	
	n	(%)	n	(%)	n	(%)	n	(%)	n	(%)
1981	292	(24.5)	545	(45.8)	104	(8.7)	196	(16.5)	54	(4.5)
1982	211	(26.0)	352	(43.2)	54	(6.6)	162	(19.9)	35	(4.3)
1983	318	(29.6)	436	(40.6)	64	(6.0)	246	(22.9)	11	(0.9)
1984	295	(27.6)	413	(38.7)	82	(7.7)	256	(24.0)	21	(2.0)
1985	355	(33.2)	374	(35.0)	53	(5.0)	252	(23.6)	36	(3.2)
1986	411	(35.1)	454	(38.8)	54	(4.6)	221	(18.9)	30	(2.6)
1987	429	(33.0)	453	(34.8)	77	(5.9)	317	(24.4)	24	(1.9)
1988	397	(38.8)	300	(29.3)	93	(9.1)	213	(20.8)	20	(2.0)
1989	484	(40.4)	377	(31.5)	75	(6.3)	237	(19.8)	24	(2.0)
1990	553	(39.0)	434	(30.6)	98	(6.9)	296	(20.9)	38	(2.7)
1991	398	(41.0)	270	(28.0)	73	(7.5)	209	(21.5)	20	(2.0)
1992	456	(37.6)	295	(24.4)	94	(7.8)	338	(27.8)	28	(2.3)

n: number of patients.

TABLE VII. Annual Changes in Resectional Procedures

Year	TP	PD	DP (t)	DP (bt)	DP (subtotal)
1981	29.4	54.9	1.7	11.9	2.1
1982	27.5	54.5	2.8	10.0	1.4
1983	26.1	56.9	1.6	12.6	0.6
1984	20.3	54.6	2.4	15.6	4.1
1985	27.9	49.9	1.3	16.9	3.7
1986	15.3	64.2	0.7	15.8	2.4
1987	14.5	58.7	2.3	19.1	2.6
1988	13.4	62.7	2.5	17.1	2.8
1989	11.0	61.2	3.1	18.4	3.9
1990	10.1	63.8	1.4	19.9	2.0
1991	9.3	65.3	0.7	18.3	3.0
1992	5.5	66.4	1.8	18.4	6.4

TP: total pancreatectomy. PD: pancreaticoduodenectomy. DP: distal pancreatectomy. (t): tail. (bt): body and tail.

TABLE VIII. Annual Changes in Dissection Extent of Lymph Nodes for Pancreatic Cancer (%)

Year	D0	D1	D2
1981	15.1	36.6	40.4
1982	15.2	23.2	53.1
1983	14.5	28.3	49.1
1984	11.9	33.9	45.8
1985	13.5	29.6	51.0
1986	13.9	26.0	53.0
1987	15.8	31.7	46.9
1988	11.3	32.5	49.6
1989	17.6	33.3	42.4
1990	14.8	32.7	44.8
1991	12.8	34.2	44.5
1992	16.4	35.9	40.4

D0: pancreatectomy without lymph node dissection.
D1: pancreatectomy with dissection of the Group 1 lymph nodes.
D2: pancreatectomy with dissection of the Group 2 lymph nodes.

increase in detection of resectable tumor and the benefit of extended surgery.

The reason for an operation not being performed in some patients was extensive growth of the cancer in 73.1%, the highest rate, followed by physical reasons other than cancer in 9.3% and patient refusal in 3.4%.

In those undergoing palliative operation, gastrojejunostomy, internal and external biliary drainage operation were performed in 47.4%, 58.4%, and 12.9%, respectively.

Among the patients with resection, 706 (15.4%), 2,810 (61.1%), and 976 (21.2%) underwent total pancreatectomy (TP), pancreaticoduodenectomy (PD), and distal pancreatectomy (DP), respectively. The annual changes in the procedures caused the proportion of patients who underwent TP, PD, and DP, 28.8%, 53.8%, and 15.4%, respectively, in 1981 to change to 5.5%, 66.4%, and 26.6%, respectively, by 1992; this was the result of a gradual decrease in TP (Table VII). At the beginning of the survey, TP tended to be actively performed to obtain radicality, but thereafter therapeutic results were reconsidered, and postoperative quality of life (QOL) was taken

TABLE IX. Annual Changes of Organs Resected in Incidence of Pancreatic Cancer (%)

Year	Colon	Liver	Spleen	Stomach	Portal vein	Artery	None
1981	4.9	0.5	25.9	5.2	15.3	3.5	27.8
1982	4.3	0.7	22.9	3.5	17.4	4.7	25.2
1983	5.2	1.2	25.9	4.4	17.7	4.4	21.3
1984	7.6	2.3	23.2	6.9	14.0	2.8	19.6
1985	6.1	1.9	22.3	5.6	17.3	3.5	14.3
1986	6.1	3.0	18.2	5.0	17.4	3.2	15.8
1987	6.2	1.3	21.3	4.3	17.5	2.5	16.8
1988	10.1	2.8	23.9	4.5	21.2	5.3	23.2
1989	7.2	1.2	27.9	5.4	26.4	7.4	22.7
1990	9.0	1.3	22.6	5.8	21.2	5.1	32.4
1991	8.3	2.3	20.9	4.3	20.9	5.5	28.6
1992	5.9	1.3	20.2	2.9	23.9	3.9	29.4

TABLE X. Frequency and Effective Rates (ER) of Chemotherapy

Combination	Pre-op.		Intra-op.		Post-op.	
	Frequency	ER	Frequency	ER	Frequency	ER
Resectional surgery	4.5%	10.2%	10.1%	6.9%	43.7%	7.4%
Bypass operation	9.2%	6.3%	14.1%	8.9%	47.3%	9.2%
Exploratory laparotomy	10.5%	4.1%	22.8%	4.3%	47.9%	10.2%
No operation			41.1%	9.5%		

TABLE XI. Frequency and Effective Rates of Radiation Therapy

Combination	Pre-op.		Intra-op.		Post-op.	
	Frequency	ER	Frequency	ER	Frequency	ER
Resectional surgery	1.1%	27.5%	10.8%	11.7%	6.1%	12.5%
Bypass operation	2.3%	22.6%	10.7%	30.7%	6.6%	23.6%
Exploratory laparotomy	2.0%	11.1%	14.8%	27.9%	9.0%	24.1%
No operation			9.0%	25.8%		

into consideration. Surgical procedures in which pancreatic function is preserved as much as possible within a range at which radicality can be maintained have become the preferred modalities.

The lymph node stations 1 to 18 according to the Japanese classification were divided into three groups, namely Group 1 of nodes closest to the tumor and Groups 2 to 3 of more distant lymph nodes. In resected cases over the 12 years the Group 1 lymph nodes were not dissected or were dissected insufficiently in 14.5% (D0), the Group 1 lymph nodes alone were dissected in 31.9% (D1), and the Group 1 and 2 lymph nodes were dissected in 46.4% (D2) (Table VIII). The organs resected with the lesion over the 12 year period were the colon in 7.8%, a portion of the liver in 1.9%, the spleen in 25.9%, the stomach (total gastrectomy) in 5.5%, portal vein in 22.0%, and artery in 4.9%. Among recent tendencies in organ resection with pancreatic lesions, the frequency of resection of the portal vein has gradually been increasing, and this combined resection seems to contribute to improvement in the rate of resection (Table IX).

As part of the multidisciplinary treatment for pancreatic cancer, the combined treatment modality of surgery with chemotherapy or radiotherapy was investigated. Frequency of this treatment was low, but there was a tendency for postoperative chemotherapy and intraoperative radiotherapy to be performed relatively actively. The effectiveness was poor, however, and both were evaluated as somewhat effective in only about 10% of cases (Tables X, XI). The usefulness and methodology of these various combined treatment modalities in resectable and unresectable pancreatic cancer should be assessed in more detail.

Survival and Factors Affecting the Prognosis

Cumulative survival rate was calculated by the actuarial method for 3,692 patients undergoing resection, 3,862 undergoing palliative operation, 736 undergoing exploratory laparotomy, and 2,444 without operation for whom follow-up data were available among those registered.

Depending on the therapeutic method used, cumulative 1-, 3-, and 5-year survival rates were 52.7%, 23.2%, and 17.5% for patients with resection, respectively. On the other hand, one-year survival rates in patients undergoing palliative operation, exploratory laparotomy and without operation were 14.0%, 12.1%, and 10.1%, respectively (Table XII). As in other gastrointestinal cancers, only those undergoing resection had the possibility of prolonged survival.

The data in 1985, when the 5-year survival rate was calculated for the first time after the start of the totalization undertaking, showed a 5-year survival rate of 10.1% in patients with resection. The recent improvement in results of surgical treatment can be attributed to the improvement in prognosis.

Histologically, patients undergoing resection with tubular adenocarcinoma, generally called ductal adenocarcinoma, constitute the majority of pancreatic cancer cases, and have the worst prognosis (Table XIII). Papillary adenocarcinoma, cystadenocarcinoma, and islet cell carcinoma showed relatively favorable prognoses, despite being in the category of pancreatic cancer. Some cases of so-called mucin-

TABLE XII. Cumulative Survival Rates of Patients with Pancreatic Cancer by Type of Treatment (%)

	n	1-Year	2-Year	3-Year	4-Year	5-Year
Resectional surgery	3,692	52.7	30.1	23.2	19.3	17.5
Bypass operation	3,862	14.0	3.5	2.0	1.6	1.6
Exploratory laparotomy	736	12.1	3.2	1.5	0.4	0.4
No operation	2,444	10.1	3.2	2.0	1.4	1.2

TABLE XIII. Postoperative Cumulative Survival Rates of Patients Who Received Resection by Histological Classification (%)

	n	1-Year	2-Year	3-Year	4-Year	5-Year
Papillary adenocarcinoma	320	66.2	46.0	36.0	32.6	32.6
Well differentiated adenocarcinoma	804	55.7	28.9	19.7	14.1	11.7
Moderately differentiated adenocarcinoma	1,172	44.8	19.8	13.4	9.8	9.1
Poorly differentiated adenocarcinoma	306	31.1	15.6	12.5	12.5	8.9
Cystadenocarcinoma	121	82.2	69.9	65.0	56.8	54.3
Islet cell carcinoma	104	89.6	85.8	82.6	75.9	65.3

producing pancreatic cancer, which is noted as one with a good prognosis, may be included in papillary adenocarcinoma because its pathologic classification has not been established.

The General Rules for the Study of Pancreatic Cancer contain rules for the description of operative findings. The stage of pancreatic cancer is expressed by peripancreatic invasion (T), hepatic metastasis (H), peritoneal dissemination(P), lymph node involvement (N), and metastasis to other distant extraperitoneal organs (M). T is also defined by infiltration to the anterior capsule of the pancreas (S), to tissue adjacent to the posterior surface of the pancreas (RP), to the intrapancreatic bile duct (CH), to the duodenal wall (DU), to the portal vein system (PV), and to the arterial system (A).

TABLE XIV. Surgical Stage Classification According to the Japan Pancreas Society (1993)

	P_0, H_0, M_0				$P_{1,2,3}$ or	$H_{1,2,3}$ M_1
	N_0	N_1	N_2	N_3		
T_{1a} Tumor size of less than 2cm and $S_0+RP_0+PV_0+A_0+DU_0+CH_{0,1}$	I	II	III			
T_{1b} Tumor size of more than 2 cm and $S_0+RP_0+PV_0+A_0+DU_0+CH_{0,1}$	II	II	III	IVa		
T_2 Regardless of tumor size and one more positive of S_1, $RP_1, PV_1, A_1, DU_{1,2,3}$, or $CH_{2,3}$	III	III	IVa		IVb	
T_3 Regardless of tumor size and one more positive of $S_{2,3}, RP_{2,3}, PV_{2,3}$, or $A_{2,3}$	IVa					

S_0: no capsular invasion. S_1: suspected invasion to the capsule. S_2: definite invasion to the capsule. S_3: invasion to the adjacent viscera. RP, PV, A, DU, and CH factors are subdivided and defined in the same manner. P_0: no evidence of peritoneal dissemination. P_1: dissemination to the peritoneum adjacent to the pancreas. P_2: sporadic dissemination to the peritoneum far from the pancreas. P_3: multiple dissemination to the peritoneum far from the pancreas. H_0: no evidence of hepatic metastasis. H_1: metastasis to a single lobe of the liver. H_2: sporadic metastases to both lobes of the liver. H_3: multiple metastases to both lobes of the liver. N_0: no evidence of lymph node involvement. N_1: evidence of lymph node involvement within Group 1. N_2: evidence of lymph node involvement within Group 2. N_3: evidence of lymph node involvement within Group 3.

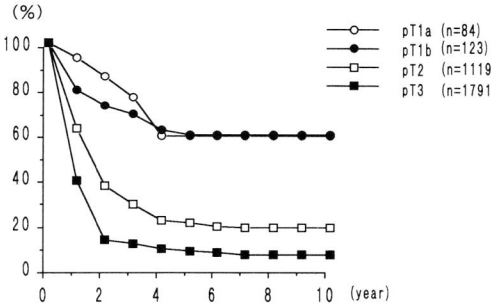

FIG. 3. Postoperative cumulative survival rates of patients who received resection according to T category proposed by the UICC

The results of calculation of the cumulative survival rate according to each factor in patients who underwent resection, except for those with cystadenocarcinoma and islet cell carcinoma, suggest that all of these are important prognostic factors. As the tumor size increased, the incidence and degree of infiltration to the pancreatic capsule and the peripancreatic tissue increased, and the incidence and extent of lymph node metastasis also increased.

Such assessments stimulated revision of the General Rules for the Study of Pancreatic Cancer and the 4th edition was published in 1993 (2). Stages of pancreatic cancer were classified as shown in Table XIV; criteria resembling the TNM classification of the Union Internationalis Contra Cancrum (UICC) were adopted for T categories, and the Japanese N classification which has conventionally been used (classification by regional lymph node group with slight modification) was adopted for N categories.

With regard to the prognosis of resected cases (except for cystadenocarcinoma and islet cell carcinoma), the cumulative survival rate was calculated according to the TNM classification of the UICC. The 1-, 3-, and 5-year survival rates were 93.3%, 75.9%, and 58.1%, respectively, for patients with pT1a, and the corresponding rates in those with pT1b were 79.1%, 67.9%, and 58.6%. Thus, the prognosis in patients without invasion to the peripancreatic tissue was good regardless of tumor size. However, the 1-, 3-, and 5-year survival rates in patients with pT2 were 61.4%, 28.2%, and 19.7%, respectively, and the corresponding rates in those with pT3 were 38.3%, 10.2%, and 7.1%, showing that the prognosis with invasion to the surrounding tissues or large vessels was very poor (Fig. 3).

Thus, the prognosis of pancreatic cancer is affected by the presence or absence of tumor infiltration to the pancreatic capsule and peripancreatic tissue, and tumor size correlates with the incidence and degree of invasion to the peripancreatic tissue. Nationwide registration now follows the new rules as of 1993, while at the same time other prognostic factors are being elucidated and various therapeutic methods evaluated for more detailed assessment.

Conclusion

The present status of pancreatic cancer registration and recent tendencies in diagnosis and treatment for the disease in Japan have been outlined. Although progress is slow, it is assumed that the rate of resection and prognosis will improve with the increase in detection of resectable pancreatic cancers and the introduction of more extensive surgery. In surgical treatment, a more rational operative procedure, which takes into consideration radicality and postoperative QOL, as well as indications for its use are under investigation. It is also urgent to evaluate the usefulness and methodology of intensive treatment which fully utilizes the various combined treatment modalities.

Acknowledgments

A part of this work was supported by a grant-in-aid for cancer research from the Ministry of Health and Welfare of Japan. The Committee appreciates the contributions of member doctors in the 345 major hospitals which are listed at the end of this book.

REFERENCES

1. Dynamic Population Statistics from 1950 to 1990, ed. The Statistical Information Division of the Secretariat of the Ministry of Health and Welfare in Japan (1950–1990). Kosei Tokei Kyokai (Welfare Statistics Association) (in Japanese).
2. General Rules for the Study of Pancreatic Cancer, ed. Japan Pancreas Society, 4th ed. (1993). Kanehara Shuppan, Tokyo (in Japanese).
3. Report of nationwide registration of pancreatic cancer patients in 1981–1992, ed. Pancreatic Cancer Registration Committee of the Japan Pancreas Society (1982–1993) (in Japanese).

TIME TRENDS AND SURVIVAL RATE OF LUNG CANCER

Lung Cancer Registration Committee*

Data in the Japanese Lung Cancer Registration by the Lung Cancer Task Force of The Japanese Committee on TNM Classification and the data of the National Cancer Center were analyzed to overview the present status of treatment and morbidity in lung cancer in Japan. It is estimated that lung cancer deaths exceeded 35,000 in 1993 and lung cancer has now become the number one killer disease in Japan.

Surgical treatment has been the number one selection for lung cancer treatment, but the actual surgical operative rate remains at approximately 40%. According to the newest data, the five-year survival rate of surgically treated patients exceeds 40%. The trend toward an increase in incidence of adenocarcinoma is pronounced and amounts to approximately 50% of the total lung cancer cases. In female lung cancer patients, adenocarcinoma accounts for 76%.

The number of lung cancer cases in 1990 in developed countries was 530,000 (3). In Japan 35,000 persons were believed to have died of this disease in 1993, and lung cancer thus held the number one position among cancer death causes. Three sets of data on lung cancer in Japan will be presented in this paper. The first has already been published in lung cancer registration program records of the Japanese Joint Committee (JJC) of TNM Classification. The second set comprises the surgical results from the Department of Thoracic Surgery in the National Cancer Center Hospital (NCCH) Tokyo. The third set is the practical data of 1991 for the same department at NCCH.

Lung Cancer Patients Registered for Analysis

From 1967 to 1983, lung cancer registration was maintained by Dr. K. Yoshimura of the Lung Cancer Task Force and accumulated reports were made every three years as shown in Tables I to V. Data of this type are believed to be exclusive to Japan. For their most recent data, the NCCH collected 1,228 cases from 1980 to 1989, a ten-year period, for statistical analysis. For analysis of stage, histological type and basic factors of surgical treatment, the newest cases from 1987 to 1991 were evaluated. Regretfully, however, the staging system for lung cancer during this period was changed three times, from JJC 1978 to UICC-TNM 1978 to UICC-

---

* Manuscript was prepared by Tomoyuki Goya, Yoshihiko Koshiishi, Tadashi Sekihara, and Ichiko Yamaoka, Department of Surgery II, School of Medicine, Kyorin University, 6-20-2 Shinkawa, Mitaka 181, Japan; Katutoshi Yoshimura, Lung Cancer Task Force, The Japanese Joint Committee on TNM Classification; and Haruhiko Nakayama, Haruhiko Kondo, Tsuguo Naruke, and Keiichi Suemasu, Department of Thoracic Surgery, National Cancer Center Hospital, 5-1-1 Tsukiji, Chuo-ku, Tokyo 104, Japan

TABLE I. Number of Registered Lung Cancer Patients

Survey	3rd(5)	4th(6)	5th(7)	6th(8)	7th(9)
Male	1,396	1,891	3,770	5,810	7,963
Female	431	562	1,161	1,677	2,381
Total	1,827	2,453	4,931	7,487	10,344
Age					
<50	19.0%	18.4%	14.0%	11.3%	9.4%
50–59	30.0%	25.7%	24.9%	23.8%	23.1%
60–69	38.8%	37.7%	39.2%	38.7%	36.0%
70<	12.2%	18.2%	21.9%	26.2%	31.5%
Mean age	—	—	61.2	62.4	63.6

3rd, 1967–69; 4th, 1972–74; 5th, 1975–77; 6th, 1978-80; 7th, 1981–83.

TABLE II. Histology of Registered Lung Cancer (%)

Survey	4th(6)	5th(7)	6th(8)	7th(9)
Adenocarcinoma	37.9	38.9	38.7	39.8
Squamous cell carcinoma	40.6	40.0	40.0	37.7
Large cell carcinoma	6.5	7.6	7.0	7.1
Small cell carcinoma	8.8	12.4	13.2	14.2
Others	6.2	1.0	1.1	1.2

TABLE III. Five-year Survival at Each Clinical Stage According to UICC-TNM 1978

Survey	3rd		4th		5th		6th		7th	
Stage	n	Survival[a]	n	Survival	n	Survival	n	Survival	n	Survival
Ia	461	25.9	827	37.1	1,251	35.4	1,842	41.5	2,412	41.9
Ib					171	22.8	196	27.0	265	22.1
II	352	10.0	332	13.0	681	13.5	807	20.1	690	21.3
III	450	4.4	584	7.9	1,443	4.3	2,559	7.4	3,698	11.0
IV	564	1.5	689	—	1,378	0.7	2,071	1.6	3,260	1.8
Total	1,827	10.0	2,432	16.3	4,924	14.9	7,475	16.1	10,325	16.3

[a] Survival rate (%) according to Japanese Clinical Staging System in 1978.

TABLE IV. Surgery and Survival

Survey	5th		6th		7th	
	n	Survival	n	Survival	n	Survival
Surgical cases	2,237	45.4%	3,393	45.3%	4,422	42.7%
5-Year survivors after resection	2,055	30.1%	3,065	36.1%	4,095	36.5%

TNM 1988, making it impossible to make exact comparisons of the stage for this period. Generally, of course, when the clinical stage and postoperative stage are compared, the staging by clinical TNM will definitely have a poor prognosis, and treatment results will unquestionably improve with time. In the data accumulated by Yoshimura, the clinical stage and postoperative stage do not agree, while the NCCH data give the survival rate based on postoperative stage alone. Therefore, simple comparisons of these three sets of data cannot be made (2).

TABLE V. Postoperative 5-Year Survival of Patients with Lung Cancer (NCCH 1980–89)

		Initial	1-Year		2-Year		3-Year		4-Year		5-Year	
		n	n	Survival	n	Survival	n	Survival	n	Survival	n	Survival
Total		1,228	947	77.8	728	62.9	548	54.2	397	48.4	291	43.8
Stage	I	447	408	91.9	369	87.1	298	80.5	231	77.0	178	72.5
	II	125	106	86.2	86	76.1	67	68.5	47	55.5	31	43.8
	IIIA	375	288	77.5	190	53.4	135	42.8	95	36.2	65	31.2
	IIIB	99	45	46.7	30	31.1	15	19.8	8	16.6	5	16.6
	IV	180	99	55.0	51	30.4	32	21.7	15	15.4	11	13.1
Adenoca		655	519	80.0	396	64.0	297	54.9	211	47.8	162	43.2
Sq		376	292	78.4	221	63.9	172	55.2	127	51.0	90	48.0
Large		88	60	68.2	47	54.4	32	49.2	22	45.7	15	38.8
Ad-sq		36	23	63.9	20	55.6	13	38.5	9	29.2	3	17.6
Small		41	25	61.0	17	41.5	12	36.1	12	36.1	11	36.1

Stage was determined postoperatively according to UICC-TNM 1988.
Adenoca, adenocarcinoma; Sq, squamous cell carcinoma; Large, large cell carcinoma; Ad-sq, adenosquamous cell carcinoma; Small, small cell carcinoma.
Total patients excluding those with 44 double primary cancers and 2 T0N0M0 cases.

TABLE VI. Postoperative Five-year Survival of Adenocarcinoma Patients with Lung Cancer (NCCH 1980–89)

		n	1-Year	2-Year	3-Year	4-Year	5-Year
Stage	I	271	93.0	90.0	85.8	81.3	76.4
	II	54	83.1	73.5	62.8	53.3	40.8
	IIIA	164	81.1	50.4	39.2	28.5	22.0
	IIIB	47	52.2	30.4	10.0	6.7	6.7
	IV	180	58.8	32.4	20.4	12.8	11.6

Stage was determined postoperatively according to UICC-TNM 1988.

TABLE VII. Postoperative Five-year Survival of Squamous Cell Carcinoma Patients with Lung Cancer (NCCH 1980–89)

		n	1-Year	2-Year	3-Year	4-Year	5-Year
Stage	I	125	94.4	87.0	76.6	73.6	68.9
	II	50	94.0	83.2	78.4	62.3	58.9
	IIIA	130	79.0	59.3	46.4	43.3	38.6
	IIIB	34	30.5	21.4	17.8	17.8	17.8
	IV	37	40.5	18.9	18.9	18.9	0

Stage was determined postoperatively according to UICC-TNM 1988.

Age and Sex

According to Yoshimura's Japan Registration, as shown in Table I, the registered cases have been increasing yearly, and it is assumed that 30% of lung cancer cases have been registered. Male to female sex ratio changed from 4.1 to 3.1 and quite a constant rising trend in the female has been suggested (Table I).

TABLE VIII. Histology of Primary Lung Cancer and Sex Distribution (NCCH 1980–89)

	Males	Females	Total
Adenocarcinoma	447	234	681 (54.2%)
Squamous cell carcinoma	358	31	389 (31.0%)
Adeno-squamous carcinoma	30	6	36
Small cell carcinoma	33	5	38
Large cell carcinoma	79	13	92
Carcinoid	9	9	18
Adenoid cystic carcinoma	2	3	5
Epidermoid carcinoma	0	1	1
Carcinosarcoma	1	1	2
Other cancer	3	3	6
Unclassified	4	1	5
Total	966	307	1,273

Including patients with double cancer ($n = 44$) and excluding those with T0N0M0 ($n = 2$).

TABLE IX. Extended Radical Surgery for Lung Cancer Invading Mediastinal Organs (NCCH 1980–89)

LA	39
SVC	26
Ao	20
Ao replacement	5
PA	3
Ao + PA	2
SVC + LA	2
Ao + LA	1
Ao + LA + PA	1
PA + LA	1
Total	100 cases

LA: left atrium. SVC: superior vena cava. Ao: aorta. PA: pulmonary artery.

TABLE X. Outcome of Extended Radical Surgery for Lung Cancer in NCCH

	No. of patients	3-Year	5-Year
Left atrium	44	8	5
Aorta	29	2	2
Aortic replacement	(5)	(1)	(1)
Superior vena cava	28	1	0
Pulmonary artery	7	0	0

The data of Yoshimura (Table I) and the most recent resected cases at NCCH (Table XI) both show a constant mean age of 62 to 63 years. Yoshimura's data includes non-resected cases, and it is thought that this is why a little difference appears.

TABLE XI. Number of Resected Primary Lung Cancer Cases (NCCH 1991)

	1987	1988	1989	1990	1991
No. of patients	154	159	138	167	168
Male/female	113/41	130/29	113/25	129/38	117/51
Age range	27–82	32–83	40–84	34–82	26–85
Mean age	63.0	62.5	62.5	60.0	62.0
Histologic type					
Adenocarcinoma	81	85	72	77	93
Squamous cell carcinoma	50	47	42	41	51
Adeno-squamous carcinoma	3	4	2	3	3
Small cell carcinoma	5	8	3	8	6
Large cell carcinoma	12	15	15	8	11
Carcinoid	3	1	4	3	3
Adenoid cystic carcinoma	1		1		2
Undifferentiated carcinoma	2	1			
Unclassified			1		
Total	157(3)	161(1)	140(2)	140	160(1)

( ) indicates number of cases with synchronous double primary carcinoma of different histology.

TABLE XII. Postoperative TNM Stage of Resected Lung Cancer Cases (NCCH 1991)

		1987	1988	1989	1990	1991
Stage	0				0	3
	I	69	52	54	58	73
	II	14	9	23	25	19
	IIIa	38	46	39	43	48
	IIIb	10	23	8	22	13
	IV	22	29	13	19	12
Total		153	159	137	167	168

TABLE XIII. Coincidence of Clinical and Pathological Stage (NCCH 1991)

p-stage/c-stage	0	I	II	IIIa	IIIb	IV	Total
Stage 0	0	0	0	2	1	0	3
Stage I	0	64	2	3	1	2	72
Stage II	1	9	7	1	1	0	19
Stage IIIa	0	11	7	22	4	4	48
Stage IIIb	0	4	0	7	2	0	13
Stage IV	0	4	4	0	0	4	12
Total	1	92	20	35	9	10	167

Accuracy of the stage in 1991; 99/167 = 59.3%.
               in 1990; 75/127 = 59.0%.
               in 1989; 86/134 = 64.2%.

One case could not be diagnosed as definite lung cancer before surgery.

TABLE XIV. Accuracy of Pre-operative Clinical N-factor (NCCH 1991)

pN/cN	cN0	cN1	cN2	cN3	cNx	Total
pN0	73	2	10	0	0	85
pN1	13	17	3	0	0	33
pN2	15	6	20	1	0	42
pN3	1	0	0	0	0	1
pNx	5	1	0	0	0	6
Total	107	26	33	1	0	167

1991: cN2 — pN2; 20/42 = 47.6%, cN1 — pN1; 17/33 = 51.5%
1990: cN2 — pN2; 21/42 = 50.0%, cN1 — pN1; 13/30 = 43.3%
1989: cN2 — pN2; 19/33 = 57.5%, cN1 — pN1; 21/33 = 63.6%

One case could not be diagnosed as definite lung cancer before surgery.

TABLE XV. Surgery for Primary Lung Cancer (NCCH 1987–91)

		1991	1990	1989	1988	1987
1)	Procedure (year)					
	Pneumonectomy	22	40	29	42	30
	Panpleuro-pneumonectomy	0	3	0	2	1
	Lobectomy	145	124	103	112	122
	Segmentectomy	1	0	1	0	0
	Partial resection	0	3	5	5	1
	Total	168	167	138	159	154
2)	Tracheo-bronchoplasty					
	Bronchoplasty	12	7	9	9	6
	Tracheal resection				2	
	Carinal resection	5	8	7	7	3
	Total	17	15	16	18	9

The number of tracheo-bronchoplastic surgery include those with wedge resection.

TABLE XVI. Curability for Resected Primary Lung Cancer (NCCH 1991)

Absolutely curative		68 (40.5%)
Relatively curative		39 (23.2%)
Relatively non-curative		36 (21.4%)
Absolutely non-curative		25 (14.9%)
Total		168
Reasons for absolutely non-curative surgery[a]		
Intrapulmonary metastasis (pm+)		9 (30%)
solitary (pm1)		6
multiple (pm2)		3
Pleural dissociation (d+)		5 (17%)
Surgical margin positive		11 (37%)
Malignant pleural effusion (E+)		4 (13%)
Distant metastasis (+)		1 (3%)
Stage	I	8 (32%)
	II	3 (12%)
	IIIA	8 (32%)
	IIIB	2 (8%)
	IV	4 (16%)

[a] In 5 cases, reason for non-curability was overlapped.

Stage

In the staging system, the JJC 1978, UICC-TNM 1978, and UICC-TNM 1988 are not in accord and the accumulation tables cannot be compared easily. The data on UICC-TNM 1978 stage I-a and UICC-TNM 1988 stage I are practically the same; accordingly, the incidence for stage I in the observations of Yoshimura was approximately 25% and unchanged during the observation period (Table III). The incidence for stage I in the NCCH data was 36% (Table V), and displays an increasing trend (Table XII).

Histology

The reports of Yoshimura show a gradually increasing trend in incidence of adenocarcinoma and a gradually decreasing trend in incidence of squamous cell carcinoma (Table II). In the NCCH data, the squamous cell carcinoma rate in resected cases is a mere 31.0%, and adenocarcinoma accounts for 54.2% (Table VIII). If one gives thought to the fact that squamous cell carcinoma patients are more apt to be targets of surgical resection than adenocarcinoma patients, the increasing trend can be readily understood. Further, adenocarcinoma accounts for 76% of lung cancer in females.

Diagnosis and Accuracy of Staging

In 1980, CT apparatus was introduced for diagnosis throughout the country and brought about remarkable improvement in accuracy in diagnosis of tumors in the lung and mediastinal lymph nodes. As can be seen in Tables XIII and XIV, the coincidence between the clinical stage and the postoperative stage is only around 60%, and the diagnostic accuracy in mediastinal lymph node metastasis remains at only 50 to 60%. The improvements in diagnostic accuracy in recent years have brought about stage immigration, and survival at each stage has been improved with the passing of years. That is to say, these improvements reflect not only improved surgical procedures but also progress in X-ray diagnosis. With the progress in CT, echography and bone scintigraphy, preoperative diagnosis has become more precise and exact and patients with occult metastasis and locally advanced unresectable lung cancer have been accurately excluded.

The surgical curability of resected cases in NCCH for 1991 is shown in Table XVI. The operation was absolutely curative or relatively curative in 107 of 168 patients (64%). It was absolutely non-curative in 25 (15%) and only 20 cases were diagnosed as having a positive surgical margin or preoperatively undetectable intrapulmonary metastases. Those cases that were diagnosed as stage IIIB to stage IV preoperatively were few, and we believe that the surgical criteria were appropriate.

Survival

The surgical cases in Yoshimura's data amounted to 42% to 45% and the five-year survival rate during this period improved from 30.1% to 36.5%. According to the NCCH data (Table V), the five-year survival rate is 43.8%. Improvement in surgical results has depended on the stage of immigration, the mediastinal lymph node dissection and the establishment of extended radical resection of lung cancer including the neighboring organs (1). The five-year survival rate according to histological type is 43.2% for adenocarcinoma (Table VI) and 48% for squamous cell carcinoma (Table VII). It is very interesting that in stage I, five-year survival was 76.4% for adenocarcinoma and 68.9% for squamous cell carcinoma. This shows that stage I of adenocarcinoma has a surprisingly good prognosis compared with squamous cell carcinoma of the lung. The five-year survival rate for adenocarcinoma stage IV is 11.6%, better than stage IIIB at 6.7%. This is due to the fact that intrapulmonary metastasis close to the primary lesion was classified as stage IV. This discrepancy was modified in 1993 in the UICC-TNM Classification.

Surgery

Major progress in lung cancer surgery has been achieved as a result of systematic mediastinal lymph node dissection, bronchoplastic procedures and extended radical resection for lung cancer including neighboring organs. Bronchoplasty was used in 10% of the surgical cases (Table XV), and has been established as a standard surgical technique. Extended radical resection including neighboring organs (Table IX) has been attempted with the left atrium, superior vena cava, aorta, and pulmonary artery. The results are shown in Table X. Tsuchiya *et al.* (4) claim that extended radical resection including the left atrium and aorta is beneficial.

Prospective

Recently, the detection of asymptomatic cases through mass screening and periodical annual check-ups has been increasing. It is definitely a favorable trend that through surgical treatment curable cases of stage I disease are increasing and this has contributed greatly to the improvement in surgical results. The issues hereafter are, first, whether limited surgery for lung cancer can be used for small lesions in the lung field. If we are able to adopt the correct criteria, it will be promising. Second, we have no effective treatment method for advanced non-small cell lung cancer. Many trials including induction chemotherapy for advanced non-small cell lung cancer have been made but, unfortunately, we do not yet have a promising procedure.

Thoracoscopic surgery has been applied aggressively for lung cancer surgery. Improvement of the instrument and devices for video-assisted thoracic surgery (VATS) makes it possible to perform lobectomy and pneumonectomy. In the near future, this should be a standard procedure for stage I disease of lung cancer. Lung Cancer Registration Committee was reorganized in 1993 under the approvement of the Japanese Lung Cancer Society, and new cancer registration program started. About 60 major institutes for lung cancer treatment agreed to provide detailed data of cancer patients to the registry.

Acknowledgments

The authors appreciate contribution of members for the Lung Cancer Registration. Drs. Shaw Watanabe and Naohito Yamaguchi, Division of Cancer Information and Epidemiology Division, National Cancer Center Research Institute, were also appreciated for their various help. A part of this work was supported by the grant-in-aid for cancer research from the Ministry of Health and Welfare.

REFERENCES

1. Naruke, T., Goya, T., Tsuchiya, R., and Suemasu, K. The importance of surgery to non-small cell carcinoma of lung with mediastinal lymph node metastasis. *Ann. Thorac. Surg.*, **46**, 603–610 (1988).
2. Naruke, T., Goya, T., Tsuchiya, R., and Suemasu, K. Prognosis and survival in resected lung carcinoma based on the new international staging system. *J. Thorac. Cardiovasc. Surg.*, **96**, 440–447 (1988).
3. Tobacco Policy Recommendations of the IASLC. A 10 point-program. 7th World Conference of Lung Cancer, June, 1994.
4. Tsuchiya, R., Asamura, H., Kondo, H., Goya, T., and Naruke, T. Extended resection of left atrium, great vessels, or both for lung cancer. *Ann. Thorac. Surg.*, **57**, 960–965 (1994).
5. Yoshimura, K. Japanese Lung Cancer Registration (3rd), Japanese Joint Committee on TNM Classification, Tokyo (1975).
6. Yoshimura, K. Japanese Lung Cancer Registration (4th), Japanese Joint Committee on TNM Classification, Tokyo (1978).
7. Yoshimura, K. Japanese Lung Cancer Registration (5th), Japanese Joint Committee on TNM Classification, Tokyo (1981).
8. Yoshimura, K. Japanese Lung Cancer Registration (6th), Japanese Joint Committee on TNM Classification, Tokyo (1984).
9. Yoshimura, K. Japanese Lung Cancer Registration (7th), Japanese Joint Committee on TNM Classification, Tokyo (1988).

BONE TUMOR REGISTRATION

Musculoskeletal Tumor Committee of the Japanese Orthopaedic Association*

The bone tumor registration system started in 1964 for primary benign and malignant bone tumors and secondary bone tumors. A total of 3,623 primary malignant bone tumors were registered during the period 1980 to 1991. Osteosarcoma (44.1%), chondrosarcoma (16.1%), multiple myeloma (13.0%), malignant fibrous histiocytoma (7.7%), Ewing's sarcoma (6.7%), and chordoma (3.8%) were common histological diagnoses. Clinicoepidemiological analyses were done on osteosarcoma cases. Ten year survival rates were 51.4% (Stage I), 43.1% (Stage II), 12.6% (Stage III), and 39.6% overall. If M factor was positive, 5 year survival rates of primary malignant bone tumors decreased to less than 10%, except for chordoma.

The bone tumor registration system was proposed by T. Amako (Kyushu University) and was initiated in western Japan in 1954. The Japanese Orthopaedic Association (JOA) decided to expand this registration system throughout the country. Nationwide registration of bone tumors in the country started in 1964, and a registry was established at the National Cancer Center (Tokyo). Maeyama and Toriyama contributed to the establishment of this registration system (8). Bone tumor registration was started to promote the study of these tumors and to record the incidence of bone tumors in Japan. Annual reports have been published since 1964, and the report for 1991 was published in April, 1993 (6). During the early years of the bone tumor registry, classification was made by the Jaffe (5) method. The Musculoskeletal Tumor Committee of the JOA proposed a new classification of bone tumors in 1969, and this was adopted for the bone tumor registration system in 1972. Several other bone tumors were added to this classification in 1982 (7). Table I shows the bone tumor classification which is used today. The registration card used was simple at the outset of the bone tumor registry, and a new card for primary malignant tumors of bone was made and distributed to hospitals and institutes in 1980. Two types of registration cards, one for benign bone tumors, tumorous conditions of bone, and secondary bone tumors, and the other for primary malignant tumors of bone are now used for the bone tumor registration.

Registered Cases

About 50,000 cases of benign and malignant tumors of bone, tumorous conditions of bone, and secondary bone tumors were registered during the period from

---

* Manuscript was prepared by Hisatoshi Fukuma, Department of Orthopaedic Surgery, National Cancer Center Hospital, 5-1-1 Tsukiji, Chuo-ku, Tokyo 104, Japan

TABLE I. Classification of Bone Tumors

I. Primary bone tumors
  1. Osteogenic
    1) Cartilaginous
      Osteochondroma (osteocartilaginous exostosis)
        Solitary
        Multiple
      Chondroma (enchondroma)
        Solitary
        Multiple
      Periosteal chondroma (ecchondroma, parosteal chondroma, juxtacortical chondroma)
      Chondroblastoma (benign chondroblastoma)
      Chondromyxoid fibroma
      Chondrosarcoma[a]
      Mesenchymal chondrosarcoma[a]
      Dedifferentiated chondrosarcoma[a]
      Clear cell chondrosarcoma[b]
    2) Osseous
      Osteoma
      Osteoid osteoma
      Osteoblastoma (benign osteoblastoma)
      Osteosarcoma[a]
      Parosteal osteosarcoma[a]
      Periosteal osteosarcoma[a]
      Telangiectatic osteosarcoma[b]
      Intraosseous well differentiated osteosarcoma[b]
    3) Fibrous
      Non-ossifying fibroma
      Desmoplastic fibroma
      Fibrosarcoma[a]
      Malignant fibrous histiocytoma[a]
  2. Vascular
    Hemangioma
    Lymphangioma
    Glomus tumor
    Hemangiopericytoma
    Hemangioendothelioma
    Angiosarcoma[a]
  3. Hematopoietic
    Myeloma[a]
      Solitary
      Multiple
    Malignant lymphoma[a]
      Non-Hodgkin's lymphoma
      Hodgkin's lymphoma
  4. Notochordal
    Chordoma[a]
  5. Lipogenic
    Lipoma
    Liposarcoma[a]
  6. Neurogenic
    Neurilemmoma (schwannoma, neurinoma)
    Neurofibroma
    Neurogenic sarcoma[a]
      Malignant schwannoma[a]
      Neurofibrosarcoma[a]
  7. Unknown or undetermined
    Giant cell tumor

        Malignant giant cell tumor[a]
        Ewing's sarcoma[a]
        Malignant mesenchymoma[a]
        Adamantinoma of long bones[a]
    8. Others
II. Secondary bone tumors
    1. Metastatic
        Carcinoma
        Sarcoma
    2. Invasive tumors of bone
        Benign
        Malignant
III. Tumorous conditions of bone
    1. Solitary bone cyst
    2. Aneurysmal bone cyst
    3. Fibrous dysplasia
        Monostotic
        Polyostotic
    4. Histiocytosis X
    5. Intra-articular bone cyst (intra-osseous ganglion)
    6. Metaphyseal fibrous cortical defect

[a] Malignant.
[b] Malignant, should be added to the classification.

1964 to 1991 with an average of 1,850 cases per year. As stated, new cards for primary malignant bone tumors have been used since 1980, and 3,623 cases of primary malignant tumors of bone were registered between 1980 and 1991 with an average of 302 cases per year. Table II shows the number of primary malignant tumors of bone by year and type of tumor. The most frequent tumor of the primary malignant tumors of bone was osteosarcoma. One thousand five hundred and ninety seven cases (44.1%) were listed in 12 years with an average of 133 cases per year. Chondrosarcoma was next in frequency of occurrence, followed by multiple myeloma, malignant fibrous histiocytoma (MFH), and Ewing's sarcoma. It is believed that the incidence of multiple myeloma is probably higher than that shown by the registered cases because this would have been treated by a physician as a blood disease in most patients.

Sex and Age Distribution

In osteosarcomas, the male-female ratio is 3:2. Osteosarcoma is most frequent in the second decade of life with 990 (62%) of the 1,957 incidences registered in this period. This age distribution essentially does not vary in any part of the world.

Ewing's sarcomas are frequent in the first and second decades, and the age distribution is similar to that of osteosarcoma.

Chondrosarcomas are frequent in the fourth, fifth, and sixth decades, and the age distribution of malignant fibrous histiocytoma (MFH) is similar to that of chondrosarcoma. Tables III-VI show the number of osteosarcomas, chondrosarcomas, MFH, and Ewing's sarcomas registered between 1980 and 1991 arranged according to sex, age, and year. Table VII shows the number of primary malignant tumors of bone registered during the period from 1980 to 1991 by sex, age, and year.

TABLE II. Number of Primary Malignant Tumor of Bone Cases Registered during 1980–1991 by Diagnosis and Year

Year	OS	Paro os	Peri os	Chon sar	Mese chon	Dedi chon	Clear chon	Fib sar	MFH	Mali gct	Ewing sar	Malig lym	Angi sar	Lipo sar	Malig schw	Chor doma	Myel oma	Adam-ant	Malig mesen	Total
1980	111	6	1	42	2	1	0	5	25	1	20	3	1	0	0	2	68	0	0	288
1981	118	3	0	33	0	0	0	5	19	2	18	12	4	2	0	10	37	0	0	263
1982	129	7	0	35	2	1	0	4	16	5	17	7	4	0	0	10	34	1	0	272
1983	147	6	0	40	1	0	0	2	30	1	24	10	2	1	0	13	52	0	0	329
1984	126	3	1	50	2	3	1	1	37	3	16	9	1	1	1	13	52	0	1	321
1985	138	4	0	57	1	0	1	3	25	6	22	6	2	0	0	16	36	1	0	318
1986	144	5	2	42	2	4	0	3	23	1	25	10	3	0	0	10	24	0	0	298
1987	126	2	0	58	0	1	1	2	25	1	22	11	1	0	2	13	33	0	0	298
1988	133	5	2	67	1	3	1	2	21	3	24	10	2	2	0	11	34	3	0	324
1989	148	4	3	50	0	5	1	4	19	0	16	12	1	0	1	14	41	4	0	323
1990	141	1	1	52	1	0	2	2	21	3	19	12	1	1	0	8	35	0	0	300
1991	136	2	2	56	1	1	1	0	17	1	19	11	1	0	0	16	25	0	0	289
Total	1,597	48	12	582	13	19	8	33	278	27	242	113	23	7	4	136	471	9	1	3,623
%	(44.1)	(1.3)	(0.3)	(16.1)	(0.4)	(0.5)	(0.2)	(0.9)	(7.7)	(0.7)	(6.7)	(3.1)	(0.6)	(0.2)	(0.1)	(3.8)	(13.0)	(0.2)		(100%)

OS: osteosarcoma; Paro os: parosteal osteosarcoma; Peri os: periosteal osteosarcoma; Chon sar: chondrosarcoma; Mese chon: mesenchymal chondrosarcoma; Dedi chon: dedifferentiated chondrosarcoma; Clear chon: clear cell chondrosarcoma; Fib sar: fibrosarcoma; MFH: malignant fibrous histiocytoma; Malig gct: malignant giant cell tumor; Ewing sar: Ewing's sarcoma; Malig lym: malignant lymphoma of bone; Angi sar: angiosarcoma; Lipo sar: liposarcoma; Malig schw: malignant schwannoma; Adamant: adamantinoma of long bones; Malig mesen: malignant mesenchymoma.

TABLE III. Number of Osteosarcoma Cases Registered during 1980–1991 by Sex, Age, and Year

	Year	Total	Age 0–4	5–9	10–14	15–19	20–24	25–29	30–34	35–39	40–44	45–49	50–54	55–59	60–64	65–69	70–
Male	1980	60	0	7	20	19	5	1	1	3	0	2	0	0	0	0	2
	1981	74	0	11	19	24	11	4	0	0	1	2	2	0	0	0	0
	1982	81	0	2	29	23	9	6	0	5	0	2	2	3	0	0	0
	1983	87	2	5	18	41	7	6	2	0	2	1	2	1	0	0	0
	1984	76	0	4	27	26	6	3	2	3	2	1	0	1	1	0	0
	1985	79	1	4	26	24	10	4	1	1	2	1	1	1	0	3	0
	1986	89	2	4	19	38	8	3	5	0	2	3	2	0	0	2	1
	1987	85	0	3	32	26	10	3	2	2	1	0	1	0	1	1	2
	1988	77	1	6	11	35	10	2	3	1	0	3	2	0	2	0	1
	1989	98	0	12	22	41	8	1	2	2	5	0	0	3	1	1	0
	1990	93	0	5	24	40	9	2	1	2	5	0	3	1	0	1	0
	1991	94	1	5	18	32	9	1	4	5	3	4	6	2	1	0	3
Subtotal		993	7	68	265	369	102	36	23	24	23	19	21	13	6	8	9
Female	1980	51	0	6	17	8	3	7	1	1	1	0	1	0	1	2	3
	1981	44	0	4	16	9	1	2	2	2	1	2	0	2	0	1	2
	1982	48	1	9	17	10	2	1	1	1	2	0	1	1	2	0	0
	1983	60	1	7	20	15	1	2	2	0	2	3	2	2	2	1	0
	1984	50	0	6	19	11	3	1	0	2	2	0	1	1	1	1	2
	1985	59	1	6	22	10	6	1	1	1	1	2	2	1	1	2	2
	1986	55	0	2	26	13	3	1	1	1	0	0	0	1	2	2	2
	1987	41	0	4	15	9	5	0	0	2	0	1	2	1	1	1	0
	1988	56	0	5	22	19	2	1	1	0	3	1	2	0	0	0	0
	1989	50	1	6	15	12	3	1	0	3	2	0	1	2	0	2	2
	1990	48	0	5	14	11	5	5	0	1	0	3	1	2	0	0	1
	1991	42	0	5	17	9	2	2	0	1	0	0	1	1	1	0	3
Subtotal		604	4	65	220	136	36	24	9	15	14	13	14	14	11	12	17
Total		1,597	11	133	485	505	138	60	32	39	37	32	35	27	17	20	26

TABLE IV. Number of Chondrosarcoma Cases Registered during 1980–1991 by Sex, Age, and Year

	Year	Total	Age 0–4	5–9	10–14	15–19	20–24	25–29	30–34	35–39	40–44	45–49	50–54	55–59	60–64	65–69	70–
Male	1980	17	0	0	1	3	0	1	2	2	3	0	2	1	0	1	1
	1981	17	0	0	0	2	2	3	1	3	2	1	2	0	0	0	1
	1982	16	0	0	0	2	1	2	2	1	5	0	0	1	2	0	0
	1983	22	0	0	0	2	0	2	0	3	2	3	4	3	0	2	1
	1984	35	0	0	0	3	2	5	3	0	2	3	7	4	1	2	3
	1985	34	0	0	0	3	4	0	2	2	4	5	1	7	3	0	3
	1986	20	1	0	0	0	1	1	2	4	3	2	1	1	1	2	2
	1987	31	0	1	1	1	0	4	1	1	5	2	2	4	5	1	4
	1988	41	0	0	1	1	0	3	5	7	3	4	2	5	3	4	2
	1989	25	0	0	2	1	1	2	2	0	4	6	3	2	2	0	1
	1990	31	0	0	2	1	2	2	1	3	3	3	3	6	1	2	2
	1991	32	0	0	0	1	1	2	3	1	5	6	4	2	2	3	2
Subtotal		321	1	1	5	20	14	27	24	27	41	35	31	36	20	17	22
Female	1980	25	0	2	0	1	0	5	3	1	1	2	1	4	3	1	1
	1981	16	0	0	0	1	2	1	0	0	2	3	0	2	0	4	1
	1982	19	1	1	0	0	1	0	2	1	3	3	1	2	1	2	1
	1983	18	0	0	0	0	0	0	4	2	2	2	2	2	4	1	1
	1984	15	0	0	0	0	0	2	0	0	0	1	2	1	6	2	1
	1985	23	0	0	0	2	0	1	2	1	3	2	3	0	3	4	2
	1986	22	0	0	2	2	1	0	2	2	2	4	1	4	2	0	2
	1987	27	0	0	0	0	2	1	2	0	1	2	4	3	6	1	3
	1988	26	0	0	0	4	3	1	2	2	1	3	2	1	3	1	3
	1989	25	0	0	0	1	2	2	2	6	0	2	1	0	5	0	4
	1990	21	0	0	0	0	1	1	1	2	2	1	5	2	2	2	2
	1991	24	0	0	0	2	1	1	1	3	2	1	2	4	1	0	6
Subtotal		261	1	3	2	13	13	15	21	20	17	26	24	25	36	18	27
Total		582	2	4	7	33	27	42	45	47	58	61	55	61	56	35	49

TABLE V. Number of Malignant Fibrous Histiocytoma Cases Registered during 1980–1991 by Sex, Age, and Year

	Year	Total	Age 0–4	5–9	10–14	15–19	20–24	25–29	30–34	35–39	40–44	45–49	50–54	55–59	60–64	65–69	70–
Male	1980	15	0	1	1	0	0	1	1	3	0	1	2	0	1	1	3
	1981	13	0	0	1	1	1	2	2	0	1	1	1	0	2	1	0
	1982	8	0	0	1	1	0	0	0	2	0	0	0	2	2	0	0
	1983	14	0	0	1	0	3	1	1	0	2	0	3	1	2	0	0
	1984	22	0	0	0	4	1	1	1	1	2	1	3	4	3	0	0
	1985	16	0	1	1	1	3	0	0	1	2	2	1	2	2	1	0
	1986	16	0	0	1	0	1	1	2	1	3	0	3	1	0	1	1
	1987	14	0	0	0	1	0	1	0	1	0	2	1	2	0	4	1
	1988	15	0	1	0	0	0	1	2	3	3	2	2	0	0	0	4
	1989	10	0	0	0	0	2	0	1	1	0	0	1	1	2	0	0
	1990	8	0	0	0	0	1	1	0	0	1	1	0	2	0	1	3
	1991	12	0	0	0	0	0	1	0	0	2	3	2	0	1	1	2
Subtotal		163	0	3	6	8	12	10	10	13	16	13	19	13	15	10	15
Female	1980	10	0	0	0	1	0	0	0	1	0	0	1	2	0	4	1
	1981	6	0	0	0	0	0	0	0	0	1	1	2	0	0	1	1
	1982	8	0	0	0	1	0	0	0	1	0	1	2	1	1	1	0
	1983	16	0	1	0	1	1	1	3	0	4	1	0	2	0	2	0
	1984	15	0	0	0	1	1	1	2	1	1	0	3	1	1	1	2
	1985	9	0	0	0	0	0	0	1	1	2	0	0	1	1	1	1
	1986	7	0	0	0	0	1	1	2	1	0	0	1	1	1	1	0
	1987	11	0	0	0	3	0	0	1	0	0	2	1	2	0	2	0
	1988	6	0	0	0	0	0	0	0	2	0	0	1	0	1	1	1
	1989	9	0	0	0	0	0	2	0	2	0	3	3	0	0	0	1
	1990	13	0	0	1	0	0	0	0	2	0	1	2	2	1	1	3
	1991	5	0	0	0	1	2	0	1	0	0	0	0	1	0	0	0
Subtotal		115	0	1	1	8	5	5	10	9	8	9	16	13	5	15	10
Total		278	0	4	7	16	17	15	20	22	24	22	35	26	20	25	25

TABLE VI. Number of Ewing's Sarcoma Cases Registered during 1980–1991 by Sex, Age, and Year

	Year	Total	Age 0–4	5–9	10–14	15–19	20–24	25–29	30–34	35–39	40–44	45–49	50–54	55–59	60–64	65–69	70–
Male	1980	12	1	2	3	3	2	0	0	0	0	1	0	0	0	0	0
	1981	14	1	2	3	5	2	1	0	0	0	0	0	0	0	0	0
	1982	7	0	0	1	3	2	0	0	0	0	0	0	0	1	0	0
	1983	13	2	2	2	4	2	1	0	0	0	0	0	0	0	0	0
	1984	12	0	1	6	5	0	0	0	0	0	0	0	0	0	0	0
	1985	14	0	0	3	8	0	0	1	1	0	1	0	0	0	0	0
	1986	15	3	3	6	2	0	0	1	0	0	0	0	0	0	0	0
	1987	11	2	1	2	4	1	0	1	1	0	0	0	0	0	0	0
	1988	16	1	1	7	2	3	1	0	0	0	0	0	0	0	0	0
	1989	8	0	0	3	3	2	0	0	0	0	0	0	1	0	0	0
	1990	8	0	0	0	7	1	0	0	0	0	0	0	0	0	0	0
	1991	14	0	0	5	2	2	2	1	1	0	0	0	0	0	0	0
Subtotal		144	10	12	41	48	17	5	4	3	0	2	0	1	1	0	0
Female	1980	8	0	4	3	0	1	0	0	0	0	0	0	0	0	0	0
	1981	4	0	1	2	1	0	0	0	0	0	0	0	0	0	0	0
	1982	10	0	4	2	2	1	1	0	0	0	0	0	0	0	0	0
	1983	11	1	4	3	2	1	0	0	0	0	0	0	0	0	0	0
	1984	4	0	0	3	1	0	0	0	0	0	0	0	0	0	0	0
	1985	8	0	2	3	3	0	0	0	0	0	0	0	0	0	0	0
	1986	10	0	0	5	4	1	0	0	0	0	0	0	0	0	0	0
	1987	11	0	2	4	3	2	0	0	0	0	0	0	0	0	0	0
	1988	8	0	0	3	3	0	2	0	0	0	0	0	0	0	0	0
	1989	8	1	2	1	2	1	0	0	0	0	0	1	0	0	0	0
	1990	11	1	0	3	5	1	0	1	0	1	0	0	0	0	0	0
	1991	5	1	0	0	2	0	1	0	0	0	0	0	0	0	0	0
Subtotal		98	4	19	32	28	8	4	1	0	1	0	1	0	0	0	0
Total		242	14	31	73	76	25	9	5	3	1	2	1	1	1	0	0

TABLE VII. Number of Primary Malignant Tumor of Bone Cases Registered during 1980–1991 by Sex, Age, and Year

	Year	Total	Age 0–4	5–9	10–14	15–19	20–24	25–29	30–34	35–39	40–44	45–49	50–54	55–59	60–64	65–69	70–
Male	1980	157	1	10	26	27	9	4	7	10	3	13	9	10	5	9	14
	1981	170	1	13	24	34	16	13	8	4	10	9	9	4	9	9	7
	1982	146	0	2	31	31	15	9	4	10	6	6	9	7	10	2	4
	1983	184	4	7	23	47	15	10	6	5	8	7	17	14	7	6	8
	1984	196	0	6	33	40	10	9	8	8	11	9	12	16	12	12	10
	1985	184	1	4	32	38	17	6	6	6	12	11	8	14	7	11	11
	1986	171	5	8	26	42	11	7	11	6	10	6	10	7	5	9	8
	1987	178	3	4	34	34	12	9	4	6	7	9	9	9	16	8	14
	1988	200	3	8	21	40	15	7	13	17	10	12	12	12	13	7	10
	1989	189	0	13	28	49	15	4	10	4	11	13	7	13	7	7	8
	1990	182	0	7	27	50	15	5	2	7	11	6	12	12	8	10	10
	1991	188	1	5	23	37	15	6	9	10	15	15	13	8	9	8	14
Subtotal		2,145	19	87	328	469	165	89	88	93	114	116	127	126	108	98	118
Female	1980	131	0	12	20	10	5	13	4	4	5	5	8	15	8	8	14
	1981	93	0	5	19	11	4	4	3	3	4	8	5	4	2	11	10
	1982	126	2	14	20	13	5	5	5	4	7	11	8	9	7	9	7
	1983	145	3	12	23	18	5	4	11	2	7	10	8	10	12	11	9
	1984	125	0	6	23	15	4	7	3	4	3	2	10	8	14	12	14
	1985	134	1	8	26	16	8	5	6	4	8	5	8	7	8	15	9
	1986	127	0	2	31	19	8	4	8	5	3	7	8	9	10	5	8
	1987	120	0	6	22	15	11	4	3	2	2	6	13	12	10	8	6
	1988	124	0	5	26	27	5	5	3	4	5	10	9	3	5	6	11
	1989	134	3	8	16	16	6	8	3	12	3	10	10	8	11	10	10
	1990	118	1	5	19	16	7	6	3	6	2	6	12	12	7	7	9
	1991	101	1	5	17	15	5	6	2	4	5	2	4	10	5	4	16
Subtotal		1,478	11	88	262	191	73	71	54	54	54	82	103	107	99	106	123
Total		3,623	30	175	590	660	238	160	142	147	168	198	230	233	207	204	241

TABLE VIII. Primary Sites of Primary Malignant Tumors of Bone Registered during 1980–1991

Diagnosis	No. of cases	Skull	Cspine	Tspine	Lspine	Sacrum	Coccyx	Sternum	Rib	Scapula	Clavicle	Humerus	Radius	Ulna	Carpal	Metaca	Phalan	Pelvis	Femur	Tibia	Fibula	Patell	Tarsal	Metata	Phalan	Multip
Osteosarcoma	1,597	6	3	4	7	7		2	11	8	3	138	7	3		2		76	858	362	75	4	2	3		16
Parosteal osteo	48											7		1				3	25	6	3		3	1		
Periosteal osteo	12											1						1	7	2	1					
Chondrosarcoma	582		7	7	6	18		12	42	41		56	5	5		8	11	148	134	44	11		9	2	6	10
Mesenchy chondroma	13				1	4			1	3								4	1	2						
Dediff chondroma	19		1						1	1		2						4	5	1	1		1			
Clear cell chondroma	8								1									1	3	1			1			
Fibrosarcoma	33				1	1			2		2	1				1		6	13	3						2
MFH	278	1		3	3	1		4	5	4	1	15	2	2	1	1	1	28	134	49	9		1	1		13
Malignant gct	27		1			1						1						6	14	3	1					
Ewing's sarcoma	242	2	3	2	5	8			16	16	10	22	2	2		1	1	61	40	24	13		3			11
Malig. lymphoma	113		1	4	6	6		2	3	2	4	10					1	17	16	15	1			1	1	25
Angiosarcoma	23				2	3			1	1		2	1	1				4	7	1						
Liposarcoma	7											1						1	5							
Malig schwannoma	4			1	1						1							1								
Chordoma	136		2		2	130	1											1								
Myeloma	471	1	13	18	14	4		2	4	4	9	16	1					16	15	1						353
Adamantinoma	9											1	1							6	1					
Malig mesenchynoma	1								1																	
Total	3,623	10	31	39	48	183	1	22	88	80	30	273	19	12	1	13	14	377	1,277	520	116	4	20	8	7	430

Cspine: cervical spine. Tspipe: thoracic spine. Lspine: lumber spine.

TABLE IX. Patient Characteristics Used for Multivariate Analysis

		No. of cases	%
Sex	Male	500	61
	Female	314	39
Age	0–9	76	9.3
	10–19	516	63.4
	20–	222	27.3
Site	Femur	458	56.3
	Tibia	180	22.1
	Humerus	73	9.0
	Fibula	37	4.5
	Others	66	8.1
Diameter	0–5 cm>	40	4.9
	5–10 cm>	319	39.2
	10–15 cm>	279	34.3
	15cm<	148	19.4
	Unknown	18	2.2
T classification	T1	51	6.3
	T2	755	92.7
	Unknown	8	1.0
Serum alkaline phosphatase	N-1.25×>	232	28.5
	2.5×>	245	30.1
	5.0×>	222	27.3
	10×>	75	9.2
	10×<	40	4.9
Mitosis rate per high power field (× 200)	0	26	3.2
	1–4	248	30.5
	5–9	221	27.1
	10≤	132	16.2
	Unknown	187	23.0
N	N0	800	98.3
	N1	11	1.4
	Unknown	3	0.4
Distant metastasis	M0	695	85.4
	M1	119	14.6
TNM stage	I	291	35.8
	II	339	41.6
	III	165	20.3
	Unknown	19	2.3

Location

The femur is the most frequent site of occurrence of primary malignant tumors of bone, and this was true in 35.3% of 3,623 cases. Each type of malignant tumor of bone has a characteristic primary site of occurrence. The most frequent site for osteosarcoma is the distal femur, followed by the proximal tibia and the proximal humerus. Chondrosarcomas occur most often in the pelvis and the femur. The most common site for MFH is the femur with an incidence rate of 48.2%, and Ewing's sarcomas occur frequently in the pelvis and the femur. Chordomas mostly occur in the sacrum. Table VIII shows the primary sites of occurrence of primary malignant tumors of bone.

TNM Classification

The International Union Against Cancer (UICC) proposed the TNM classification of malignant tumors of bone in 1987 (15). Primary tumors were classified into two categories: T1: tumor confined within the cortex, and T2: tumor invades beyond the cortex. Most of the osteosarcomas were included in the T2 category, and 92.7% of 814 cases of osteosarcoma in our data were in this category. Eight hundred and fourteen cases of osteosarcoma registered between 1980 and 1989 were analyzed for prognostic factors of osteosarcoma; patient details of these cases are shown in Table IX. The nine variables used were sex, age, primary site, maximal diameter, T classification (UICC), alkaline phosphatase level, mitotic rate in high power field ($\times$ 200), regional lymph node metastasis, and distant metastasis. Results of multivariate analysis showed that the most important prognostic factors for osteosarcoma were distant metastasis, serum level of alkaline phosphatase, regional lymph node metastasis, mitotic rate, and tumor size. The prognostic significance of each variable can be estimated by its ratio of risks as determined by multivariate analysis. Table X shows the ratio of risks of each variable. Distant metastasis at diagnosis posed the worst threat to patients with osteosarcoma. Alkaline phosphatase level ranked 2nd in the ratio of risks. Reverse-correlation was found between the survival rate and the serum level of alkaline phosphatase. Regional lymph node metastasis was prognostically significant.

TABLE X. Prognostic Factors in Osteosarcoma

Patient characteristics (prognostic factors)	Relative risk				Ratio of risk
	Favorable		Unfavorable		
Sex	Female	0.95815043	Male	1.02743008	1.07230560
Age	0–9	0.70545342	20–	1.27483991	1.80712131
Location	Others	0.91277125	Femur	1.02559514	1.12360587
Tumor size	5 cm>	0.63845422	15cm<	1.40808002	2.20545181
Tumor extent (T)	T1	0.88960859	T2	1.00816072	1.13326325
SAP	×1.25>	0.68288538	×10≤	2.15618840	3.15746749
Regional node (N)	N0	0.98482673	N1	2.94877234	2.99420421
Distant metastasis	M0	0.72132875	M1	6.46135605	8.95757452
Mitotic rate	0	0.53617179	10≤	1.59335443	2.97172375

TABLE XI. TNM Classification of Osteosarcoma (JJC)

T: primary tumor	T1: maximal diameter < 15cm
	T2: maximal diameter ≥ 15cm
A: alkaline phosphatase	A0: normal value × 2.5 >
	A1: normal value × 2.5 ≤
N: regional lymph node	N0: no regional lymph node metastasis
	N1: regional lymph node metastasis
M: distant metastasis	M0: no distant metastasis
	M1: distant metastasis
G: mitotic rate in HPF (× 200)	G1: 0–9 / 1 HPF
	G2: 10 ≤ / 1 HPF

TABLE XII. Nunber of Osteosarcoma Cases Registered during 1980–1991 by TNM(JJC) Classification and Year

	TNM	n	Total	1980	81	82	83	84	85	86	87	88	89	90	91
Stage I	T1A0N0M0G1		355 (35.6%)	28	30	35	21	20	29	26	26	35	45	29	31
Stage II	T1A0N0M0G2	74		11	12	9	6	4	2	4	1	2	7	8	8
	T1A1N0M0G1-2	275	434 (43.5%)	14	21	21	22	28	29	24	32	18	20	24	22
	T2A0N0M0G1-2	85		4	8	7	13	8	9	6	6	6	7	11	0
Stage III	T2A1N0M0G1-2	60		5	2	3	3	6	12	7	2	1	6	6	7
	T1-2A0-1N1M0G1-2	5	208 (20.9%)	0	0	0	1	0	0	1	1	2	0	0	0
	T1-2A0-1N0-1M1G1-2	143		6	7	14	18	8	13	19	8	18	8	14	10
	Total		997	68	80	89	84	74	94	87	76	82	93	92	78

TABLE XIII. Treatment for Patients with Extremity Osteosarcoma by Stage (JJC)

Stage	No. of cases	LS	LS+C	LS+C+R	Amp	A+C	A+C+R	Rot+C	No surg
I	325	11	149	16	1	128	10	1	9
	(100%)	(3.4%)	(45.8%)	(4.9%)		(39.4%)	(3.1%)		(2.8%)
II	418	0	144	17	1	229	8	1	18
	(100%)		(34.4%)	(4.1%)		(54.8%)	(1.9%)		(4.3%)
III	175	1	43	7	4	77	2	0	41
	(100%)		(24.6%)	(4.0%)	(2.3%)	(44.0%)			(23.4%)
Total	918	12	336	40	6	434	20	2	68
	(100%)	(1.3%)	(36.6%)	(44.4%)	(0.7%)	(47.3%)	(2.2%)	(0.2%)	(7.4%)

LS: limb salvage operation; C: adjuvant chemotherapy; R: radiation; Amp, A: amputation; Rot: rotation plasty; No surg: no surgical treatment.

Multivariate analysis indicated that regional lymph node metastasis was also an important prognostic factor, ranking 3rd in the ratio of risks. However, N1 cases of osteosarcoma were very rare, and only 1.4% of all cases were classified in the N1 category. Mitotic rate ranked 4th in the ratio of risks, and the survival rate for patients with grade 4 (10≤ in high power field) was the poorest of all groups. Multivariate analysis of prognostic factors of osteosarcoma shows that there is no significant difference in survival rate between the T1 and T2 (UICC) groups. However, the tumor size was an important prognostic factor, and the survival rate for patients with a tumor 15 cm or larger was poorer than those with a tumor less than 15 cm. The TNM classification and staging system of osteosarcoma based on this study as shown in Table XI were proposed by the Japanese Joint Committee (JJC) of JOA (4).

Table XII shows the number of osteosarcoma cases registered during the period from 1980 to 1991 by TNM classification (JJC) and year. Three hundred and fifty five (35.6%) were classified in Stage I, 434 (43.5%) in Stage II, and 208 (20.9%) in Stage III.

Treatment of Osteosarcoma

Since the late 1970s intensive chemotherapy has been used as adjuvant chemotherapy for patients with osteosarcoma. Amputations for osteosarcomas of the extremities have been reduced, and limb salvage operations have been widely performed. Table XIII shows the treatment methods in each stage of osteosarcoma of

TABLE XIV. Treatment of Osteosarcoma by Stage, Surgery, and Year

Year	Stage I				Stage II				Stage III			
	LS (%)	Amp (%)	Others	Subtotal	LS (%)	Amp (%)	Others	Subtotal	LS (%)	Amp (%)	Others	Subtotal
1980	8 (30.8)	18 (69.2)	0	26	3 (10.3)	25 (86.2)	1	29	1 (10.0)	5 (50.0)	4	10
1981	6 (20.7)	18 (62.1)	5	29	7 (18.0)	29 (74.4)	3	39	0	6 (75.0)	2	8
1982	9 (29.0)	22 (71.0)	0	31	5 (14.3)	29 (82.9)	1	35	1 (7.1)	9 (64.3)	4	14
1983	9 (47.4)	10 (52.6)	0	19	15 (37.5)	25 (62.5)	0	40	6 (33.3)	9 (50.0)	3	18
1984	10 (52.6)	9 (47.4)	0	19	18 (45.0)	19 (47.5)	3	40	2 (18.2)	6 (54.6)	3	11
1985	16 (64.0)	9 (36.0)	0	25	12 (33.3)	22 (61.1)	2	36	8 (33.3)	12 (50.0)	4	24
1986	16 (69.6)	6 (26.1)	1	23	17 (50.0)	16 (47.1)	1	34	9 (40.9)	11 (50.0)	2	22
1987	17 (68.0)	7 (28.0)	1	25	19 (51.4)	16 (43.2)	2	37	1 (12.5)	7 (87.5)	0	8
1988	19 (57.6)	12 (36.4)	2	33	16 (61.5)	8 (30.8)	2	26	8 (40.0)	7 (35.0)	5	20
1989	29 (69.1)	13 (30.9)	0	42	16 (48.5)	15 (45.5)	2	33	4 (36.4)	5 (45.5)	2	11
1990	19 (73.1)	6 (23.1)	1	26	25 (61.0)	14 (34.2)	2	41	6 (37.5)	3 (18.8)	7	16
1991	18 (66.7)	9 (33.3)	0	27	8 (28.6)	20 (71.4)	0	28	5 (38.5)	3 (23.1)	5	13
Total	176 (54.1)	139 (42.8)	10	325	161 (38.5)	238 (56.9)	19	418	51 (29.2)	83 (47.4)	41	175

LS: limb salvage operation; Amp: amputation.

TABLE XV. Survival Rates of Patients with Osteosarcoma by Stage (JJC)

Stage	No. of cases	1	2	3	4	5	6	7	8	9	10 years
Stage I	355	93.4	78.1	69.3	63.5	59.8	58.2	56.3	54.1	52.4	51.4%
Stage II	434	83.4	64.1	54.2	50.6	47.8	45.7	44.2	43.1	43.1	43.1%
Stage III	208	52.7	23.2	13.9	12.6	12.6	12.6	12.6	12.6	12.6	12.6%
Total	997	80.5	60.5	51.1	47.2	44.7	43.2	41.9	40.6	40.0	39.6%

TABLE XVI. Cumulative Survival Rates of Patients with Primary Malignant Tumors of Bone Registered during 1972–1991

| Diagnosis | TNM | Survival rates (%) | | | | | Cases |
		1	2	3	4	5 years	
Chondrosarcoma	Total	89.5	80.4	73.0	68.5	65.6	753
	M0	93.8	85.8	77.6	74.0	71.1	681
	M1	48.6	30.0	30.0	16.0	12.0	72
Osteosarcoma	Total	79.3	58.0	49.1	44.1	40.9	2,181
	M0	86.0	65.8	56.5	50.9	47.3	1,824
	M1	45.4	18.8	12.0	9.9	9.1	357
Fibrosarcoma	Total	83.2	68.4	59.9	52.0	49.7	95
	M0	88.8	76.3	68.6	60.6	57.8	80
	M1	53.3	26.7	13.3	6.7	6.7	15
MFH	Total	79.0	65.4	59.6	53.3	50.4	277
	M0	82.3	70.0	65.0	58.4	55.1	244
	M1	53.9	29.5	16.9	12.7	12.7	33
Chordoma	Total	92.4	87.6	84.3	76.7	66.7	171
	M0	93.3	88.3	84.9	77.0	66.7	165
	M1	66.7	66.7	66.7	66.7	66.7	6
Ewing's sarcoma	Total	72.4	45.6	35.5	30.5	27.4	308
	M0	80.1	54.4	43.3	36.9	33.0	242
	M1	43.9	13.6	7.2	7.2	7.2	66

the extremities registered between 1980 and 1991. Three hundred and eighty eight (42.3%) of 918 patients were treated by limb salvage surgery, and 460 (50.1%) were treated by amputation. Table XIV shows the surgical procedures for osteosarcoma. Since 1984 the number of limb salvage operations was higher than that of amputations in the Stage I group, with about 60 to 70% of patients with osteosarcomas of the extremities being treated by this means.

Treatment Results

Table XV shows the survival rates of patients with osteosarcoma according to JJC staging. These cases were registered during the period from 1980 to 1991 and were available for the analysis of the prognostic factors of osteosarcoma. In the Stage I group, 59.8% had a 5-year survival rate, while 47.8% in the Stage II group, and 12.6% in the Stage III group showed the same survival rate. The 10-year survival rate was seen in 51.4%, 43.1%, and 12.6% of Stage I, II, and III, respectively. The 5-year cumulative survival rates of patients with primary malignant tumors of bone registered between 1972 and 1991 by distant metastasis are shown in Table XVI. These rates in the M0 group were 71.1% for chondrosarcoma, 47.3% for osteosarcoma,

TABLE XVII. Estimated Number of Malignant Bone Tumor by Age and Sex in Japan

Site	Year	Total n	Age 0–4	5–9	10–14	15–19	20–24	25–29	30–34	35–39	40–44	45–49	50–54	55–59	60–64	65–69	70–
Male																	
	1984	351	0	5	41	40	28	8	10	5	14	8	31	16	18	19	108
	1985	447	0	13	36	50	25	12	5	16	27	16	31	20	21	28	145
	1986	436	7	21	45	44	33	16	9	11	9	8	32	38	39	20	105
Female																	
	1984	284	4	21	34	43	12	0	9	5	19	4	4	11	21	21	78
	1985	339	0	4	54	52	8	4	13	5	23	4	28	29	12	19	84
	1986	278	7	8	34	23	8	4	13	11	17	0	24	29	16	20	66

57.8% for fibrosarcoma, 55.1% for malignant fibrous histiocytoma, 66.7% for chordoma, and 33.0% for Ewing's sarcoma. The survival rate of Ewing's sarcoma was thus the poorest of all tumors.

Discussion

There are several reports on the incidence of primary malignant tumors of bone. Fraumeni and Boice (3) reported that the annual age adjusted incidence rate (per 100,000 population) was 0.9 for white males, 0.7 for white females, 1.0 for black males, and 0.5 for black females in the United States. Nilsonne (10) reported that in Sweden 242 cases of osteosarcoma were registered (28.8% of all bone tumors) in 10 years (1958–1968) and the incidence of osteosarcoma was calculated at 2–3 cases per one million a year. Maeyama (8) indicated that the incidence of osteosarcoma is presumed to be one in 100,000–200,000 persons in Japan. The estimated number of primary malignant tumors of bone from 1984 to 1986 in Japan is shown in Table XVII(16). The incidence of such tumors is estimated at an average of 411 cases a year for males and 300 cases for females. Registered cases in these three years were 321, 318, and 298 cases, respectively, with an average of 312 cases a year. These correspond to 44% of the estimated incidence of primary malignant tumors of bone.

Osteosarcoma was the most frequent (44.1%) of the primary malignant tumors of bone registered within 12 years in Japan, followed by chondrosarcoma (16.1%), multiple myeloma (13.0%), MFH (7.7%), and Ewing's sarcoma (6.7%). Except for multiple myeloma, histological distribution of primary malignant tumors of bone is similar to the reports from other countries (2, 10, 12).

Age distribution of osteosarcoma is characteristic, and the peak of occurrence is in the second decade. A second peak during advanced age has not been found, because Paget's disease is very rare in Japan compared with its incidence in Europe (1) or in the United States (2).

The most common locations of osteosarcoma are the distal femur, the proximal tibia, and the proximal humerus. These findings are similar to the reports from other countries (1, 12).

There are many prognostic factors considered significant in relation to the survival of patients with osteosarcoma. The multivariate analysis of prognostic factors in osteosarcoma shows that the most important of these are distant metastasis, serum level of alkaline phosphatase, lymph node metastasis, mitotic rate, and tumor size.

However, our study shows that there is no significant difference of survival rate between the T1 (UICC) and the T2 groups. Furthermore, the histologic response to preoperative chemotherapy and serum level of lactate dehydrogenase should be studied to evaluate the prognostic significance.

Treatment of osteosarcoma has been advanced using intensive adjuvant chemotherapy with adriamycin and high dose methotrexate (HD-MTX) with citrovorum factor (CF) rescue. The 5-year survival rate of osteosarcoma was only 10–15% in the 1960s. In the 1970s adriamycin and HD-MTX with CF rescue were used for this treatment (*11*). Cisplatinum and ifosfamide were also added to the adjuvant chemotherapy. Almost all patients with osteosarcoma registered from 1980 to 1991 were treated by intensive adjuvant chemotherapy and surgery. Since the 1980s limb salvage operations for osteosarcoma of the extremities have been widely performed, and our results show that the number of these operations is more than that of amputations in Stage I osteosarcoma. The 5-year survival rate for osteosarcoma registered between 1972 and 1991 is 40.9% for all cases and 47.3% for the M0 group. The 5-year survival rates of osteosarcoma registered during the period 1980 to 1991 are 59.8% for Stage I, 47.8% for Stage II, 12.6% for Stage III, and 44.7% for all cases. In 1984 Maeyama (*8*) reported that the 5-year survival rate was 53.0% for patients with osteosarcoma treated by adriamycin alone, and 68.5% for those who received multiagent therapy. Meyers *et al.* (*9*) reported that the 5-year disease free survival rate was 70% for patients less than 21 years of age who had primary tumors of the extremity and were treated with T10 protocol. The 5-year survival rate for osteosarcoma is about 60–70% in the leading hospital in Japan (*13, 14, 17*). The data from the nationwide bone tumor registration in Japan show the incidence, age distribution, location, survival rate of primary malignant tumors of bone and the prognostic factors of osteosarcoma.

Acknowledgments

A part of this work was supported by the Ministry of Health and Welfare. The registration committee is grateful to the member doctors who contributed to this registry.

REFERENCES

1. Campanacci, M. Classic osteosarcoma. *In* "Bone and Soft Tissue Tumors," pp. 455–505 (1990). Springer-Verlag, Vienna.
2. Dahlin, D.C. and Unni, K.K. Osteosarcoma. *In* "Bone Tumors," 4th ed., pp. 269–307 (1986). Charles C Thomas, Springfield.
3. Fraumeni, J.F. Jr. and Boice, J.D. Jr. Bone. *In* "Cancer Epidemiology and Prevention," ed. D. Schottenfeld and J.F. Fraumeni, Jr., pp. 814–826 (1982). Saunders, Philadelphia.
4. Fukuma, H. Bone and soft tissue tumors. *In* "Staging of Cancer," Progress in Cancer Clinics, No. 34, ed. N. Hattori and Y. Koyama, pp. 76–84 (1990) (in Japanese). Medical View, Inc., Tokyo.
5. Jaffe, H.L. Classification of primary tumors of bone. *In* "Tumors and Tumorous Conditions of Bones and Joints," pp. 7–16 (1961). Lea and Febiger, Philadelphia.
6. Japanese Orthopaedic Association, Musculoskeletal Tumor Committee: Bone Tumor Registry in Japan–1991. National Cancer Center, Tokyo (1993) (in Japanese).

7. Japanese Orthopaedic Association, Musculoskeletal Tumor Committee: General Rules for Clinical and Pathological Studies on Malignant Bone Tumors, 2nd ed., pp. 1–4 (1990) (in Japanese). Kanehara Shuppan, Tokyo.
8. Maeyama, I. Bone tumors in Japan. *Clin. Orthop.,* **184**, 23–29 (1984).
9. Meyers, P.A., Heller, G., Healey, J. *et al.* Chemotherapy for nonmetastatic osteogenic sarcoma; The Memorial Sloan-Kettering experience. *J. Clin. Oncol.,* **10**, 5–15 (1992).
10. Nilsonne, U. Epidemiology and prognostic factors in osteosarcoma in Sweden. *Sem. Hop. Paris,* **58**, 1727–1728 (1982).
11. Rosen, G., Murphy, M.L., Huvos, A.G. *et al.* Chemotherapy, en bloc resection, and prosthetic bone replacement in the treatment of osteogenic sarcoma. *Cancer,* **37**, 1–11 (1976).
12. Schajowicz, F. Classification of bone tumor. *In* "Tumors and Tumor-like Lesions of Bone and Joints," pp. 17–23 (1981). Springer-Verlag, New York.
13. Tomita, K., Aotake, Y., Sugihara, M., and Tsuchiya, H. Overall results and functional evaluation of limb salvage for osteosarcoma. *In* "New Developments for Limb Salvage in Musculoskeletal Tumors," ed. T. Yamamuro, pp. 53–57 (1989). Springer-Verlag, Tokyo.
14. Tsuchiya, H. and Tomita, K. Members of the Ten-year Intergroup. Prognosis of osteosarcoma treated by limb-salvage surgery: The Ten-year Intergroup Study in Japan. *Jpn. J. Clin. Oncol.,* **22**, 347–353 (1992).
15. UICC International Union Against Cancer: TNM Classification of Malignant Tumours, 4th ed., pp. 75–79 (1987). Springer-Verlag, Berlin.
16. Watanabe, S. Cancer of Japanese (1995) (in Japanese). Kanehara-Shuppan, Tokyo.
17. Yamawaki, S., Isu, K., Ubayama, Y. *et al.* Adjuvant chemotherapy for osteosarcoma. *Jpn. J. Cancer Chemother.,* **17**, 180–188 (1990) (in Japanese).

STATISTICS OF MALIGNANT MELANOMA

The Japanese Skin Cancer Society*

The Prognosis and Statistical Investigation Committee of the Japanese Skin Cancer Society has periodically conducted a nationwide survey of skin malignancies. This report analyzed 1,717 cases of malignant melanoma among 9,439 malignant skin cancers registered in 1993 (1987–1991 cases) in comparison to those in 1987 (1975–1986 cases).

Acral lentigenous melanoma (42.2%) and nodular melanoma (29.0%) were still predominant, but melanoma in sunburned areas seemed to be increasing. Five-year survival rates of Stages I and II were more than 90%, while Stages II, III-1, III-2, IV, and (M1a and M1b) were 81.2, 51.0, 37.5, 15.4, respectively. Nodular melanoma and melanoma more than 3mm thick showed poorer prognosis.

The Prognosis and Statistical Investigation Committee, a part of the Japanese Skin Cancer Society, has for some years conducted a statistical investigation on the prognosis for malignant skin tumors. This investigation was previously conducted in 9 institutions, but in the most recent 5-year investigation made between 1987 and 1991, the scale of the survey was expanded to include institutions nationwide. Tumors investigated in this survey were: malignant melanoma, squamous cell carcinoma, basal cell carcinoma, mycosis fungoides, and carcinoma *in situ* (Bowen's disease, Paget's disease, and actinic keratosis). This is the first attempt to statistically investigate these tumors using registration forms (case cards). In this report, we only present findings relating to malignant melanoma, which is known to have the poorest prognosis among the aforementioned tumors. Results of a previous investigation (1975–1986) will be used as a comparison to the findings in the current investigation.

Data Collection

Registration forms (case cards) for this survey were distributed to 111 institutions (usually to the Department of Dermatology) in June 1992, and collected in May 1993. Cards were collected from 76 institutions (53 universities, 23 hospitals: collection rate 69.1%). Another 25 universities' replies only indicated the incidence of tumors by type and year. We were able to obtain some type of reply from 101 institutions in all. Overall collection rate was 91%.

Collected case cards numbered 15,091, of which 5,552 cases were in the prodromal stage and 9,439 cases were malignant tumors. Malignant melanoma was reported in 1,717 cases (18.2%). The incidence of each type of tumor by year is

---

* Manuscript was prepared by Kazuyuki Ishihara, Dermatology Division, National Cancer Center Hospital, 5-1-1 Tsukiji, Chuo-ku, Tokyo 104, Japan

TABLE I. Incidence of Malignant Skin Tumors in Japanese Subjects
(Jan. 1987–Dec. 1991, 101 institutions)

Tumor/year	1987	1988	1989	1990	1991	Total
Malignant melanoma	338	322	361	341	355	1,717
Squamous cell carcinoma (SCC)	521	491	461	508	526	2,507
Basal cell carcinoma (BCC)	866	805	940	926	940	4,477
Paget's disease	179	173	199	180	222	953
Bowen's disease	375	381	454	454	466	2,130
Actinic keratosis	438	411	526	533	561	2,469
Mycosis fungoides	78	67	64	59	49	317
Adult T-cell leukemia/lymphoma (ATLL)	25	35	37	31	35	163
Other malignant lymphoma	64	59	86	74	75	358
Total	2,884	2,744	3,128	3,106	3,229	15,091

TABLE II. Number of Patients with Melanoma by Year and by Status of Registration

	1987	1988	1989	1990	1991	Total
Registered patients	217	197	229	212	216	1,071
Non-registered patients	121	125	132	129	139	646
Total	338	322	361	341	355	1,717

summarized in Table I. The largest number of cases was reported for basal cell carcinoma (4,477 cases, 47.4%), followed by squamous cell carcinoma (2,507 cases, 26.6%). In the following parts of this report, we will only give findings for malignant melanomas.

Data Analysis

As shown in Table I, cases with malignant melanoma numbered 1,717, and among these 1,071 patients replied to questions on the case cards. These 1,071 cases became part of the statistical analysis (registered). The other 646 case cards reported only the year of disease appearance, and these cases are not part of this analysis (non-registered). Table II summarizes the annual incidence of malignant melanoma in registered and non-registered patients. Among the 1,071 registered cases, we analyzed the following check-items, and each will be discussed in detail below. The list of participating institutions is given at the end of this book.

1. Incidence by gender and year.
2. Incidence by age group and gender.
3. Five-year-survival rate by disease type (in new and previously treated cases).
4. Site of melanoma.
5. Five-year survival rate by disease stage (in new and previously treated cases).
6. Five-year survival rate by Clark's level (in new and previously treated cases).
7. Five-year survival rate by tumor thickness (Breslow's depth) (in new and previously treated cases).
8. Five-year survival rate by clinical symptom (in new and previously treated cases).
9. Treatment by disease stage.

Basic Data of the Registered Patients

1. Incidence by gender and age

During the 5-year period between January 1987 and December 1991, the total number of reported malignant melanomas was 1,717, and the annual incidence was almost constant at the 300 level. For the 1,071 registered cases, incidence by gender and by year is summarized in Table III. The 1,071 cases consisted of 522 males and 549 females. In the previous data concerning Japanese subjects (4, 5), male cases tended to outnumber females, while for Caucasians females outnumbered males (1).

2. Incidence by age group and by gender

Table IV shows the number of patients by age and by gender. The incidence of malignant melanoma is quite low in those younger than 19 years old, then starts to increase from 20, and markedly increases from 40: 0.3% in the group 0–9 years old, 1% in the 10–19 years, 3.1% in the 20s, 8.7% in the 30s, 16.1% in the 40s, 17.3% in the 50s, 23.1% in the 60s, and 30.5% in the 70s.

3. Incidence by disease type

Malignant melanoma can be classified into 4 types: lentigo malignant melanoma (LMM), superficial spreading melanoma (SSM), acral lentiginous melanoma (ALM), and nodular melanoma (NM). The incidence of each type in the Japanese population differs from the rates in Caucasians. For example, sunlight is the most predominant cause of melanoma in Caucasians, and the incidence is high on bare parts of the body. On the other hand, in Japanese subjects, the highest incidence has been recorded on the planta, which is a subtype of ALM, even though the incidence

TABLE III. Number of Registered Patients with Melanoma

Year	Males	Females	Total
1987	112	105	217
1988	92	105	197
1989	121	108	229
1990	93	119	212
1991	104	112	216
Total	522	549	1,071

TABLE IV. Number of Patients with Melanoma by Age

Age (years)	Males	Females	Total (%)
0–9	2	1	3 (0.3)
10–19	3	8	11 (1.0)
20–29	16	17	33 (3.1)
30–39	38	55	93 (8.7)
40–49	75	97	172 (16.1)
50–59	96	89	185 (17.3)
60–69	133	114	247 (23.1)
70 or over	159	168	327 (30.5)
Total	522	549	1,071 (100.0)

TABLE V. Number of Patients by Disease Type in the Two Investigations

Years of investigation	Disease type	No. of patients	(%)	Total
1975–1986 (9 institutions)	LMM	21	(4.0)	529
	SSM	67	(12.7)	
	ALM	229	(43.3)	
	NM	212	(40.0)	
1987–1991 (75 institutions)	LMM	85	(9.1)	926
	SSM	151	(16.3)	
	ALM	391	(42.2)	
	NM	269	(29.0)	
	Unevaluable	30	(3.4)	

LMM: lentigo malignant melanoma.
SSM: superficial spreading melanoma.
ALM: acral lentiginous melanoma.
NM: nodular melanoma.
Unevaluable: type was not clearly stated on the case cards.

on arms and legs has been increasing. ALM is found only in a small percentage of Caucasians. SSM is another type with a high incidence in Caucasians, but is rare in the Japanese population.

Table V presents incidence by tumor type in the present investigation and findings in the previous study (9 institutions, 1975–1986). Type of melanoma was not reported in 30 cases, the most recent study, and those were excluded from this analysis. The slightly increased incidence of LMM suggests the effect of sunlight has become more harmful, even in Japan. SSM incidence has also increased, while that of ALM has remained constant. NM incidence, on the other hand, has decreased even though this ratio was not very small. Because malignancy is high in NM and ALM, melanoma patients in Japan may have greater possibility of poor prognosis.

4. Site of melanoma

Incidence at major sites of lesions by gender and overall incidence are summarized in Table VI. After excluding 46 cases, whose sites were not listed on the case cards, incidence was calculated for 1,025 cases.

Overall incidence in the present study was higher in females than males (51% vs. 49%), but the previous study showed the opposite findings (males had a higher rate). When we observe the male-female differences by site, the total number of female patients with lesions on the face (61 cases), upper limbs (19 cases) and lower limbs (65 cases) is 170, which is approximately 2 times larger than in males (44 on the face, 19 on the upper limbs, and 27 on the lower limbs). These 3 parts of the body are normally bare (uncovered) sites. In contrast, the total number of male patients with lesions on the shoulders/body trunk (45 cases) and planta (163 cases) is 208, which is 1.3 times larger than in females (24 on the shoulders/trunk and 136 on the planta). In total, the highest incidence is recorded on the planta (299 cases, 28.4%), followed by the face (105 cases, 10%), knee/shin/calf (92 cases, 8.7%), shoulder/body trunk (69 cases, 6.6%), palm (66 cases, 6.3%), upper limbs (63 cases, 6.0 %), and toes (61 cases, 5.8%). When summing up the numbers for the hand (55 cases) and for the foot (22 cases), subungual showed a high incidence, 74 cases (7.1%). Cases with melanoma on the bare parts of the body, or the total of the head, face, ear, neck, and knee/shin/calf

TABLE VI. Sites of Melanoma

Site of lesion	Males (%)	Females (%)	Total (%)
Scalp	14 (2.7)	9 (1.7)	23 (2.2)
Face	44 (8.5)	61 (11.4)	105 (10.0)
Ear	5 (0.9)	4 (0.7)	9 (0.9)
Neck	5 (0.9)	3 (0.6)	8 (0.7)
Chest/abdomen	25 (4.8)	21 (3.9)	46 (4.4)
Shoulder/trunk	45 (8.7)	24 (4.7)	69 (6.6)
Upper limbs	19 (3.7)	44 (8.2)	63 (6.0)
Hand: dorsum	5 (0.9)	3 (0.6)	8 (0.7)
Hand: palmar	37 (7.2)	29 (5.4)	66 (6.3)
Finger: subungual	24 (4.7)	28 (5.2)	52 (5.0)
Buttock	6 (1.2)	7 (1.3)	13 (1.2)
Inquinal/thigh	27 (5.2)	20 (3.7)	47 (4.5)
Vulva	0 (0.0)	7 (1.3)	7 (0.7)
Knee/shin/calf	27 (5.2)	65 (12.1)	92 (8.7)
Toes	39 (7.6)	22 (4.1)	61 (5.8)
Toe: subungual	11 (2.1)	11 (2.0)	22 (2.1)
Foot: dorsum	7 (1.4)	17 (3.2)	24 (2.3)
Foot: edge	9 (1.7)	2 (0.3)	11 (1.0)
Foot: planta	163 (31.6)	136 (25.3)	299 (28.4)
Unknown	10 (1.9)	36 (6.6)	46 (4.3)
Total	522 (49)	549 (51)	1,071 (100)

is high (237 cases, 22.5%). However, incidence on the ear, neck, vulva, or dorsal surface of hands is low ($\leq 0.9\%$). Remarkable contrast in incidence is observed between the palmar surface of the hand (66 cases) and the dorsal surface of the hand (8 cases), and between the planta (299 cases) and the dorsal surface of the foot (24 cases). Therefore, we conclude that, in Japan, the highest incidence of melanoma occurs on the planta of the foot, and the second highest on bare parts of the body.

Disease Stage and Related Matters

This study followed the UICC classification of disease stage in melanoma (8). Because these stages will be referred to in the analysis of factors which influence prognosis, their descriptions are summarized in Table VII referring to the TNM classification.

1. Incidence by disease stage

Table VIII summarizes the number of patients entered in the previous study (1975–1986) and in the present study (1987–1991) by disease stage. In the previous study, incidence in Stage I was high, possibly because that investigation was conducted in university hospitals which have high identification rates of melanoma. The more recent study, however, included many institutions other than universities, and these institutions usually take longer for disease identification; it is therefore not surprising that the number of Stage II patients is larger than that of Stage I.

The decreased ratio of Stage IV patients in this study indicates there has been progress and improvement in treatment methods for melanoma.

TABLE VII. Classification of Disease Stage in Malignant Melanoma

Stage I (primary site only)
 pT1: tumor thickness is less than 0.75mm, and the tumor invades the papillary dermis (level 2).
 pT2: tumor thickness is more than 0.75mm but less than 1.5mm, and/or the tumor invades the papillary-reticular dermal interface (level 3).

Stage II (primary site only)
 pT3: tumor thickness is more than 1.5mm but less than 40mm, and/or the tumor invades the reticular dermis (level 4). pT3 could be subclassified into 2 groups: pT3a (tumor thickness is more than 1.5mm and less than 3.0mm) and pT3b (thickness is more than 3.0mm and less than 4.0mm).

Stage III (primary site only, or primary site and lymph node metastasis)
 pT4: tumor thickness is more than 4.0mm, and/or the tumor invades subcutaneous tissues and/or satellites within 2cm from the primary lesion (level 5). pT4 could be subclassified into 2 groups: pT4a (thickness>4.0mm and/or there is invasion to subcutaneous tissues (level 5)) and pT4b (associated with invasion to satellites within 2 cm from the primary lesion).
 N1: there is evidence of involvement of regional lymph node(s) within 3 cm or less from the primary lesion.
 N2: there is evidence of involvement of regional lymph node(s) located 3 cm or further away, and/or in transit metastasis.

Stage IV (distant metastasis)
 M1: there is evidence of distant metastasis. This category can be further classified into 2 groups: (i) M1a: there is an involvement of skin or subcutaneous tissues, and lymph nodes beyond the site of primary lymph drainage (other than regional drainage), and (ii) M1b: there is visceral metastasis.

2. Guidelines for treatment of melanoma

Table IX summarizes the guidelines for treatment of malignant melanoma. Chemotherapy which is used for Stage II and III patients is usually DAV therapy (dacarbazine, nimustine, and vincristine), whereas in Stage IV patients, CDV therapy (cisplatin, dacarbazine, and vindesine) is usually used. For skin metastasis in all disease stages, interferon (IFN)-β is administered intra-tumorally. Besides these therapies, adoptive immunotherapy has also been administered. In Stage II and III patients, complete extirpation of regional lymph nodes has been actively performed, and improvement of the prognosis has been reported.

3. Method of diagnosis

Diagnosis of the primary lesion of melanoma is determined by histopathological examination. Recently, identification of 5-S-cystenyldopa in serum has been reported as highly useful for patients having advanced stages of the disease. As in many other tumors, various physiological equipment has also been utilized in making a diagnosis.

Survival

There are various factors which influence a patient's prognosis. Examples are disease stage, disease type, Clark's level, maximal thickness of a melanoma (Breslow's thickness), and clinical symptoms.

If therapy is administered without seriously considering the patient's condition, the disease prognosis will be poor. Therefore, we investigated the state of prognosis for new cases and for cases who had undergone previous treatment. Survival rates were calculated using the life table method.

TABLE VIII. Number of Patients by Disease Stage in the Two Investigations

Investigation	Disease stage	No. of patients (%)	Total
1975–1986 (9 institutions)	I	149 (24.7)	604
	II	116 (19.2)	
	III-1 (pT4N0M0)	126 (20.8)	
	III-2 (anyTN1+2M0)	132 (21.9)	
	IV	81 (13.4)	
1987–1991 (75 institutions)	I	206 (21.7)	948
	II	236 (25.0)	
	III-1 (pT4N0M0)	206 (21.7)	
	III-2 (anyTN1+2M0)	218 (23.0)	
	IV	82 (8.6)	

TABLE IX. Guidelines for Treatment of Malignant Melanoma

Stage I:	extensive resection (skin grafting starting 2–3 cm from the edge of the tumor)
Stage II:	extensive resection (skin grafting starting 3–5 cm from the edge of the tumor, and wide dissection of the regional lymph nodes with administration of chemotherapy and immunotherapy.
Stage III:	similar treatments to those for Stage II.
Stage IV:	multidisciplinary treatment.

1. *Five-year survival rate by disease stage of a malignant melanoma (3–5)*

All subjects were categorized either as new cases or cases having had previous treatment. New cases consisted of 651 subjects (not including 56 whose disease courses were not reported), and 323 cases had had previous treatment (excluding 41 whose disease course was unknown).

1) *New cases (Table X):*

There were 173 Stage I patients whose 5-year survival rate was 99%, and 163 Stage II patients with a 93% rate. Among the Stage III subjects, there were 140 under the subclassification of pT4aN0M0, whose 5-year survival rate was 81.2%, and 130 patients in the TN1+2aM0 subclassification, whose 5-year survival rate was 51%. In Stage IV, the 8 patients who had skin metastasis only (M1a) had a 37.5% rate, while the survival rate for 37 patients with remote metastasis (M1b) was 15.4%.

Among these data, it should be noted that approximately half of the new cases (*i.e.*, 315 patients, 48.4%) were those who already had an advanced disease in Stage III or IV.

2) *Cases having had previous treatment (Table XI):*

After excluding 40 cases whose treatment course was not clear on the case cards, 323 patients were evaluated. There were 33 Stage I cases with a 93% 5-year survival rate, 73 Stage II cases with 82.7%, 160 cases in the pT4aN0M0 subcategory of Stage III with 48.2%, and 88 cases in the TN1+2aM0 subcategory of Stage III with 49.1%. This suggests that, in Stage III patients with previous treatment but without any lymph node metastasis, treatment given without serious consideration of the patient's condition will result in a poor prognosis. In Stage IV, 26 cases who had skin metastasis only (M1a) had a 31% 4-year survival rate (5-year survival rate was not obtained), but this rate decreased to 12.1% in the 37 cases who had associated remote metastasis (M1b). For patients having had previous treatment, 5-year survival rates

TABLE X. Survival Rate in New Cases by Disease Stage and Year

Disease stage	No. of new cases	Survival rate (%)				
		1 year	2 years	3 years	4 years	5 years
I	173	100.0	100.0	99.0	99.0	99.0
II	163	100.0	98.6	96.9	95.6	93.0
III-1 (pT4aN0M0)	140	95.7	92.2	87.5	81.2	81.2
III-2 (anyTN1+2a)	130	92.1	78.7	63.5	57.5	51.0
IV (M1a)	8	75.0	37.5	37.5	37.5	37.5
IV (M1b)	37	48.5	43.1	30.8	15.4	15.4

Note: for the description of disease stage, please refer to Table VII.

TABLE XI. Survival Rates in Previously Treated Cases by Disease Stage

Disease stage	No. of new cases	Survival rate (%)				
		1 year	2 years	3 years	4 years	5 years
I	33	97.0	97.0	93.0	93.0	93.0
II	73	97.0	92.0	87.6	87.6	82.7
III-1 (pT4aN0M0)	66	92.4	76.4	67.0	53.0	48.2
III-2 (anyTN1+2a)	88	82.0	67.9	62.2	49.1	49.1
IV (M1a)	26	57.7	43.3	31.0	31.0	31.0
IV (M1b)	37	32.4	24.3	24.3	12.1	N.A.

Note: for the description of disease stage, please refer to Table VII.
N.A.: 5-year observation has not yet been completed in most of the patients in this category.

in all stages were lower than in new cases, and 217 of the 323 cases (67.2%) were in the advanced disease stage.

2. *Five-year survival by disease type*

Malignant melanoma was subclassified into 4 types, *i.e.*, LMM, SSM, ALM, and NM. From the total number of subjects (1,071), 175 cases were excluded because of insufficient recording on the case cards, and the remaining 896 cases were classified into either new cases or those having had previous treatment for this analysis. In the following, we report only the rate for new cases.

New cases numbered 707, from which 67 were excluded because of insufficient information. The remaining 640 cases were then subclassified into one of the 4 types and analyzed for the 5-year survival rate (Fig. 1). Among LMM, SSM, and ALM, there were no significant differences in rate. NM showed a much faster decreasing rate tendency compared to the other 3 types ($p < 0.56$). Therefore, we presume that if complete and appropriate therapy were administered in the first treatment, there would be no significant difference in prognosis by disease type.

Prognosis was the poorest in NM, and improved in order from ALM, SSM to LMM. In cases having had previous treatment (data not presented), the 5-year survival rate became markedly lower in ALM and NM. Therefore, again, the first treatment is a very important factor in determining the disease course for a patient.

3. *Five-year survival rate by Clark's level in new cases*

Clark's level indicates the depth of infiltration of tumor cells (see Table VII).

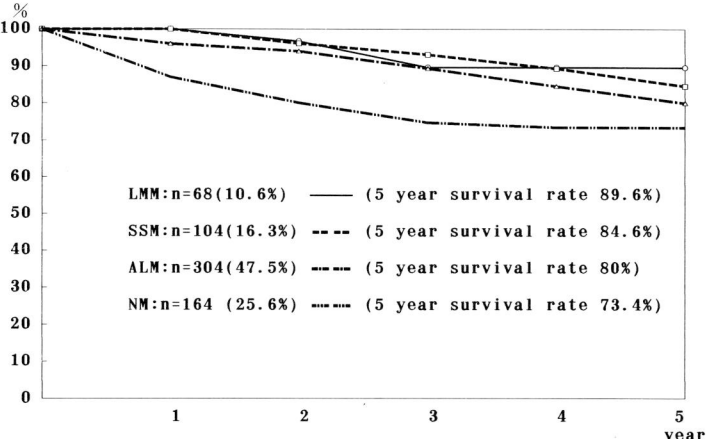

FIG. 1. Survival rate by disease type of melanoma and by year in 640 new cases (Jan. 1987–Dec. 1991)

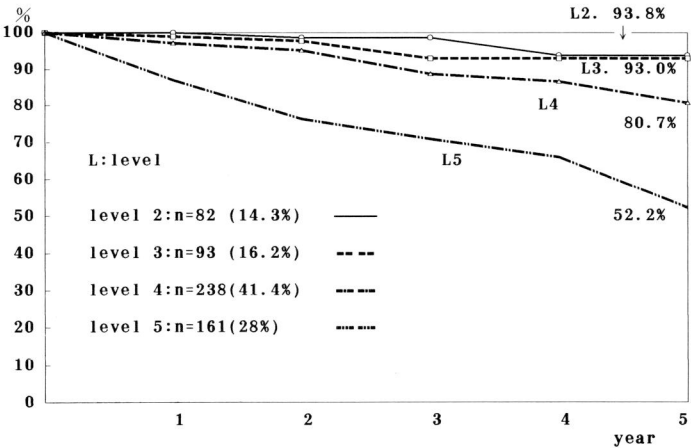

FIG. 2. Survival rate by Clark's level of melanoma and by year in 574 new cases (Jan. 1987–Dec. 1991)

Depth of infiltration is expressed in levels, and the higher the level (deeper the infiltration), the poorer the prognosis. Findings in new cases are presented below.

From the 707 new cases, 133 were excluded from this analysis. As shown in Fig. 2, the 5-year survival rate for levels 2 and 3 were nearly the same, while the rate for level 4 tended to decrease and the rate for level 5 decreased significantly ($p < 0.01$).

4. *Five-year survival rate by tumor thickness (Breslow) in new cases (2, 6, 7, 9)*

Thickness of the tumor is considered to be a factor influencing the prognosis of melanoma. For an explanation of the thickness, please refer to Table VII (9). We categorized patients into 5 groups by thickness: ≦0.75 mm, 0.76–1.5 mm, 1.6–3.0 mm, 3.1–4.0 mm, and ≧4.1 mm.

Among 707 new cases, 220 were not evaluable. The remaining 487 were classified into one of 5 groups, and their 5-year survival rates are shown in Fig. 3. When tumor

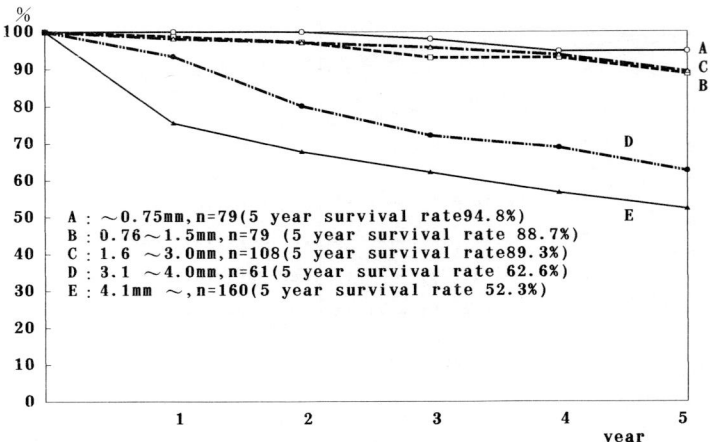

FIG. 3. Survival rate by tumor thickness of melanoma and by year in 487 new cases (Jan. 1987–Dec. 1991)

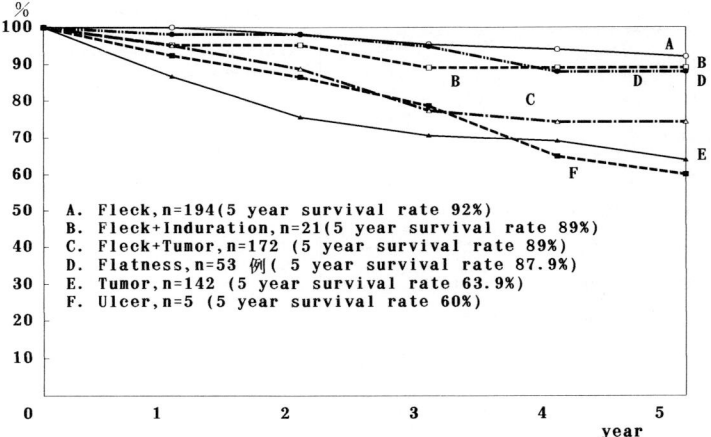

FIG. 4. Survival rate by clinical symptom of melanoma (647 new cases, Jan. 1987–Dec. 1991)

thickness was 3 mm or more, prognosis became poorer. Patients with 4 mm or deeper infiltration should be monitored very carefully. In cases having had previous treatment (data not shown), the prognosis for patients with tumors 4 mm or thicker became even worse.

5. *Five-year survival by clinical symptoms in new cases*

In malignant melanoma, it is known that changes in clinical symptoms correlate with the prognosis. Major symptoms are tachetic lesions, tachetic and indurated lesions, tachetic and tumor lesions, flattened lesions, swelling, and ulceration. For new cases, 5-year survival rates were analyzed for each of these symptoms.

After excluding 60 unevaluable cases, the survival rates were analyzed for 647 new cases (Fig. 4). The best prognosis was obtained in those who had tachetic lesions, and prognosis was poor in patients whose lesions were associated with induration, swelling or ulceration. Specifically, lesions which formed tumors or ulcerated resulted in a poor prognosis.

Acknowledgments

A part of this work was supported by the Ministry of Health and Welfare and the Foundation of Electronic Industries of Japan. The registration committee is grateful to the dermatologists in 76 major hospitals who contributed to this registry.

REFERENCES

1. Beardmore, G.I. The epidemiology of melanoma in Australia. *In* "Melanoma and Skin Cancer, Proceedings of the International Cancer Conference, Sydney," pp. 39–64 (1972).
2. Breslow, A. Thickness, cross-sectional areas and depth of invasion in the prognosis of cutaneous melanoma. *Ann. Surg.*, **172**, 902–908 (1970).
3. Ikeda, S., Suzuki, T., and Kiyohara, Y. TNM classification and prognosis for skin cancer. *Prog. Cancer Clin.*, **20**, 154–157 (1988) (in Japanese).
4. Ishihara, K., Ikeda, S. Mori, S. *et al.* Prognostic factors for malignant melanoma. *Skin Cancer*, **4**, 349–360 (1989).
5. Ishihara, K. Statistics of prognostic factors for malignant melanoma. *Dermat. Mook.*, **18**, 159–167 (1992).
6. Jones, S. K., Pocock, P.V., and Briggs, J.C. Tumor thickness is not a prognostic factor in thin melanoma. *Arch. Dermatol. Res.*, **281**, 81–82 (1989).
7. Salman, S.M. and Rogers, G.S. Prognostic factors in thin cutaneous malignant melanoma. *J. Dermatol. Surg. Oncol.*, **16**, 413–418 (1990).
8. UICC. "Melanoma of the Skin: TNM Classification of Malignant Tumors," 3rd ed., pp. 141–144 (1987). Springer-Verlag, Berlin.
9. Worth, A.J., Gallagher, R.P., Elwood, J.M., Yang, P.C., Lamb, C., Spinelli, J.J., Wood, W.S., Threlfall, W.J., and Hill, G.B. Pathologic prognostic factors for cutaneous malignant melanoma. *Int. J. Cancer,* **43**, 370–375 (1989).

CLINICAL STATISTICS ON REGISTERED BREAST CANCER PATIENTS IN JAPAN

Registration Committee of the Japanese Breast Cancer Society*

The multi-institutional registry of mammary cancer patients was begun in 1975 and a total of 45,667 females and 218 males were registered during the subsequent 11 years until 1985. Mammography and echography have been common diagnostic tools. The Halsted operation was the most common procedure as of 1985 and adjuvant chemotherapy and endocrinetherapy have increased. Five-year survival rates of patients in the 1980s were 94.1% (Stage I), 86.2% (Stage II), 62.8% (Stage IIIa), 49.41% (Stage IIIb), and 23.6% (Stage IV).

The number of breast cancer deaths in Japan has steadily increased (3, 7). The mortality rate in 1960 was 3.5/100,000, but this had increased to 10.1 by 1991 (Table I). Female breast cancer mortality rates in Western countries, however, were 30–40/100,000, so the Japanese mortality rate as of 1991 was still just one third to one fourth of that (Table II). The multi-institutional registry of mammary cancer patients was begun in 1975. With the establishment of the Japanese Breast Cancer Society in 1992, the registration committee was reorganized and registration was taken over by the Society in 1993. The number of patients registered from 1975 to 1985 was 45,885, 218 of which were males (Table III). The estimated number of new patients with breast cancer in 1985 was 18,964, so that the rate documented by the registry was about one fourth of them (Table IV).

Clinicopathological Features of Registered Patients

1. Age distribution
Age distribution of registered breast cancer patients was similar throughout the study period with the age group of 45–49 being the greatest (Table V). Registered patients tended to be younger than those in the population based registry.

2. Tumor location and size
Left breast was slightly dominant in location of the mammary tumor: 51.5–52.5% in the left and 47.5–48.9% in the right by year. Tumor site was also stable by year: 43.2% in the upper-outer, 19.0% in the upper-inner, 9.7% in the lower-outer, 5.5% in the central, and 4.7% in the lower-inner portion (Fig. 1). Tumor size by palpation was

---

* Manuscript was prepared by Takeshi Nanasawa, National Cancer Center Hospital, 5-1-1 Tsukiji, Chuo-ku, Tokyo 104, Japan; Fujio Kasumi, Cancer Institute Hospital, 1-37-1 Kami-Ikebukuro, Toshima-ku, Tokyo 170, Japan; Suketami Tominaga, Aichi Cancer Center, 1-1 Kanokoden, Chikusa-ku, Nagoya 464, Japan; and Masaru Izuo, Tokyo Women's Medical College, 8-1 Kawada-cho, Shinjuku-ku, Tokyo 162, Japan

TABLE I. Number of Deaths and Death Rate from Female Breast Cancer in Japan

Year	No. of deaths	Death rate (per 100,000)[a]	Age-adjusted
1960	1,683	3.5	5.1
1965	1,966	3.9	5.2
1970	2,486	4.7	5.8
1975	3,262	5.8	6.5
1980	4,141	7.0	7.2
1985	4,922	8.0	7.6
1990	5,848	9.4	8.2

[a] Crude rate. From Statistics and Information Department, Minister's Secretariat, Ministry of Health and Welfare.

TABLE II. Comparison of Breast Cancer Death Rates[a]

Country	1978	1988	1989	1990
England	47.3	53.2	54.1	56.1
West Germany	36.5	45.9	45.7	45.6
Sweden	33.4	36.9	35.0	34.1
Italy	28.1	35.9	36.8	36.9
France	29.7	34.8	35.2	34.9
U.S.A.	30.6	33.5	33.7	34.0
Czechoslovakia		30.8	30.9	31.4

[a] Crude rate. From World Health Statistics Annual, Geneva, 1994.

TABLE III. Annual Registration of Breast Cancer Patients in Japan

Year	No. of institutes	Male	Female	Total
1975	189	20	3,455	3,475
1976	145	9	3,000	3,009
1977	200	18	3,619	3,637
1978	219	20	4,103	4,123
1979	185	22	4,123	4,145
1980	155	19	4,144	4,163
1981	157	28	4,709	4,737
1982	137	16	4,493	4,509
1983	138	28	4,704	4,732
1984	118	13	4,477	4,490
1985	122	25	4,840	4,865
Total		218	45,667	45,885

TABLE IV. Estimated Annual Number of New Breast Cancer Patients in Japan

Year	No. of patients
1984	15,780
1985	18,964
1986	19,026
1987	20,155
1988	20,903

TABLE V. Age Distribution of Female Breast Cancer Patients

Age	1975	'76	'77	'78	'79	'80	'81	'82	'83	'84	'85	Total
–19	1	0	9	4	2	2	0	1	3	0	0	22
20–24	8	10	16	11	11	9	13	15	10	7	14	121
25–29	56	50	58	72	69	56	61	66	63	43	43	637
30–34	169	150	177	201	194	205	278	225	215	211	186	2,211
35–39	317	242	318	344	388	405	437	412	485	386	452	4,159
40–44	476	429	505	567	565	603	703	613	693	713	688	6,555
45–49	573	525	673	661	660	745	838	795	828	739	885	7,922
50–54	434	393	412	553	581	563	623	647	654	598	617	6,075
55–59	308	259	352	449	434	490	525	544	550	518	591	5,020
60–64	255	236	281	302	301	347	472	390	420	441	472	3,917
65–69	163	176	212	257	263	286	334	282	297	310	295	2,875
70–74	129	103	123	134	172	169	220	210	220	211	234	1,925
75–79	57	51	78	116	81	100	130	120	109	104	140	1,086
80–84	23	9	26	31	65	140	76	142	45	50	67	674
85–89	1	3	2	7	5	8	16	20	14	11	15	102
90–	2	0	2	3	8	4	9	7	2	1	4	42
Unknown	160	75	62	24	21	1	2	0	113	104	107	669

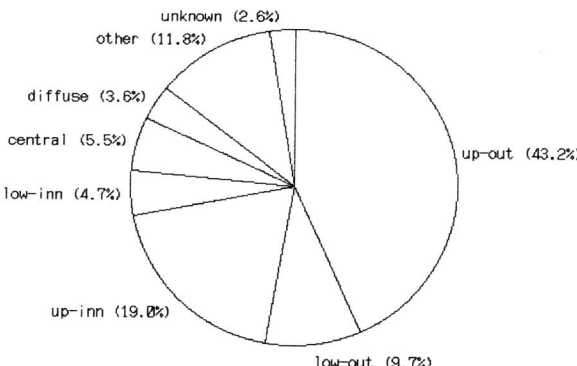

FIG. 1. Site of the breast cancer
The most common site of breast cancer is the upper-outer quadrant. Diffuse type accounts for 3.6% and central type 5.5%.

usually less than 5 cm, and the number of those under 2 cm had increased as of 1985; mammary tumors more than 10 cm diameter were still present in 14% of the cases in 1985. Incidence of breast cancer of less than 2 cm diameter was 33.8% and of 2–5 cm in diameter was 49.9%. Cancer sizes among 40,096 resected cases excluding 3,591 size-unknown cases was less than 1 cm (10.8%), 1–1.9 cm (31.3%), 2–2.9 cm (27.0%), 3–3.9 cm (12.7%), 4–4.9 cm (7.1%), and more than 5.0 cm (10.9%) (Table VI).

3. Diagnosis

Fifty-four and nine-tenths percent of cases were diagnosed as malignant by palpation, 38.3% were suspected to be malignant and 7.0% cases were considered to be benign tumor (2,898/41,326). Application of mammography increased to 85.7% in 1985 from 71.9% in 1975 (Fig. 2); 2,407 out of 27,913 cases were misdiagnosed as

TABLE VI. Size of the Breast Cancer (Cut Surface)

Year	−1cm	−2.0	−3.0	−4.0	−5.0	5.1−	Unknown
1975	194	721	625	401	321	413	434
1976	243	711	634	329	236	328	205
1977	280	842	733	420	257	368	367
1978	350	962	831	524	309	389	340
1979	324	991	897	502	316	438	322
1980	407	1,194	973	489	354	387	314
1981	502	1,309	1,124	538	338	482	383
1982	458	1,280	1,089	536	340	436	324
1983	446	1,347	1,169	575	369	422	334
1984	424	1,337	1,104	523	307	438	296
1985	486	1,415	1,219	575	321	494	272
Total	4,114	12,109	10,398	5,412	3,468	4,595	3,591

benign tumors during that period, while 59.6% cases were correctly diagnosed as malignant and 31.8% cases remained suspicious.

Echography gradually increased after 1980, and 66.3% of cases (3,095/4,669) were diagnosed by this means in 1985 (Fig. 2). Rate of misdiagnosis as benign tumor was 22.4% in the 1975–1977 period, but decreased to 12.6% in the 1984–1985 period. Rate of correct diagnosis as malignant tumor increased from 60.5% to 65.6% (3,776/5,752) during the latter period.

Diagnosis by xero-radiography was still minimal (10.6%), but the correct diagnosis was made in 59.6% of cases (Fig. 2), while misdiagnosis as benign tumor occurred in 18.3%.

Tumor biopsy was taken in 53.9% of cases and aspiration biopsy was done in 4.3% of cases during the 11 year period (Fig. 3). Development of graphic diagnosis and serological diagnosis with tumor markers seemed to reduce unnecessary diagnostic biopsy, and surgical diagnosis during operation became preferential.

Treatment and Survival

1. Operation and other treatment methods

There were 43,985 operated cases between 1975 and 1985. The Halsted operation was the most common method, while Auchincloss and Patey operations gradually increased in popularity (Fig. 4). The former was used 45.6% of the time and the latter two methods were used in 34.6% of the instances in 1985. Extended radical mastectomy, radical mastectomy with supraclavicular node dissection and super-extended radical mastectomy were done in 15.8% of the cases in 1985.

Radiotherapy was done in 40.4% of the patients in 1975, but by 1985 its use had gradually decreased to 10.5% (Fig. 5). Adjuvant chemotherapy increased from 53.1% in 1975 to 75.0% in 1985. Hormonal therapy increased after 1981, and was used in 42.1% of patients in 1985.

Data about immunotherapy has been gathered since 1980, and this was used for 14.4% of the patients between that year and 1985.

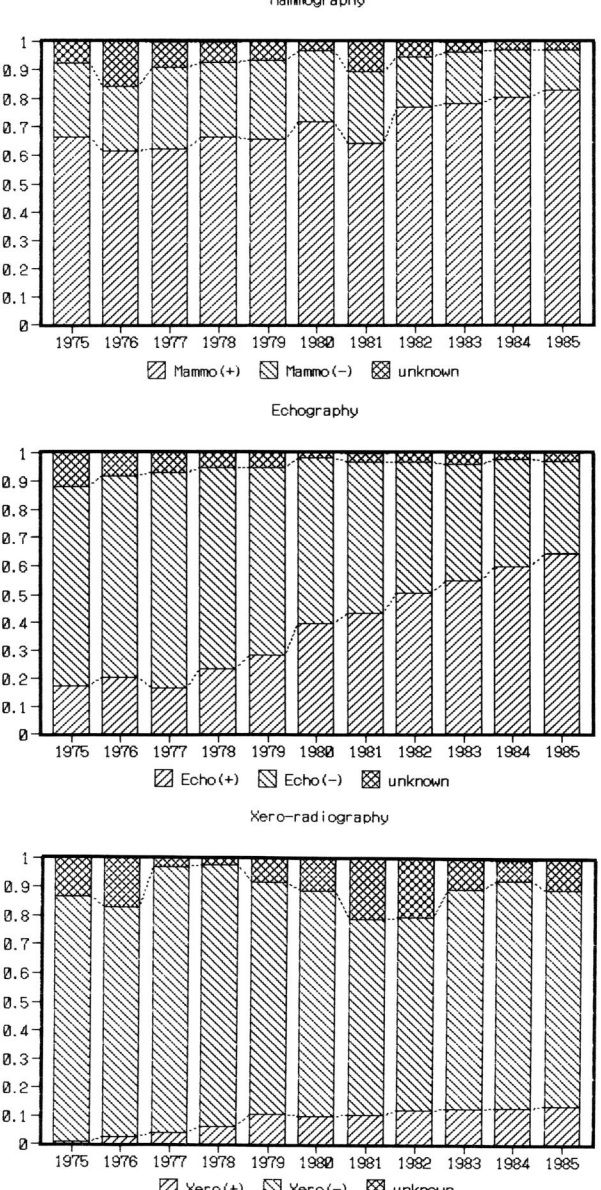

FIG. 2. Changes in diagnostic methods
Echography became the most popular diagnostic tool after 1980.

2. Histological type and TNM stage

In 1975 common type of invasive adenocarcinoma accounted for 83.2% of the cases, in 1985 87.9% of the cases and over the 1975–1985 period it averaged 87.1%. Special types of carcinoma accounted for 6.0% in 1975 and had increased slightly to 7.5% by 1985. An increasing trend of lobular carcinoma was recognized in urban

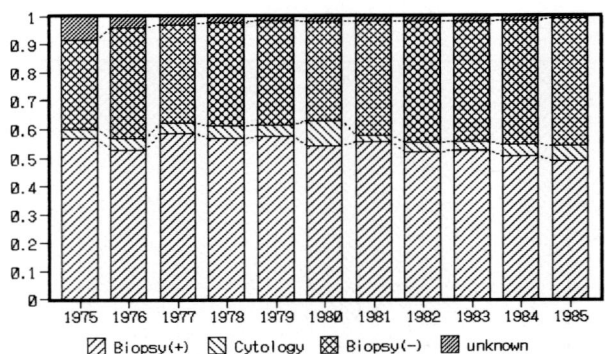

FIG. 3. Frequency of biopsy and aspiration cytology as clues to diagnosis
Biopsy is decreasing, and surgical diagnosis during the operation is preferential.

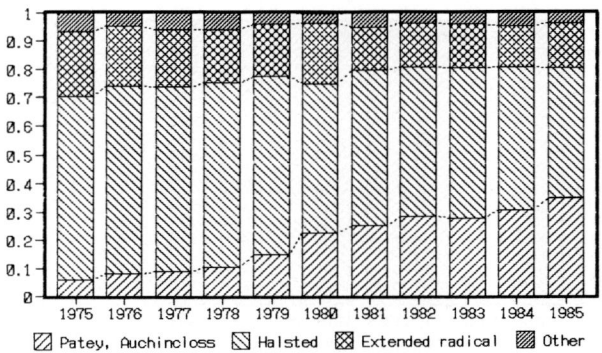

FIG. 4. Changes in surgical procedure by year
Although the Halsted operation is the most frequent operation procedure, partial glandectomy is steadily increasing.

areas. Sarcoma such as sarcoma phyllodes and malignant lymphoma was rare, but in 1985 it accounted for 0.6% of the total.

3. Hormone receptors

Presence or absence of estrogen and progesterone receptors have been reported to the registry since 1980. Estrogen receptors were present in an average of 61.5% of cases during the six year period, while progesterone receptors were detected in 45.3% of cases (Table VII).

4. Lymph node involvement

In 1975 44.8% of cases showed no lymph node involvement and in 1985 56.0% did not (Fig. 6). Thus, the proportion of lymph node involvement did not greatly differ during the years 1975–1985.

5. TNM stage and survival

The TNM stages of 43,984 cases were : 2.9% in Tis, 0.8% in T0, 26.6% in Stage I, 45.8% in Stage II, 16.8% in Stage III, and 3.1% in Stage IV (Table VIII).
Changes of 5-year survival rates by stage did not significantly improve over the

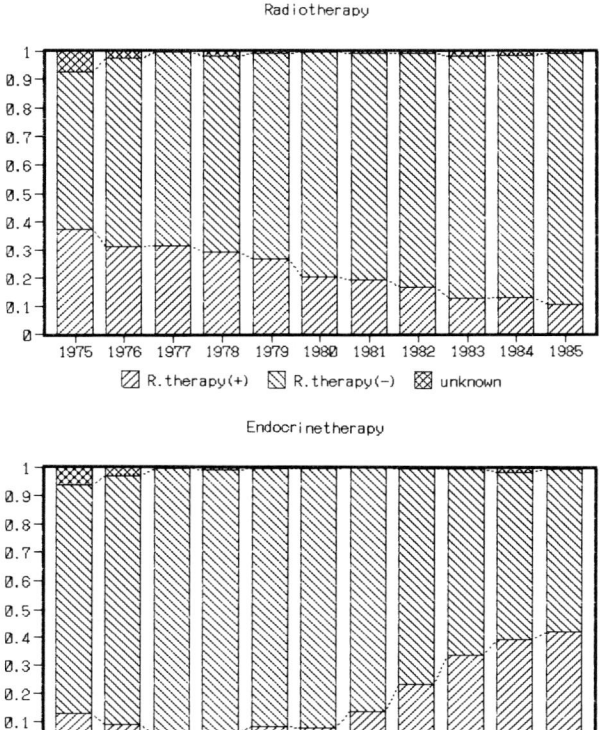

FIG. 5. Changes in treatment methods by year
Decreased irradiation therapy and increased endocrinetherapy are noted.

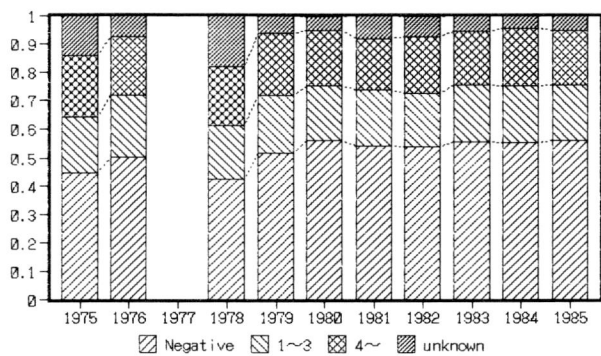

FIG. 6. Changes in lymph node involvement
More than half of the cases since 1980 have not shown lymph node metastasis.

period (Table IX): the 10-year survival rate of Stage I was 85%, that of Stage II was 68%, Stage III was 42%, and Stage IV was 13% (Fig. 7).

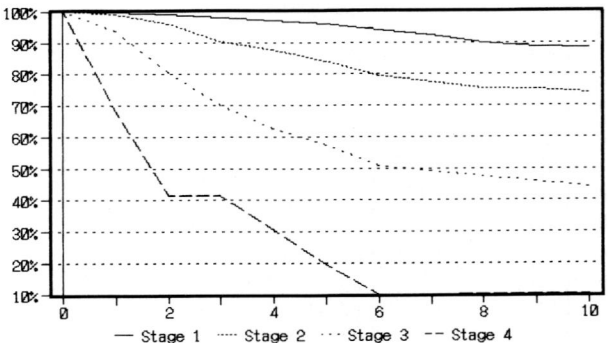

FIG. 7. Ten-year survival rates by TNM stage
More than 80% of the Stage I cases have survived more than 10 years.

TABLE VII. Presence of Hormone Receptor

Year	Estrogen receptor		Progesterone receptor	
	(+)	(−)	(+)	(−)
1980	498	394	172	231
1981	779	574	323	392
1982	1,120	639	497	583
1983	1,459	796	656	762
1984	1,394	971	721	932
1985	1,718	997	862	919

TABLE VIII. Changes in TNM Stage by Year

Year	Tis	T0	I	II	III	IV	Unknown	Total
1975	7	112	719	1,300	632	92	270	3,132
1976	38	30	696	1,213	476	79	177	2,709
1977	456	21	829	1,402	617	102	290	3,306
1978	48	16	929	1,681	691	136	236	3,737
1979	145	13	950	1,762	716	131	103	3,820
1980	135	19	1,144	1,957	668	102	108	4,133
1981	122	35	1,347	2,154	715	152	178	4,703
1982	172	26	1,234	2,082	720	137	115	4,486
1983	171	19	1,300	2,222	735	153	92	4,692
1984	181	19	1,211	2,130	683	143	89	4,456
1985	208	39	1,348	2,256	750	135	74	4,810
Total	1,272	349	11,707	20,159	7,403	1,362	1,732	43,984

TABLE IX. Changes in 5-Year Survival Rate (%)

Stage	1975	1976	1977	1978	1979	1980
Stage I	91.6	92.8	93.0	94.3	91.6	94.1
Stage II	79.9	80.6	82.1	83.8	84.5	86.2
Stage III	55.9	53.9	55.9	63.3	62.1	
Stage IIIa						62.8
Stage IIIb						49.4
Stage IV	18.7	24.8	24.5	20.2	19.5	23.6

Comments and Discussion

The incidence rate of breast cancer among Japanese is about one-half or one-third that among Caucasians (*1*). Comparative studies are being carried out on many phases such as differences in life style and in hormonal level or tissue types. Breast cancer in Japan has shown a continuous increase throughout the post-Second World War years. The number of patients in 1965 was estimated to be 4,300 and the number of deaths 1,995, and this increased respectively to 12,250 and 4,185 in 1980, and to 15,840 and 4,922 in 1985. Based on changes in mortality of breast cancer between 1960 and 1990 broken down by sex and age group, the increase after menopause was evident as true in the industrialized countries of the West. Mortality rates in Japan increased 75% or more among women aged 35–64, and 46% among those aged 65–74 between 1960 and 1990. The breast cancer registry information was contributed mostly by surgeons, and registered cases tended to be younger patients and operated cases.

The 5-year survival rate of breast cancer patients between 1975 and 1980 was 73.3% among inpatients at the National Cancer Center, 96.3% for Stage I patients and 36.2% for Stage IV patients among those registered with the Breast Cancer Study Group (*5, 9*). This cancer is thought to be curable if recognized in the early stage. Studies on the treatment of breast cancer are now tending toward minimal surgical operation and improved quality of life (QOL) for the patient. Mass-screening for breast cancer mandated by the Law on Health and Medical Service for the Aged was introduced in 1987 (*8*). The sensitivity of the screening at that time by visual and palpatory examinations varied extensively from 53% to 95%. Even though the specificity is 95% to 96%, however, the positive predictive value is between 3% and a little less than 9%.

Mammography or ultrasonic imaging diagnosis to improve the accuracy of breast cancer mass screening is recommended. Introduction of the imaging process now enables the detection of early cancer.

Among the common type duct carcinomas, the differentiated type is more predominant among Japanese than Caucasians, and it is often accompanied by the infiltration of lymphocytes (*2*). Precancerous lesions for duct carcinoma include intraductal papilloma and hyperplastic ducts, but the latter is found less frequently among Japanese patients upon autopsy, indicating differences in the incidence of precancerous lesions from those of Caucasians (*4*).

The expression of c-erbB-2 genes was recently found to be a poor prognostic factor (*6*). In addition to the TNM staging, such a molecular marker could be utilized in the decision for post-operative adjuvant therapy.

Acknowledgments

The committee appreciated the contributions of member doctors at the 345 major hospitals as listed at the end of this book. We also thank Drs. Naohito Yamaguchi and Shaw Watanabe, Cancer Information and Epidemiology Division, National Cancer Center Research Institute for their technical advice and statistical analyses.

A part of this work was supported by a grant-in-aid for cancer research from the Ministry of Health and Welfare of Japan.

REFERENCES

1. Henderson, B.E. and Bernstein, L. The international variation in breast cancer rates: an epidemiological assessment. *Breast Cancer Res. Treat.,* **18**, Suppl. 1, 11–17 (1991).
2. Sakamoto, G. and Sugano, H. Pathology of breast cancer: present and prospect in Japan. *Breast Cancer Res. Treat.,* **18**, Suppl. 1, 81–83 (1991).
3. Statistics and Information Department. Vital Statistics of Japan. Minister's Secretariat, Ministry of Health and Welfare, Japan (1992).
4. Stemmermann, G.N. The pathology of breast cancer in Japanese women compared to other ethnic groups: a review. *Breast Cancer Res. Treat.,* **18**, Suppl. 1, 67–72 (1991).
5. The Report of Clinical Statistical Studies on Registered Breast Cancer Patients in Japan. Vols. 1–13, Japanese Breast Cancer Society (in Japanese).
6. Tsuda, H., Hiroshi, S., Shimosato, Y. *et al.* Correlation between histological grade of malignancy and copy number of c-erbB-2 gene in breast carcinoma. A retrospective study. *Cancer,* **65**, 1794–1800 (1990).
7. Tsukuma, H. Future trend of cancer incidence. Nationwide estimates up to the year 2015. *Jpn. J. Cancer Clinics,* **38**, 1–9 (1992) (in Japanese).
8. Watanabe, S. Breast cancer in Japan. Trends and recent research in biology and epidemiology. *Asian Med. J.,* **36**, 486–494 (1993).
9. Watanabe, S., Oshima, A., Fujimoto, I., Wada, T., and Maruyama, K. Workshop for the evaluation of survival trends for cancer patients. *Jpn. J. Clin. Oncol.,* **19**, 178–180 (1990).

REGISTRATION OF GYNECOLOGIC MALIGNANCIES

The Japan Society of Obstetrics and Gynecology*

The Japan Society of Obstetrics and Gynecology started registration of uterine cervical and corpus cancer in 1952. Periodic detailed surveys have been conducted by a subcommittee on uterine cervical cancer, corpus cancer, ovarian cancer, and vulvar cancer. The mass-screening program for cervical cancer begun in 1961 shows that the proportion of Stage I has continuously increased, and in 1991 was 56%. The overall 5-year survival rate reached 66.5%, although the 5-year survival by stage did not greatly differ between 1970 and 1983. Recent population-based survival data showed better results.

Corpus cancer has shown on increasing trend and now accounts for about 30% of all uterine cancer. About three fourths of corpus cancer is found in Stage I. The number of ovarian cancers is also increasing. Complete resection resulted in 60–70% 5 year survival but incomplete resection resulted in a poor prognosis of 10–20%. Number of choriocarcinoma deaths was about 300 in the 1960s, but it decreased to only 20 or less by the established treatment method during the last 20 years.

Ovarian cancers also showed an increasing time trend. More than half of the ovarian cancer cases were discovered at an advanced stage, so the overall prognosis is not satisfactory. The 5-year relative survival rate of clear cell adenocarcinoma was only 45.7%, and the average age of onset was the youngest among gynecologic malignancies.

The first survey of vulvar cancer in 1994 registered 331 patients. Squamous cell carcinoma (73.3%) was the most frequent cancer, and Paget's disease (14.8%), adenocarcinoma (4.5%), and melanoma (2.6%) followed. These figures showed the time trends in gynecological malignancies for cancer etiology, diagnosis, and treatment.

Uterine cervical cancer was the most frequent gynecologic cancer in Japan in the 1950s and 1960s. The Japan Society of Obstetrics and Gynecology (JSOG) started registration of uterine cancer in 1952. The number of registration hospitals is about 200, and the rate covered is estimated from the number of deaths among these hospitals and that of all Japan to be 38.5% of the population. Number of patients registered in the annual reports is shown in Table I. A more detailed national survey was also conducted by a subcommittee of JSOG of expert gynecologists for patients treated in 1983. Patient data in a standardized format, including age, histologic diagnosis, clini-

---

* Manuscript was prepared by Takahiko Sonoda, Department of Gynecology, National Cancer Center Hospital, and Naohito Yamaguchi, Cancer Information and Epidemiology Division, National Cancer Center Research Institute, 5-1-1 Tsukiji, Chuo-ku, Tokyo 104, Japan

TABLE I. Number of Patients with Uterine Cervical Cancer and Their Clinical Stage by Year

Period	Stage I	Stage II	Stage III	Stage IV	Total
1953–57	2,909 (21)	5,319 (39)	4,268 (31)	1,226 (9)	13,722 (100)
1958–62	3,885 (23)	6,792 (40)	5,052 (30)	1,094 (7)	16,823 (100)
1963–67	5,905 (29)	8,214 (40)	5,458 (27)	891 (4)	20,468 (100)
1968–72	7,252 (37)	7,458 (38)	4,442 (22)	698 (4)	19,850 (100)
1973–77	9,264 (53)	5,899 (34)	2,207 (13)	118 (7)	17,488 (100)
1978–82	11,395 (44)	7,709 (30)	5,465 (21)	1,083 (4)	25,652 (100)
1983	2,476 (47)	1,572 (30)	1,034 (19)	240 (5)	5,322 (100)
1991	2,477 (56)	1,071 (24)	635 (14)	214 (5)	4,397 (100)

From JSOG. Percent in parenthesis.

cal and post-surgical stages, method of treatment and prognosis were sent to the JSOG tumor committee, and 4,663 patients were registered. So, for uterine cervical cancer two sources of information are dealt with in this report, one is an annual report and the other is the national survey.

Uterine corpus cancer and ovarian cancer have also been registered because of their increasing trends in Japan. In addition to the annual reports to JSOG from the hospitals, a more detailed national survey was conducted in 1983 for patients with corpus cancer treated between 1966 and 1976 to learn their prognosis. Two national surveys were conducted for patients with ovarian cancer treated from 1971 to 1977 and from 1978 to 1983. Recently uterine corpus cancer has accounted for about 30% of all uterine cancer. In 1994, vulvar cancer was first registered to determine the status of this rare disease.

The Tumor Registration Committee was reorganized in 1993, and the above gynecological malignancies are now being registered by a new format from JSOG gynecologists in the member hospitals listed at the end of this book.

Uterine Cervical Cancer

The number of registered uterine cervical cancers was 4,000–5,000 in the 1960s but was only half that in the 1980s, reflecting a substantial decreasing trend in incidence (*3, 7*). Mortality of cervical cancer has also greatly decreased in Japan, being 6,373 in 1970, 5,465 in 1980, and 4,600 in 1990. This decrease is mainly due to early detection of the disease. Doctors of JSOG and the Japan Association of Obstetricians and Gynecologists cooperate in the mass screening program, which has been conducted by the government since 1961. This program asks that women over the age of 35 have a pap smear test, and about 20% of the target population is believed to have this examination (*3*). According to the Japanese Cancer Association, the number screened for cervical cancer was more than 4 million from 1986 to 1994. Health education for women alerted them to cervical cancer, and resulted in an increased proportion of early cervical cancer discovery (Fig. 1). Stage I cervical cancer in the recent registry accounted for 56% of all cases (Table I). The 1988 JSOG survey showed that patients detected by mass screening at an earlier stage had a higher 5-year survival rate than those found at hospital. The proportion of carcinoma *in situ* (CIS) in the former group was 50.0%, Stage I 40.7%, Stage II 7.5%, and Stages III

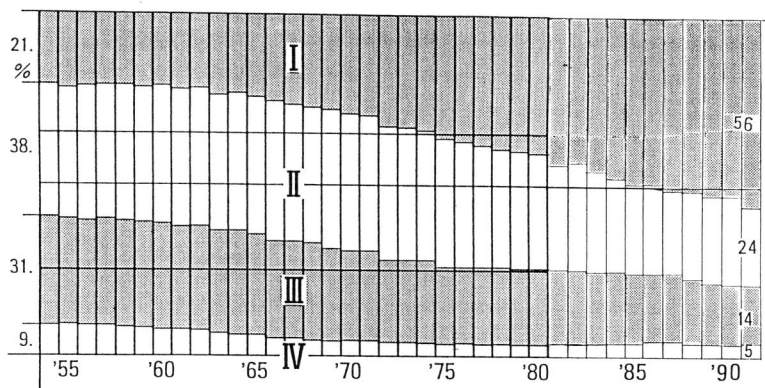

FIG. 1. Trend of stage distribution (%) of cervical cancer (JSOG Annual Report)

TABLE II. Treatment of Uterine Cervical Cancer by Stage

Stage	Conization	TAH	MRH	ARH	Exenteration	Operation rate (%)
0	87	813	317	7	—	98.7
Ia	5	168	404	63	—	91.0
Ib	—	54	102	674	—	
II	—	7	32	636	1	63.8
III	—	2	—	35	2	5.4
IV[a]	—	—	2	5	1	5.2

From the National Survey for patients treated in 1983.
TAH: total abdominal hysterectomy. MRH: modified radical hysterectomy. ARH: abdominal radical hysterectomy. Exenteration: resection of pelvic organ.
[a] Multidisciplinary treatment is usual.

TABLE III. Radiation Therapy for Uterine Cervical Cancer by Stage

Stage	n	External radiotherapy						Intra-cavitary irradiation
		<29 Gy	30–39 Gy	40–49 Gy	50–59 Gy	60< Gy	Subtotal	
0	15	1	—	2	4	1	8	13
Ia	12	—	—	3	3	3	9	11
Ib	136	3	11	38	66	8	126	128
II	385	7	19	67	221	67	381	357
III	717	21	30	134	353	169	707	650
IV	144	8	7	19	65	41	140	111
Total	1,409	40	67	263	712	289	1,371	1,270

Number of patients with only external radiation is 139, only intracavitary irradiation 38, and both 1,231. From the National Survey for patients treated in 1983.

and IV 1.1%. In the hospital group, CIS was 20.0%, Stage I 32.1%, Stage II 25.2%, and Stages III + IV 17.2%.

The average patient age rose from 1966 to 1983: during 1966–1968 it was between 40 and 65, but in 1983 it was 40 to 75. Longer life expectancy is the reason for this change. Older patients were usually found in an advanced stage, so their mortality rate was inevitably high.

The general principle of cervical cancer treatment is surgical resection for Stage I and II patients, and radiotherapy for Stages III and IV. Rate of operation for Stage I patients was 91%, Stage II was 63.8%, and Stage III was 5.4% (Tables II and III). Intracavitary radiation therapy was often used for Stage II and III patients. The 5-year survival by stage has been relatively stable during the 20 years from 1974 to 1994 (Fig. 2). Slight improvement is observed in Stage III patients. Overall 5-year survival was 66.5%, although Stage I patients showed 82.8% actuarial survival. Ten-year survival differed only slightly (about 5% less) from the 5-year survival rate, because of early detection and treatment and improved care to prevent complications. Administration of new anti-cancer drugs and more accurate diagnosis for the spread of cancer by new imaging techniques such as ultrasonography, computed tomography, and magnetic resonance imaging have contributed to the improvement of survival data.

Medical data such as age, clinical and post-surgical stage, histological diagnosis, and prognosis of registered patients are analyzed and the results are reported in the *Acta Obstetrica et Gynecologica Japonica* by the JSOG Committee every year (4). In addition to these reports, the results of the national survey are periodically published with the support of a Grant-in-Aid for Cancer Research from the Ministry of Health and Welfare. Each volume contains various data on past history, pathology of surgical materials, method of treatment, complications before and after the treatment, and recurrence data including sites.

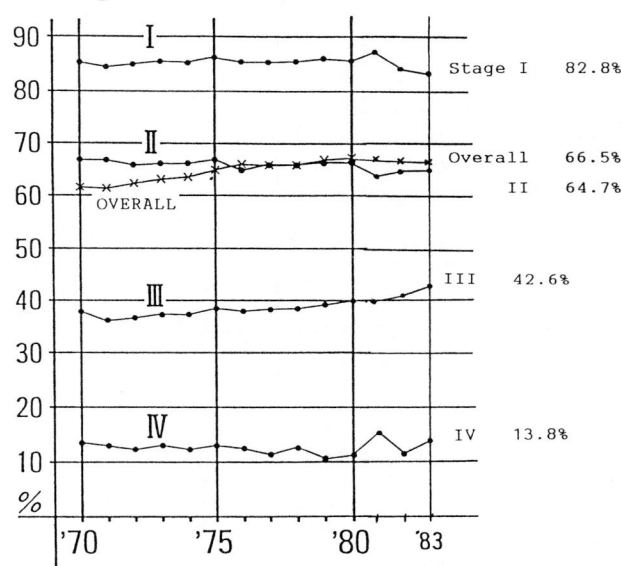

FIG. 2. Trend of five-year survival of cervical cancer by stage (JSOG Annual Report)

TABLE IV. Five-year Survival Rate (%) of Uterine Cervical Cancer Patients

Stage	n	1	2	3	4	5 years
I	1,242	99.6	98.1	96.7	95.8	94.8
II	855	95.3	88.3	83.5	80.6	77.5
III	608	86.1	73.6	63.6	59.2	53.4
IV	105	59.8	36.2	27.6	24.6	23.8

From the National Survey for patients treated in 1983. n(I–IV) = 2,810.

TABLE V. Time Trends in Five-year Survival Rate (%) of Cervical Cancer Patients by Stage

Period	Stage I	Stage II	Stage III	Stage IV	Total
1953–57	77.5	57.5	29.2	9.9	48.7
1958–62	80.4	63.8	32.0	14.0	54.8
1963–67	83.5	65.9	36.2	10.7	60.6
1968–72	86.6	66.4	36.9	13.3	65.3
1973–77	86.2	66.3	38.3	11.7	66.2
1978–82	86.1	66.1	41.1	13.7	67.5
1983	82.8	64.7	42.6	13.8	66.5

TABLE VI. Survival Rate (%) of Uterine Cervical Cancer Patients by Histological Diagnosis

Histology	n	1	2	3	4	5 years
Squamous cell carcinoma	2,592	94.5	88.7	84.6	82.3	79.7
Adenocarcinoma	185	87.9	79.3	69.3	66.3	63.0
Adenosquamous carcinoma	44	91.3	72.6	62.9	63.5	58.2

From the National Survey for patients in 1983. n(I–IV 2,810 + CIS11) = 2,821.

The prognosis of patients by stage in 1983 and time trend are shown in Tables IV and V. Five-year survival of Stage I patients was 94.8%, Stage II 77.5%, Stage III 53.4%, and Stage IV 23.8%. Survival rate by histological diagnosis that year is shown in Table VI. Five-year survival rates were 79.7% in squamous cell carcinoma, 63.0% in adenocarcinoma, and 58.2% in adenosquamous carcinoma. The stage distribution by histology of the cervical cancer from the 1983 data was as follows: squamous cell carcinoma was composed of 26.8% CIS, 45.4% Stage I, 29.5% Stage II, 21.2% Stage III, and 4.1% Stage IV; in adenocarcinoma it was 3.1% in CIS, 49.9% in Stage I, 31.7% in Stage II, 14.2% in Stage III, and 4.1% in Stage IV. The 5-year survival of squamous cell carcinoma *vs.* adenocarcinoma was 90.1% *vs.* 86.2% in Stage I, 73.7% *vs.* 56.0% in Stage II, 42.9% *vs.* 25.5% in Stage III. The poor prognosis of Stage II and III adenocarcinoma was remarkable and presumably explains the poor prognosis of cervical adenocarcinoma in general. Number of cases of stump cancer of the cervix was 340 out of 13,004 cases of squamous cell carcinoma (2.61%), while that of adenocarcinoma was 33 out of 795 (4.15%).

The difference in the occurrence of stump cancer was significant by chi-square test ($\chi^2 = 6.7$). Location of the lesion may explain this difference, since the adenocarcinoma was more frequent in the cervical canal.

Carcinoma of the Corpus Uteri

The number of corpus cancers is increasing in Japan (*3, 5, 7*). About 4,500 corpus carcinomas were estimated in 1990 with 1,034 deaths from this cause. About 75% of all corpus cancer in Japan occurs after age 50: 5.7% in the under 39-year old category, 6.6% from age 40 to 44, 11.5% from age 45 to 49, 68.1% from age 50 to 69, 5.5% from age 70 to 74, 2.0% from age 75 to 79, and 0.7% over age 80; 21.1% occurred in pre-menopausal period, 5.3% in climacteric, 69.0% in post-menopausal state, and 4.4% was unknown for menstruation.

About three fourths of corpus carcinoma was found to be 75% at Stage I and 15%

TABLE VII. Number of Patients with Corpus Carcinoma by Stage and Year

Period	Stage I	Stage II	Stage III	Stage IV	Total
1953–62	307 (69)	87 (20)	41 (9)	7 (2)	442 (100)
1963–72	410 (74)	82 (15)	45 (8)	15 (3)	552 (100)
1973–82	568 (65)	192 (22)	75 (9)	36 (4)	871 (100)
1983	542 (71)	140 (18)	54 (7)	31 (4)	767 (100)

Percent in parenthesis.

TABLE VIII. Survival Rates (%) of Patients with Corpus Carcinoma

Stage	n	1	2	3	4	5 years
I	1,372	95.4	91.3	89.2	87.6	84.8
G1	720	96.7	93.6	91.9	91.2	89.0
G2	240	94.8	91.7	90.4	86.7	83.0
G3	107	87.2	77.2	68.4	66.9	65.1
G(unknown)	365	95.6	90.4	89.0	87.0	83.8
II	324	90.5	78.3	71.6	68.8	65.2
III	164	73.0	57.8	48.4	44.4	42.6
IV	63	38.0	21.6	18.2	13.0	13.0
Overall	1,983	87.7	81.4	78.0	75.9	73.3

Stage I was further subclassified by G grade.
From the National Survey for patients treated from 1966 to 1976.

TABLE IX. Five-year Survival Rate (%) of Corpus Cancer Patients by Year

Period	Stage I	Stage II	Stage III	Stage IV	Total
1953–62	79.8	51.7	24.4	0.0	67.6
1963–72	84.9	59.8	46.7	20.0	76.3
1973–82	87.5	74.0	46.7	5.6	77.3
1983	79.0	65.0	46.3	9.7	71.3

TABLE X. Five-year Survival Rates (%) of Corpus Carcinoma by Various Prognostic Factors

	G1	G2	G3
Lymph node involvement			
0	89.1	86.5	73.9
1	4.7	6.2	6.5
2,3	4.0	5.1	7.6
4<	2.3	2.2	12.0
Depth of muscle invasion			
superficial	22.1	21.9	12.1
<1/3	53.2	52.9	43.9
1/3–2/3	12.8	13.9	14.6
2/3<	11.9	11.2	29.3
Location of the lesion			
Fundus	45.9	45.2	35.9
Side wall	21.2	22.8	16.3
Isthmus	3.9	4.2	6.5
Fundus-Isthmus	29.2	27.9	41.3
Size of tumor			
≦8 cm	94.5	88.6	68.2
>8 cm	93.1	82.7	61.5

From the National Survey for patients treated from 1966 to 1976.

TABEL XI. Frequency of Cervical Involvement of Corpus Carcinoma (%) by Clinical Stage and Histological Grade

	I (G1)	I (G2)	I (G3)	I (G?)	II	III	IV	Overall
Cervix (−)	628	187	82	284	71	46	8	1,306
Cervix (+)	31	14	8	16	176	47	6	298
Cervix (unknown)	41	19	11	42	40	15	8	176
Positive %	4.8	7.0	8.9	5.3	71.3	51.7	42.9	18.6

From the National Survey for patients treated from 1966 to 1976.

at Stage II (Table VII). So-called corpus cancer syndrome like hypertension, obesity, diabetes mellitus or heredity was not significantly observed among Japanese patients.

The prognosis of corpus cancer ranged from 84.8% to 13% by stage and grade, 73.3% on the average (Tables VIII and IX). Grade 3 group showed the poorest prognosis among G1, G2, and G3 (Table VIII).

The 5-year survival rate of corpus carcinoma is shown in Table III. As Stage I and II patients were 90%, the resultant overall survival rate is better than that of cervical cancer.

Corpus carcinoma is usually resistant to irradiation and surgical operation is carried out even for Stage III and IV patients: 67.1% of Stage III and 33.3% of Stage IV patients. Preoperative irradiation, teletherapy, or brachytherapy has rarely been employed. After evaluation of the surgical specimen, post-operative irradiation is planned for cases with deep muscle invasion, positive lymph node metastasis, positive vaginal stump, and cervical involvement in whom the radial operation has been unsuccessful.

Various prognostic factors and 5-year survival rates are shown in Table X. Since almost all cases were of endometrial adenocarcinoma and belong to Stage I or II, the grade becomes the most important prognostic factor. Stage migration from clinical Stage I to Stage II (pTII) is not rare in G3 cancer which often locates at the isthmus. Radical hysterectomy should be employed in cases which have reached that stage. Incidental cervical involvement of corpus cancer is shown in Table XI.

Ovarian Cancer

The number of ovarian cancer deaths in Japan was 1,129 in 1970, 2,098 in 1980, and 3,297 in 1990, while the estimated number of patients with the condition was 1,700, 3,510, and 6,030, respectively (*6, 7*). Rapid increase of the disease was thus noteworthy during the last 10 year period. Number of ovarian cancer patients registered between 1971 and 1977 was 1,060, and that between 1978 and 1983 was 1,311. Total registered as of 1991 was 1,954: 184 low potential malignancy, 169 germ cell tumors, 1,291 adenocarcinoma, 31 dermoid carcinoma, 49 embryonal cancer, and others, including 166 metastatic cancer cases.

Age of these patients was characteristic. Average age of embryocarcinoma, dysgerminoma, and immature teratoma was in the 20s, that of adenocarcinoma was 40 to 50 years, and that of sarcoma was in the 60s (Table XII).

The clinical FIGO stage distribution of the patients treated during 1971 and 1977 and of those during 1978–1983 was almost the same. In the former period,

TABLE XII. Age and Relative 5-Year Survival Rates (%) in Ovarian Cancer Registry

Histology	n	Average age	Survival rate
LPM serous	40	49.6 ± 15.6	96.2
mucinous	121	49.5 ± 17.4	100.9
endometrioid	1	51.0	101.7
clear cell	2	55.5 ± 3.5	—
Pseudomyxoma peritonei	20	56.5 ± 10.1	59.4
Dysgerminoma	57	24.3 ± 9.9	81.1
Granulosa cell tumor	62	46.5 ± 15.6	77.1
Stromal cell tumor	7	34.4 ± 19.4	102.9
Immature teratoma	31	24.1 ± 10.5	87.7
Other germ cell tumor	12	54.4 ± 19.7	99.0
Adenocarcinoma, NOS	186	52.2 ± 12.8	35.3
serous	576	51.8 ± 12.0	42.6
mucinous	238	46.9 ± 15.5	64.9
endometrioid	122	48.7 ± 10.6	51.9
clear cell	119	50.5 ± 10.2	45.7
Undifferentiated carcinoma	50	54.1 ± 11.7	28.7
Dermoid carcinoma	31	44.5 ± 16.8	48.0
Embryonal carcinoma A[a]	29	22.0	100.0 (4 years)
B	6	25.3 ± 10.7	28.3
C	13	26.0 ± 7.4	83.6
NOS	1	28.3	
Choriocarcinoma	0		
Sarcoma	9	63.7 ± 5.6	31.0 (4 years)
Metastatic carcinoma	166	44.7 ± 11.0	13.2
Others	24	26.5 ± 11.4	69.1
Unknown	31	53.0 ± 15.7	24.5
Total	1,954		

LPM: low potential malignancy. NOS: not otherwise specified.
From the National Survey for patients treated from 1978 to 1983.
[a] JSOG classification.

39.1% were in Stage I, 17.3% in Stage II, 32.6% in Stage III, and 11.6% in Stage IV, and in the latter period, 38.9%, 16.2%, 33.9%, and 11.6%, respectively.

The relative 5-year survival rate of the completely resected cases was 66–69%, and that of the incompletely resected patients was 16–19%. In completely resected cases, relative 5-year survival rates were 66–69%. Patients with incomplete resection showed poor prognosis; their 5-year survival rates were 19% and 16%, respectively, in the two terms. It is clear that the complete surgical operation is mandatory in the management of ovarian cancer. Total abdominal hysterectomy and bilateral salpingo-ophorectomy are essential and curative for Stage I and II patients. Staging or second-look operation to determine the effectiveness of prior treatment is useful.

The migration from Stage I or II to III was 5.9% and 32.3%, respectively, mostly due to unexpected retroperitoneal lymph node metastases. The development of radical surgery for Stage III patients is important. *Cis*-platin containing regimen is strongly effective for adjuvant chemotherapy. The CDDP containing regimens were administered to 393 out of 1,511 patients with ovarian malignancies in this series (The National Survey of Ovarian Cancer in 1992 by JSOG). The number of patients is not sufficient to analyze the chemotherapeutic effect at the present time.

The survival rates of ovarian cancer by histological types and stage are shown in

TABLE XIII. Five-year Survival Rates (%) of Ovarian Cancer by Histology

	n	1	2	3	4	5 years
Cystadenocarcinoma, NOS						
Stage I	50	89.6	79.6	71.9	71.9	71.9
II	31	82.5	61.8	61.8	56.9	56.9
III	70	58.8	37.6	25.5	12.7	9.9
IV	23	52.4	29.1	23.3	16.6	—
Serous cystadenocarcinoma						
Stage I	181	92.3	86.2	82.8	78.1	78.1
II	84	89.9	73.0	67.0	54.6	51.1
III	225	73.6	44.5	28.9	22.5	16.9
IV	83	51.3	24.1	17.2	13.2	13.2
Mucinous cystadenocarcinoma						
Stage I	140	93.0	90.1	90.1	86.7	86.7
II	26	87.7	64.0	51.8	51.8	51.8
III	46	66.3	36.3	23.1	23.1	11.5
IV	15	42.9	25.7	17.1	17.1	17.1
Endometrioid carcinoma						
Stage I	50	97.9	81.8	78.5	78.5	78.5
II	23	86.3	76.5	70.8	63.3	50.7
III	33	63.1	42.6	34.1	28.4	28.4
IV	11	36.4	15.6	15.6	—	—
Clear cell carcinoma						
Stage I	53	91.9	75.4	69.4	69.4	69.4
II	30	85.7	67.7	60.2	45.1	45.1
III	27	60.8	26.1	15.6	7.8	7.8
IV	5	60.0	36.0	36.0	—	—
Unclassified carcinoma						
Stage I	6	100.0	100.0	75.0	45.0	—
II	10	80.0	58.8	58.8	45.6	45.6
III	25	56.5	25.7	25.7	25.7	25.7
IV	9	41.2	13.7	13.7	—	—

From the National Survey for patients treated from 1978 to 1983.

TABLE XIV. Number of Patients with Ovarian Cancer by Histology and Stage and Their 5-Year Survival Rates

	Stage I	Stage II	Stage III	Stage IV
Dysgerminoma	32 (94)	8 (87)	6 (33)	5 (0)
Granulosa cell tumor	37 (83)	4 (61)	9 (69)	0
Stromal cell tumor	5 (100)	0	1	0
Immature teratoma	15 (100)	3 (67)	4 (72)	1
Dermoid carcinoma	14 (60)	4 (51)	9 (28)	0
Embryonal carcinoma A[a]	10 (31)	6 (45)	11 (24)	0
B	2 (100)	3 (100)	0	1
C	6 (46)	1 (0)	3 (0)	0
Sarcoma	1 (0)	2 (0)	4 (0)	0

Number of patients and 5-year survival rates (%).
From the National Survey for patients treated from 1978 to 1983.
[a] JSOG classification.

TABLE XV. Histological Distribution of Vulvar Carcinoma

Squamous cell carcinoma	228	73.3%
CIS	17	
poor to moderately differentiated	145	
well differentiated	66	
Adenocarcinoma	14	4.5%
adenocarcinoma	13	
adenosquamous carcinoma	1	
Melanoma	8	2.6%
Paget's disease	46	14.8%
Basal cell carcinoma	7	2.3%
Verrucous carcinoma	4	1.3%
Undifferentiated carcinoma	2	0.7%
Sarcoma	2	0.7%
Total	311	100.0%

Patients were treated between 1986 and 1988 in 133 registry hospitals.

Tables XIII and XIV. Clear cell carcinoma showed the poorest prognosis, although the cystadenocarcinoma showed 70% to 80% 5-year survival in Stage I. Most frequent histology of ovarian tumor was serous cystadenocarcinoma, and 300 cases out of 576 were found in Stage III or IV. It is noteworthy that more than half the cases with ovarian cancer were found at the advanced stage.

A multi-institutional study group has recently started a phase III study of retroperitoneal lymph node dissection in cytoreductive surgery. The effect of high dose chemotherapy as the phase III trial has been analyzed as well.

Carcinoma of the Vulva

The mortality rate of vulvar carcinoma was 0.19 per 100,000 females in 1990, while that of uterine cancer was 7.4; vulvar cancer is very rare in Japan as in most other countries. The Japan Vulvar Cancer Study Group collected the cases in 1975, and 259 cases treated between 1968 and 1970 were registered at that time. Patient age ranged from 25 to 94 with an average age of 60.9 ± 4.87 years. Number of patients by clinical stage was 7 in Stage 0, 66 in Stage I, 81 in Stage II, 67 in Stage III, and 38 in Stage IV.

The tumor committee of the JSOG planned to register the vulvar cancer again as well as other gynecological cancers in 1994 (Preliminary Report of the Vulvar Cancer in Japan, unpublished data). The preliminary registration was done by members of the uterine cancer registration committee to finalize the registration format. It covered age, histology, stage, type of treatment, and prognosis.

Survival rates have not yet been analyzed, so the histological frequency is shown in Table XV. Squamous cell carcinoma was the most frequent, with Paget's disease, adenocarcinoma, melanoma, and basal cell carcinoma following.

Choriocarcinoma

The JSOG tumor committee will take over registry of trophoblastic disease from the Trophoblastic Tumor Registry Committee in JSOG. Prof. T. Tomoda, Nagoya

University, was the chairman of the committee and twenty-two registry centers participate in the registry. The number of deaths from choriocarcinoma reached 300 in the 1960s but recently it has been less than 20 per year. Well established control for hydatidiform moles is believed to have contributed to this decrease. From January to December 1992 1,144 moles, 44 invasive moles, and 18 choriocarcinoma were registered.

Comments and Discussion

The mortality of uterine cervical cancer has been continuously decreasing in Japan, and this is believed to be the result of mass-screening to detect the condition early. The incidence rate of invasive cervical cancer is also decreasing, but early detection seems to be making the greatest contribution, because of the different proportion of clinical stage among mass-screenees and hospital patients. Improved hygiene in individual homes and the habit of taking a hot bath should also contribute to reducing incidence of this cancer. The increase of uterine corpus cancer and ovarian cancer, however, has become a problem. Westernization of dietary habits such as greater intake of animal protein and fat is thought to be the reason for this. As ovarian cancer is found at an advanced stage, development of a method for early detection is necessary. Ultrasonography has recently been employed by some doctors for mass-screening.

Choriocarcinoma has been separately registered in Nagoya University. The number of choriocarcinomas reached 300–500 a year in the 1960s but in recent years has been less than 30 (*2*). Well established control for hydatidiform moles is believed to have contributed to this decrease. The number of choriocarcinomas after hydatidiform mole decreased but that after normal delivery or abortion remains unchanged.

Acknowledgments

The Tumor Committee of the Japan Society of Obstetrics and Gynecology is grateful to the members who have contributed many years to the registry. The authors thank Dr. Shaw Watanabe, Chief of the Cancer Information and Epidemiology Division, National Cancer Center Research Institute, for his support of this work. A part of this work was supported by a Grant-in-Aid for Cancer Research from the Ministry of Health and Welfare of Japan.

REFERENCES

1. Suemori, U. Report of villous disease registry. *Jpn. J. Obst. Gynecol.*, **45**, 957–964 (1993) (in Japanese).
2. Suemasu, K. (ed.). The Report of the 5th Surveillance on Malignant Neoplasms. Sogo-Igaku-Sha, Tokyo, 1990 (in Japanese).
3. The Japan Society of Obstetrics and Gynecology. *Acta Obst. Gynecol. Jpn.*, **11** (1995) to **47** (1995) (in Japanese).
4. The Japan Society of Obstetrics and Gynecology. The National Survey of Uterine Cervical Cancer in Japan. Vol. 4 (1978), Vol. 5 (1988), and Vol. 6 (1995) (in Japanese).
5. The Japan Society of Obstetrics and Gynecology. The National Survey of Uterine Corpus Cancer in Japan. Vol. 1 (1980), Vol. 2 (1981), and Vol. 3 (1984) (in Japanese).

6. The Japan Society of Obstetrics and Gynecology. The National Survey of Malignant Ovarian Tumors in Japan. Vol. 1 (1980) and Vol. 2 (1982) (in Japanese).
7. Tominaga, S., Aoki, K., Fujimoto, I., and Kurihara, M. (eds.). "Cancer Mortality and Morbidity Statistics: Japan and the World — 1994," Gann Monograph on Cancer Research No. 41 (1994). Japan Sci. Soc. Press, Tokyo.
8. Watanabe S. Mass-screening program as a cancer control strategy. *Asian Med. J.*, **36**, 341–350 (1993).

STATISTICS OF BLADDER CANCER REGISTRY, 1982–1987

Bladder Cancer Registry, Japanese Urological Association*

Twelve thousand bladder cancer patients were registered by the Japanese Urological Association between 1982 and 1987. This was about one fourth of all new cases in Japan. About 60% of these patients were in clinical stage Tis-T1, whereas 13% in T2, 11% in T3, and 4% in T4. Surgical treatment for the primary tumor was TUC/TUR-Bt in 62.7%, radical cystectomy in 17.1%, simple cystectomy in 5.0%, and partial cystectomy in 4.5%. The ileal conduit has been commonly used, but the continent reservoir and the orthotopic neobladder have recently appeared. More than 60% patients received combined chemotherapy. Histological grades were about 40% in G2 and 25% in both G1 and G3. Five-year survival rates were 88.1% in G1, 77.8% in G2, and 48.1% in G3. In terms of pT, these were 83.1% in pT1, 62.3% in pT2, 47.7% in pT3a, 35.5% in pT3b, 28.3% in pT4a, and 18.7% in pT4b.

Bladder cancer has been the most common malignant disease of the urogenital tract in Japan. The estimated total number of new bladder cancer patients in 1990 was 8,400, 6,300 males and 2,100 females.

In 1980 the Japanese Urological Association and the Japanese Pathological Association jointly published the booklet "General Rules for Clinical and Pathological Studies of Bladder Cancer" which defined the biological characteristics, pathological findings, and treatment relating to each type of bladder cancer. On the basis of these guidelines, the Japanese Urological Association in 1982 established an annual register of new cases of bladder cancer in Japan. Since then, approximately 2,000 cases annually have been registered by around 200 hospitals. The central office for this project is located in the National Cancer Center to take advantage of the Center's main computer, and has since produced yearly data analyses and reports.

In 1991, the Japanese Urological Association published a Japanese summary of 12,000 bladder cancer patients registered between 1982 and 1987. This is an English translation of that summary, including survival data for the year 1982 which was reviewed for the first time in 1993.

Method of Registration

In November each year the Registration Office in the National Cancer Center mails registration forms to 674 institutions including university hospitals, national and other public hospitals, prefectural cancer centers and others for completion and

---

* Manuscript was prepared by Tadao Kakizoe, National Cancer Center Hospital, 5-1-1 Tsukiji, Chuo-ku, Tokyo 104, Japan

return. Those which are returned are checked by a specialist and, if they contain ambiguous descriptions or insufficient data, are sent back to the responsible institution for correction. The final accepted data then is coded and input into the main computer, analyzed, and an annual report prepared. The published report is distributed to all participating institutions and board members of the Japanese Urological Association in April of the following year.

Follow-up Study on Survival

Of 2,743 patients registered in 1982, data pertaining to 1,567 survivals (53%) was collected. Follow-up forms were sent in 1993 to the hospitals which cooperated in the 1982 registration, and 195 of them returned the completed forms. Survival statistics were calculated by actuarial SAS (Statistical Analysis System).

Summary of 1982 to 1987 Registered Cases

1. *Male to female ratios and age distribution of patients (Tables I and II)*

The annual, and highest, number of registered patients was 2,943 in 1982. Since then, about 2,000 patients have consistently been registered each year. The top age group is believed to be in the 60s, but in this series the 70–79 age group accounted for 30%, and the 60–69 age group 25–28%. The average male to female ratio of 77.4:22.6, *i.e.,* 3.4:1 has been constant for the past six years.

2. *Clinical diagnoses (data not shown)*

Papillary carcinoma accounted for an average 70.8% of cases and non-papillary carcinoma for an average 20.9%. There was no change in this ratio from 1982 to 1987.

TABLE I. Male to Female Ratio

	1982	1983	1984	1985	1986	1987
Male	2,257 (76.7)	1,616 (77.3)	2,081 (76.5)	1,581 (77.6)	1,570 (79.0)	1,679 (77.3)
Female	686 (23.3)	474 (22.7)	640 (23.5)	457 (22.4)	417 (21.0)	492 (22.7)
Total	2,943	2,090	2,721	2,038	1,987	2,171

Number in parentheses shows percentage.

TABLE II. Age Distribution

Age	1982	1983	1984	1985	1986	1987
0–9	2 (0.1)	—	—	—	—	—
10–19	6 (0.2)	1 (0.0)	3 (0.1)	2 (0.1)	2 (0.1)	1 (0.0)
20–29	22 (0.7)	24 (1.1)	15 (0.6)	21 (1.1)	21 (1.1)	11 (0.5)
30–39	105 (3.6)	67 (3.2)	84 (3.1)	69 (3.4)	60 (3.0)	61 (2.8)
40–49	176 (6.0)	151 (7.2)	177 (6.5)	127 (6.2)	127 (6.4)	143 (6.6)
50–59	581 (19.7)	435 (20.8)	534 (19.6)	426 (20.9)	379 (19.1)	382 (17.6)
60–69	850 (28.9)	603 (28.9)	772 (28.4)	523 (25.7)	534 (26.9)	604 (27.8)
70–79	915 (31.1)	605 (28.9)	858 (31.5)	638 (31.3)	633 (31.9)	726 (33.4)
80–	286 (9.7)	204 (9.8)	278 (10.2)	232 (11.4)	231 (11.6)	243 (11.2)
Total	2,943	2,090	2,721	2,038	1,987	2,171

TABLE III. Clinical T Classification

Stage	1982	1983	1984	1985	1986	1987
Tis	54 (1.8)	56 (2.7)	64 (2.4)	47 (2.3)	54 (2.7)	75 (3.5)
Ta	590 (20.0)	376 (18.0)	473 (17.4)	388 (19.0)	335 (16.9)	421 (19.4)
T0	47 (1.6)	45 (2.2)	31 (1.1)	49 (2.4)	17 (0.9)	35 (1.6)
T1	1,026 (34.9)	723 (34.6)	968 (35.6)	758 (37.2)	781 (39.3)	831 (38.3)
Tis-T1	1,717 (58.3)	1,200 (57.4)	1,536 (56.4)	1,242 (60.9)	1,187 (59.7)	1,362 (62.7)
T2	368 (12.5)	292 (14.0)	354 (13.0)	272 (13.3)	281 (14.1)	287 (13.2)
T3a	222 (7.5)	153 (7.3)	225 (8.3)	158 (7.8)	130 (6.5)	143 (6.6)
T3b	161 (5.5)	113 (5.4)	157 (5.8)	119 (5.8)	133 (6.7)	106 (4.9)
T4a	71 (2.4)	64 (3.1)	82 (3.0)	54 (2.6)	44 (2.2)	53 (2.4)
T4b	44 (1.5)	36 (1.7)	39 (1.4)	38 (1.9)	36 (1.8)	32 (1.5)
T2-T4b	866 (29.4)	658 (31.5)	857 (31.5)	641 (31.5)	624 (31.4)	621 (28.6)
TX	360 (12.2)	232 (11.1)	328 (12.1)	155 (7.6)	176 (8.9)	188 (8.7)
Total	2,943	2,090	2,721	2,038	1,987	2,171

TABLE IV. Surgery for Primary Cancer

Surgery	1982	1983	1984	1985	1986	1987
None	251 (8.5)	141 (6.7)	241 (7.9)	149 (7.3)	145 (7.3)	181 (8.3)
TUC/TUR-Bt	1,764 (59.9)	1,260 (60.3)	1,581 (58.1)	1,275 (62.6)	1,274 (64.1)	1,362 (62.7)
SVR[a]	72 (2.4)	26 (1.2)	47 (1.7)	22 (1.1)	23 (1.2)	25 (1.2)
Partial cystectomy	274 (9.3)	166 (7.9)	192 (7.1)	108 (5.3)	94 (4.7)	98 (4.5)
Subtotal cystectomy	4 (0.1)	13 (0.6)	7 (0.3)	5 (0.2)	5 (0.3)	3 (0.1)
Simple cystectomy	229 (7.8)	164 (7.8)	233 (8.6)	125 (6.1)	90 (4.5)	109 (5.0)
Radical cystectomy	313 (10.6)	288 (13.8)	410 (15.1)	321 (15.8)	330 (16.6)	371 (17.1)
Pelvic exenteration	2 (0.1)	1 (0.0)	3 (0.1)	5 (0.2)	3 (0.2)	—
Others	32 (1.1)	28 (1.3)	32 (1.2)	27 (1.3)	18 (0.9)	20 (0.9)
Not identified	2 (0.1)	3 (0.1)	2 (0.1)	1 (0.0)	5 (0.3)	2 (0.1)
Total	2,943	2,090	2,721	2,038	1,987	2,171

[a] SVR: supravesical resection.

Carcinoma *in situ* (CIS) accounted for 1.7% in 1982 but gradually increased to 3.1% in 1987. It is difficult to judge from the data whether this increase in CIS was due to an actual increase in patients or was a diagnostic increase in line with rule book definition and broadening recognition in Japan of the concept of CIS.

3. *Clinical classification (Table III)*

The most frequent T stage annually was T1 (34–39%). When Tis, Ta, T0, and T1 were combined as superficial bladder cancers, the total increased to 56.4–62.7% (mean 59.1%). Invasive bladder cancer such as T2-T4b accounted for 28.6–31.5% (mean 30.6%).

4. *Clinical N classification (data not shown)*

In this series, superficial bladder cancer accounted for more than half the total cases. Consequently, N0 accounted for 44.2–56.1% and NX was 40.6–52.3% of such cases.

5. *Clinical M classification* (*data not shown*)

There were 4.0–7.4% M1 cases. Distant metastases to bones accounted for 16.4%, to the lungs 11.8%, and to the intestinal tract/liver 3.6%.

6. *Surgery for primary cancer* (*Table IV*)

TUC/TUR-Bt were the most commonly performed operations (mean, 61.0%). The number of radical cystectomies gradually increased from 10.6% in 1982 to 17.1% in 1987. No surgery was performed in 7.7% of cases, but it is unclear whether this was due to excessively advanced cancer or to the patient's general physical condition.

7. *Urinary diversion* (*Table V*)

An annual average 24.6% of patients underwent urinary diversion. This was a little higher than the 21.4% resulting from simple and radical cystectomy. The difference may be accounted for by the cases which underwent urinary diversion alone.

TABLE V. Urinary Diversion

Diversion	1982	1983	1984	1985	1986	1987
Conducted	658 (22.4)	536 (25.7)	738 (27.2)	494 (24.3)	466 (23.5)	524 (24.3)
Not conducted	2,279 (77.6)	1,547 (74.3)	1,971 (72.8)	1,538 (75.7)	1,513 (76.5)	1,629 (75.7)
Not determined	6	7	12	6	8	18
Nephrostomy	16 (2.4)	10 (1.9)	16 (2.2)	15 (3.0)	25 (5.4)	23 (4.4)
Ureterostomy	262 (39.8)	215 (40.1)	316 (42.8)	178 (36.0)	150 (32.2)	148 (28.2)
Ileal conduit	303 (46.0)	261 (48.7)	354 (48.0)	267 (54.0)	236 (50.6)	272 (51.9)
Colonic conduit	14 (2.1)	2 (0.4)	11 (1.5)	8 (1.6)	3 (0.6)	10 (1.9)
Ureterosigmoidostomy	34 (5.2)	24 (4.5)	27 (3.7)	11 (2.2)	10 (2.1)	10 (1.9)
Rectal bladder	2 (0.3)	1 (0.2)	5 (0.7)	—	—	—
Others	27 (4.1)	23 (4.3)	9 (1.2)	15 (3.0)	42 (9.0)	61 (11.7)
Total	658	536	738	494	466	524

TABLE VI. Pathological T Classification

Age	1982	1983	1984	1985	1986	1987
pTis	65 (2.3)	49 (2.4)	62 (2.3)	51 (2.5)	50 (2.5)	66 (3.1)
pTa	651 (22.7)	447 (21.5)	536 (19.9)	452 (22.5)	399 (20.3)	460 (21.3)
pT0	49 (1.7)	28 (1.3)	36 (1.3)	43 (2.1)	34 (1.7)	27 (1.3)
pT1	862 (30.1)	677 (32.6)	901 (33.5)	650 (32.4)	658 (33.5)	762 (35.3)
pTis-pT1	1,627 (56.8)	1,201 (57.9)	1,535 (57.1)	1,196 (59.6)	1,141 (58.1)	1,315 (61.0)
pT2	313 (10.9)	202 (9.7)	227 (8.4)	178 (8.9)	172 (8.8)	191 (8.9)
pT3a	164 (5.7)	123 (5.9)	140 (5.2)	94 (4.7)	91 (4.6)	107 (5.0)
pT3b	135 (4.7)	115 (5.5)	170 (6.3)	122 (6.1)	117 (6.0)	102 (4.7)
pT4a	66 (2.3)	51 (2.5)	51 (1.9)	48 (2.4)	36 (1.8)	37 (1.7)
pT4b	49 (1.7)	34 (1.6)	45 (1.7)	38 (1.9)	26 (1.3)	30 (1.4)
pT2-pT4b	727 (25.4)	525 (25.3)	633 (23.5)	480 (23.9)	442 (22.5)	467 (21.7)
Others	10 (0.3)	3 (0.1)	7 (0.3)	2 (0.1)	6 (0.3)	6 (0.3)
pTX	498 (17.4)	346 (16.7)	514 (19.1)	330 (16.4)	376 (19.1)	368 (17.1)
Total	2,862	2,075	2,689	2,008	1,965	2,158

Nephrostomy was an almost constant average 3.2%. Ureterocutaneostomy accounted for a mean of 37.3% but decreased remarkably in 1986 and 1987. The ileal conduit was utilized in a mean 49.6% of cases, indicating that this had been accepted as the most reliable urinary diversion in Japan. There was a sharp decrease in uterosigmoidostomy from 5.2% in 1982 to 1.9% in 1987. Miscellaneous urinary diversions accounted for a mean of 5.1% but increased sharply in 1986 (8.8%) and 1987 (11.1%), probably indicating the spread of continent urinary reservoir and orthotopic neobladder.

8. Pathological T classification (Table VI)

Superficial bladder cancer, such as pTis-pT1, accounted for 56.8–61.0% of cases, not much different from that of clinical T, whereas invasive bladder cancer such as pT2-pT4b accounted for 28.6–31.5%. The difference between clinical T and pathological T is attributable to the increase in pTX(16.4–19.1%).

9. Predominant histological grade (Table VII)

G2 was predominant throughout the subject period and accounted for between

TABLE VII. Predominant Histological Grade

Grade	1982	1983	1984	1985	1986	1987
G0	86 (3.0)	47 (2.3)	77 (2.9)	48 (2.4)	50 (2.5)	34 (1.6)
G1	747 (26.1)	555 (26.7)	644 (23.9)	513 (25.5)	469 (23.9)	532 (24.7)
G2	1,087 (38.7)	802 (38.7)	1,055 (39.0)	835 (41.6)	842 (42.8)	897 (41.6)
G3	732 (25.6)	537 (25.9)	716 (26.6)	514 (25.6)	485 (24.7)	554 (25.7)
Combination of any G	189 (6.6)	134 (6.5)	202 (7.5)	98 (4.8)	119 (6.0)	139 (6.4)
Total	2,862	2,075	2,689	2,008	1,965	2,156

TABLE VIII. Radiotherapy

Radiotherapy	1982	1983	1984	1985	1986	1987
Conducted	383 (13.5)	322 (15.7)	327 (12.3)	248 (12.4)	260 (13.4)	262 (12.3)
with surgery	371	282	278	209	211	215
without surgery	12	39	49	38	48	46
Not conducted	2,454 (86.5)	1,725 (84.3)	2,331 (87.7)	1,751 (87.6)	1,677 (86.6)	1,872 (87.7)
Not determined	106	43	63	39	50	37
Total	2,837	2,047	2,685	1,999	1,937	2,134

TABLE IX. Chemotherapy

Chemotherapy	1982	1983	1984	1985	1986	1987
Conducted	1,858 (66.5)	1,328 (64.2)	1,777 (65.8)	1,263 (62.2)	1,246 (63.1)	1,336 (61.9)
with surgery	1,817	1,263	1,675	1,192	1,182	1,252
without surgery	40	64	101	71	61	83
Not conducted	935 (33.5)	742 (35.8)	922 (34.2)	769 (37.8)	729 (36.9)	822 (38.1)
Not determined	150	20	22	6	12	13
Total	2,793	2,070	2,699	2,032	1,975	2,158

38.7 and 42.8%. G3 remained at an almost constant value of about 25%, which is similar to that of pT2-pT4b.

10. Radiotherapy (Table VIII)

An almost constant 12.3–15.7% of patients underwent radiotherapy during the period under review. In most cases this was as a modality combined with surgery. There were 37–106 cases annually in which treatment with radiotherapy was undetermined, indicating a somewhat negative credibility of such data.

11. Chemotherapy (Table IX)

Chemotherapy was administered to 61.9–66.5% of patients, a majority of whom also underwent surgery. Most of these patients probably had superficial bladder cancer because, as Table III indicates, 60% of cases were of the superficial type, in which cases the chemotherapy applied may have been intravesical instillation therapy. The application of chemotherapy gradually decreased from 66.5% in 1982 to 61.9% in 1987, which probably indicates the increasing popularity of BCG instillation therapy.

TABLE X. Predominant Grade and Survival

Grade	No. of patients	Survival (%)				
		1	2	3	4	5 years
G0	26	100.0	100.0	100.0	100.0	100.0
G1	422	95.7 (93.7–97.7)[a]	94.9 (92.7–97.1)	92.6 (89.9–95.2)	90.4 (87.4–93.4)	88.1 (84.7–91.5)
G2	650	93.9 (92.0–95.8)	88.0 (85.3–90.6)	83.0 (79.9–86.1)	80.1 (76.8–83.5)	77.8 (74.2–81.3)
G3	389	75.2 (70.8–79.6)	59.8 (54.6–64.9)	55.9 (50.7–61.2)	49.5 (44.2–54.9)	48.1 (42.7–53.5)
GX	80	77.4 (68.0–86.9)	73.0 (62.9–83.1)	68.4 (57.6–79.1)	68.4 (57.6–79.1)	61.8 (50.3–73.3)

[a] 95% confidence limit.

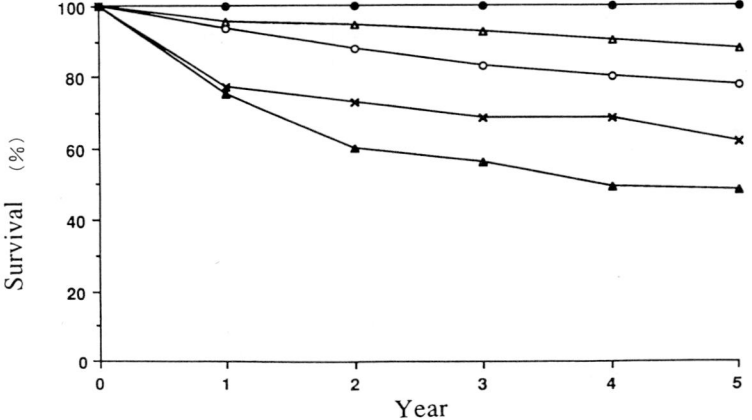

FIG. 1. Survival according to the most predominant grade
● G0, △ G1, ○ G2, ▲ G3, × GX.

TABLE XI. Pathological T Classification (pT) and Survival[a]

Depth of invasion	No. of patients	Survival (%)				
		1	2	3	4	5 years
pTis	18	93.5 (81.3–10:00)[a]	93.5 (81.3–100.0)	93.5 (81.3–100.0)	84.1 (63.6–100.0)	84.1 (63.6–100.0)
pTa	388	96.2 (94.3–98.1)	95.0 (92.8–97.3)	93.2 (90.6–95.8)	90.6 (87.5–93.7)	88.5 (85.1–92.0)
pT0	24	100.0 (100.0–100.0)	100.0 (100.0–100.0)	89.7 (76.2–100.0)	84.4 (68.2–100.0)	84.4 (68.2–100.0)
pT1	494	124 (96.5–99.1)	97.8 (92.4–96.7)	94.5 (87.6–93.2)	90.4 (83.1–89.7)	86.4 83.1 (79.4–86.8)
pT2	167	84.8 (79.2–90.4)	71.6 (64.4–78.8)	68.7 (61.2–76.1)	63.2 (55.3–71.1)	62.3 (54.4–70.3)
pT3a	94	82.4 (74.5–90.2)	63.4 (53.3–73.5)	55.8 (45.2–66.4)	50.5 (39.7–61.3)	47.7 (36.8–58.5)
pT3b	74	76.6 (66.6–86.6)	51.6 (39.2–64.0)	41.3 (28.9–53.6)	39.4 (27.1–51.8)	35.5 (23.2–47.7)
pT4a	36	53.6 (36.9–70.2)	28.3 (12.9–43.8)	28.3 (12.9–43.8)	28.3 (12.9–43.8)	28.3 (12.9–43.8)
pT4b	27	29.4 (11.7–47.0)	18.7 (2.3–35.0)	18.7 (2.3–35.0)	18.7 (2.3–35.0)	18.7 (2.3–35.0)
pTX	245	77.8 (73.4–84.1)	72.1 (66.1–78.0)	67.6 (61.2–73.9)	65.8 (59.2–72.3)	63.7 (57.0–70.5)
Total	1,567					

[a] 95% confidence limit.

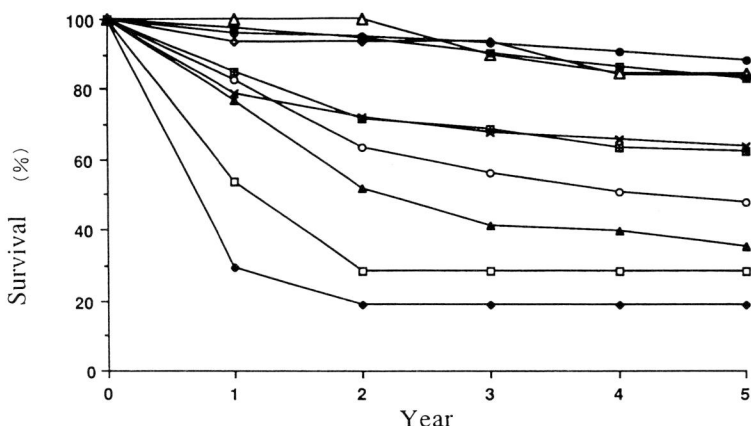

FIG. 2. Survival according to pT stage
◇ pTis, ● pTa, △ pT0, ▲ pT1, ■ pT2, ○ pT3a, ▲ pT3b, □ pT4a, ◆ pT4b, × pTX.

12. Survival and grade

Survival in accordance with the most predominant grades is indicated in Table X and Fig. 1.

13. Survival and pT stage

Survival in accordance with the pT stage is illustrated in Table XI and Fig. 2. The five-year survival rates of pTis, pTa, pT1, pT2, pT3a, pT3b, pT4a, and pT4b were, respectively, 84, 86, 83, 62, 48, 36, 28, and 19%.

Discussion

This is a summary of the nationwide registry of new cases of bladder cancer in Japan in the years from 1982 to 1987. Each year about 2,000 new cases of bladder cancer were registered, or about 25% of the estimated annual figure of 8,400. The Central Office of Cancer Registry at the National Cancer Center deals with 16 organs and collects data on 16,000 cases of cancer every year. The 25% coverage in the case of bladder cancer is the average for the 16 organ-registries. Should greater coverage be sought, there might well be a decrease in data quality, while decreased coverage could void any significance as a national registry. Consequently, this creates a dilemma. Under this present system of data collection and analysis, we are able to determine the situation in Japan with respect to bladder cancer and to more clearly judge its changing patterns and changes in treatment during specific time spans. For example, as described in the Summary section, CIS is increasing, ureterostomy and ureterosigmoidostomy are decreasing, the ileal conduit is frequently used, but recently use of the continent reservoir and the orthotopic neobladder appears to be increasing. These facts constitute very important information with respect to bladder cancer in Japan. However, the biggest problem faced by this project is that the true annual incidence of bladder cancer in the country remains unknown.

The true incidence of cancer can only be determined by a population-based

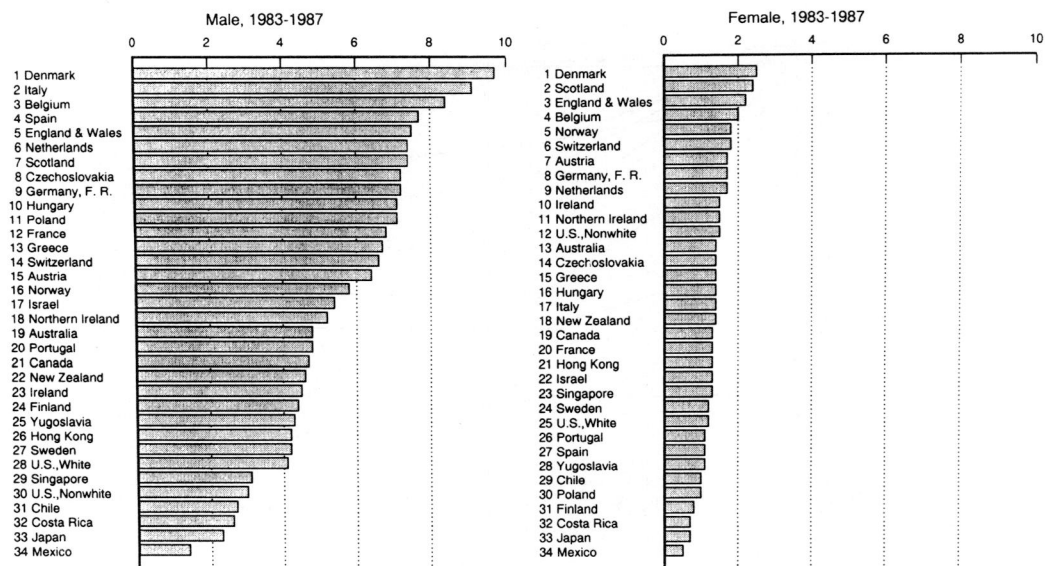

FIG. 3. Age-adjusted death rates of bladder cancer in 1983–1987 in 34 countries of the world
(From ref. 4, with permission)

cancer registry covering all people living in a specific area (*3*). There is no national cancer registry system in Japan but, since 1975, the Osaka Cancer Registry Office has collected data from prefectural registration systems and published an annual estimate of cancer incidence (*1, 2*).

The database for a population-based registry must have certain features to be truly useful: 1) it must contain all cases of cancer occurring within the population of interest during a specified period of time; 2) all relevant demographic information such as sex, race, age and residence at time of diagnosis, diagnosis data, and type of cancer is required to produce meaningful but crude age-specific and age-adjusted cancer incidence rates for specific types of cancer; 3) the stage at time of diagnosis must be carefully and consistently recorded for each new primary case of cancer; and, 4) such data must be reasonably accessible to end-users. All new primary cases of cancer must be accurately, consistently, and completely recorded in the registry data system.

Death rates based on a model population in 1985 were calculated and published in Japanese (*4*). This book also contains age-adjusted 1983–1987 bladder cancer (*4*) death rates in 34 countries of the world (Fig. 3). It is interesting to compare the data described in this paper with that of the book.

As was described in the Summary section, there are several problems of description in the registry documents which should be corrected. We also require some ethical guidelines on use of the data collected in the registration. The registration does appear to be gaining acceptance among Japanese urologists and is becoming routine. Nonetheless, further improvement and refining of the system are required.

Acknowledgments

Sincere appreciation is expressed for the efforts of Dr. Keiichi Matsumoto who made this registration applicable at its onset, and for the great contributions of Ms. Yasuko Ishida and Mr. Takashi Yoshida in data management and publication of annual reports. Dr. Naohito Yamaguchi, head of the Cancer Information and Biometry Section, Cancer Information and Epidemiology Division, National Cancer Center Research Institute, planned and analyzed the survival data, and the Japanese Urological Association wishes to express its appreciation.

REFERENCES

1. The Research Group for Population-based Cancer Registration in Japan. Cancer Incidence in Japan, 1975—Cancer Registry Statistics. *In* "Cancer Mortality and Morbidity Statistics, Japan and the World." Gann Monograph on Cancer Research No. 26, ed. M. Segi, S. Tominaga, K. Aoki, and I. Fujimoto, pp. 92–116 (1981). Japan Sci. Soc. Press, Tokyo.
2. The Research Group for Population-based Cancer Registration in Japan. Cancer incidence and incidence rates in Japan in 1987. *Jpn. J. Clin. Oncol.*, **22**, 437–442 (1993).
3. Tucker, T.C. and Friedell, G.H. Using cancer registry data in primary care practice. *Primary Care and Cancer*, **14**, 33–36 (1994).
4. "White Papers on Cancer Statistics—Incidence, Death and Prognosis—1993," ed. S. Tominaga, K. Aoki, A. Hanai, and M. Kurihara, p. 30 and p. 255 (1993). Shinohara Press, Tokyo (in Japanese).

STATISTICS OF BRAIN TUMORS, 1969–1987: GENERAL FEATURES

The Committee of the Brain Tumor Registry of Japan*

Forty-six thousand and two primary and 7,772 metastatic brain tumors were registered in the Brain Tumor Registry of Japan from 1969 to 1987, accounting for nearly one third of all brain tumors in the country. The most frequent type was glioma (30.1%), meningioma (26.1%), schwannoma (10.5%), pituitary adenoma (18.1%) in adults, and glioma (61.1%), craniopharyngioma (11.0%), germinoma (8.3%), teratoma (3.5%), and meningioma (2.8%) in children. The proportion of glioma has recently been decreasing, while meningioma and pituitary adenoma have increased. CT scanning diagnosis and the microsurgical method for pituitary tumor could be contributing factors. Frequency of craniopharyngioma and germinoma of the pineal body was high compared to western countries. Five-year survival of benign tumors was more than 90%, while those of astrocytoma and glioblastoma were 61.1% and 7.1%, respectively. Detailed clinicopathological analyses were done and factors for prognosis determined.

The Brain Tumor Registry of Japan was organized in 1975 with the purpose of supplying vital information which could prove beneficial in the development of treatment for brain tumor patients as well as revealing the actual characteristics of their disease. The Committee of Registry is comprised of 81 professors from departments of neurosurgery in all universities and colleges throughout Japan. The secretariat office is located in the Department of Neurosurgery, National Cancer Center Hospital, Tokyo. The first chairman of the Registry from 1979 to 1991 was Dr. K. Sano, presently Professor Emeritus of University of Tokyo, Department of Neurosurgery; he was succeeded in 1992 by the current chairman, Dr. K. Takakura, Professor of Tokyo Women's Medical University, Department of Neurosurgery. In 1993 the Registry published its eighth report, containing a statistical analysis of 53,774 patients registered from 1969 to 1987 inclusive (Report of the Committee of the Brain Tumor Registry of Japan, 1993). The present paper is an excerpt from that report, presenting data on the frequency and anatomical distribution of brain tumors, patient age and sex, and changes in these factors during these years.

Data Collection

The registered institutions recruited for the acquisition of the statistics reported

---

* Manuscript was prepared by Kazuhiro Nomura, Department of Neurosurgery, National Cancer Center Hospital, 5-1-1 Tsukiji, Chuo-ku, Tokyo 104, Japan

herein numbered 412 as of 1984, and consisted of most universities, colleges, and hospitals with a board authorized by the Japan Neurological Society. Prior to 1983, only universities, colleges, and their affiliate hospitals (247 institutes in total) had been enrolled with the Registry. The method of investigation was questionnaire forms included with their case registration forms, which were sent by the secretariat to all of the above-referenced institutions. The completed registration forms provide information regarding patient birthplace and present residential area, occupation, age, tumor pathology, tumor sites, diagnostic method employed, clinical grade (performance state), therapies (surgery, radiation, chemo- or immunotherapy), and the outcome of these treatments. All registration forms returned to the secretariat were thoroughly reviewed by the editors and then by neurosurgeons at the National Cancer Center. A follow-up study was conducted prior to the publication of each report presenting the result of analysis of the collected data. Analysis of case data collected between 1988 and 1991 is still in progress. Brain tumors were classified mainly on the basis of histological findings using the classification system developed by the Union Internationale Contre le Cancer (Unio Internationalis Contra Cancrum, 1965).

Cases of brain abscesses, arterio-venous malformations, and skull tumors were excluded from this research.

General Features of Brain Tumor Statistics

1. Number of cases per year

There were a total of 53,774 cases registered during the period between 1969 and 1987; they consisted of 46,002 primary and 7,772 metastatic brain tumors. The number of cases of primary brain tumor registered each year from 1974 to 1985 is shown in Fig. 1. The registered cases of brain tumors are estimated to represent 30–40% of the total number of such cases in Japan. This was estimated from the proportion of registered deaths of brain tumor patients reported in the statistics registry of national investigation by the Japanese Ministry of Health and Welfare (8).

2. Frequency of primary brain tumors by type

The frequencies of the various types of primary brain tumors in adults, children,

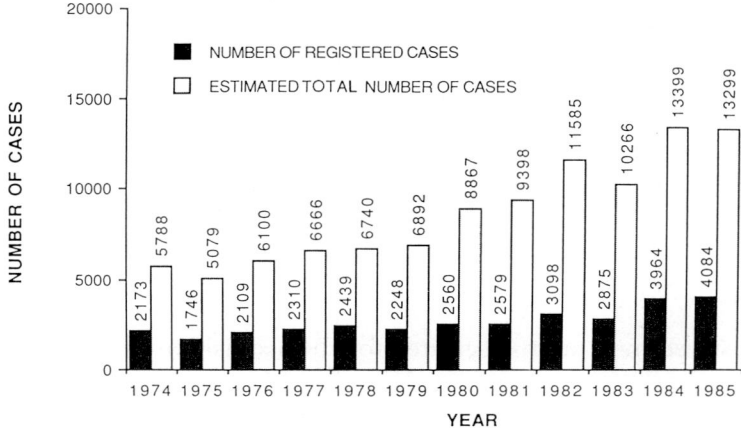

FIG. 1. Number of cases of primary brain tumor registered each year from 1974 to 1985

TABLE I. Frequency of Various Types of Primary Brain Tumor by Patient Age

Type of tumor	All ages (%)	Adult (%)	Child (%)	Aged (%)
Glioma	33.8	30.1	61.1	28.4
Meningioma	23.4	26.1	2.8	45.4
Schwannoma	9.4	10.5	1.3	6.7
Pituitary adenoma	16.2	18.1	1.6	8.8
Germinoma	2.3	1.5	8.3	0.1
Craniopharyngioma	4.5	3.6	11.0	1.2
Dermoid, epidermoid	1.5	1.5	1.3	0.8
Teratoma	0.8	0.3	3.5	0
Chordoma	0.5	0.5	0.3	0.2
Hemangioblastoma	2.3	2.6	0.2	1.6
Sarcoma	0.4	0.3	0.7	0.1
Malig lymph	1.4	1.6	0.4	4.5
Others	3.5	3.3	7.5	2.2
Total	100% (N=42,628)	100% (N=37,544)	100% (N=5,084)	100% (N=2,218)

Adult: ≧15, child: <15, aged: ≧70.
Abbreviations: malig lymph, malignant lymphoma.

TABLE II. Frequency of Glioma by Type

Type of glioma	All ages (%)	Adult (%)	Child (%)	Aged (%)
Glioblastoma	28.9	35.2	6.7	54.5
Astrocytoma	29.5	28.5	31.3	18.6
Anaplastic astrocytoma	15.9	18.0	8.7	20.2
Oligodendroglioma	6.2	7.4	2.2	1.7
Ependymoma	5.7	3.7	12.8	1.4
Choroid plexus papilloma	1.4	1.0	2.9	0.0
Medulloblastoma	6.8	1.6	25.7	0.2
Others	5.6	4.2	9.7	3.4
Total	100% (N=14,419)	100% (N=11,178)	100% (N=3,107)	100% (N=629)

Adult: ≧15, child: <15, aged: ≧70.

and the aged are listed in Table I. In adults (≧15 to <70 years) and children, glioma was noted at the highest frequency, while in the aged, meningioma (45.4%), followed by glioma (28.4%) was highest.

The frequency of various types of gliomas in the 3 age groups is shown in Table II. Glioblastoma showed the highest frequency in both adult and aged groups, while in children, astrocytoma followed by medulloblastoma was most often seen. The annual frequency of major brain tumors as a percent of all primary brain tumors is shown in Fig. 2. Glioma showed an annual percentage decrease, from 34% in 1969 to 28% in 1987, while meningioma and pituitary adenoma markedly increased from 15% and 11% in 1969 to 25% and 16% in 1987, respectively.

3. Anatomical site

The frequencies for representative gliomas in patients of all ages are shown in Table III. Oligodendroglioma was located predominantly in the frontal lobe (50.5%), and ependymomas in the lateral ventricle (17.2%) or fourth ventricle (33.3%).

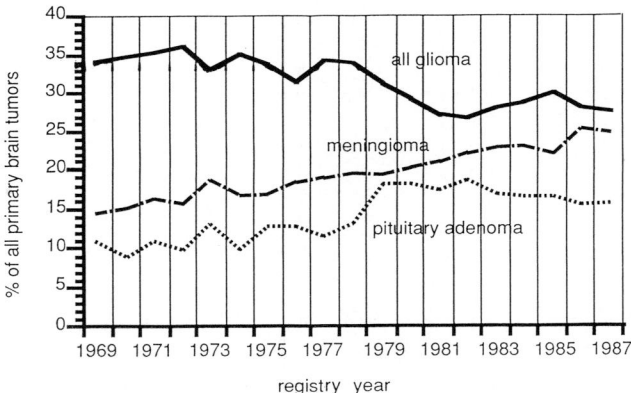

Fig. 2. Annual frequency of major brain tumors as a percent of all primary brain tumors

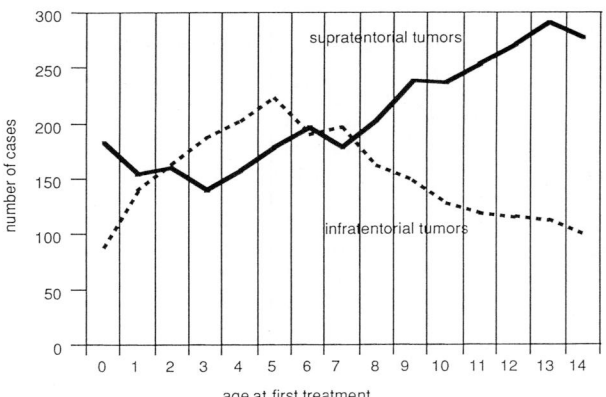

Fig. 3. Frequencies of supratentorial and infratentorial pediatric brain tumors

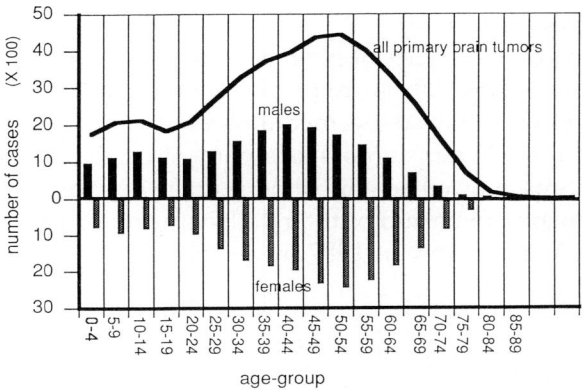

Fig. 4. Patient age and sex distribution for all registered primary cases

Glioblastoma was most frequently located in the frontal lobe (35.2%), followed by the temporal lobe (24.4%).

The frequencies of supratentorial and infratentorial pediatric brain tumors in children are shown in Fig. 3.

4. Age distribution

The patient age and sex distribution for all these registered primary cases is given in Fig. 4. The age-specific distribution for both genders (solid line in Fig. 4) shows two peaks, between the ages of 10 and 14 years and 50 and 54 years, indicating that these age groups show the highest incidence. Children comprised 13% of the 44,530 patients (3,393 boys and 2,552 girls), a male preponderance of 1.3 to 1. Analysis of the frequency of pediatric brain tumors by age revealed that the lowest was observed between the ages of one and two years and was almost uniform after 4 years old (data not shown).

The annual age distribution was also studied for each registry year. The peak of the age distribution of the brain tumor patients was 45–49 years in 1969–1973 but

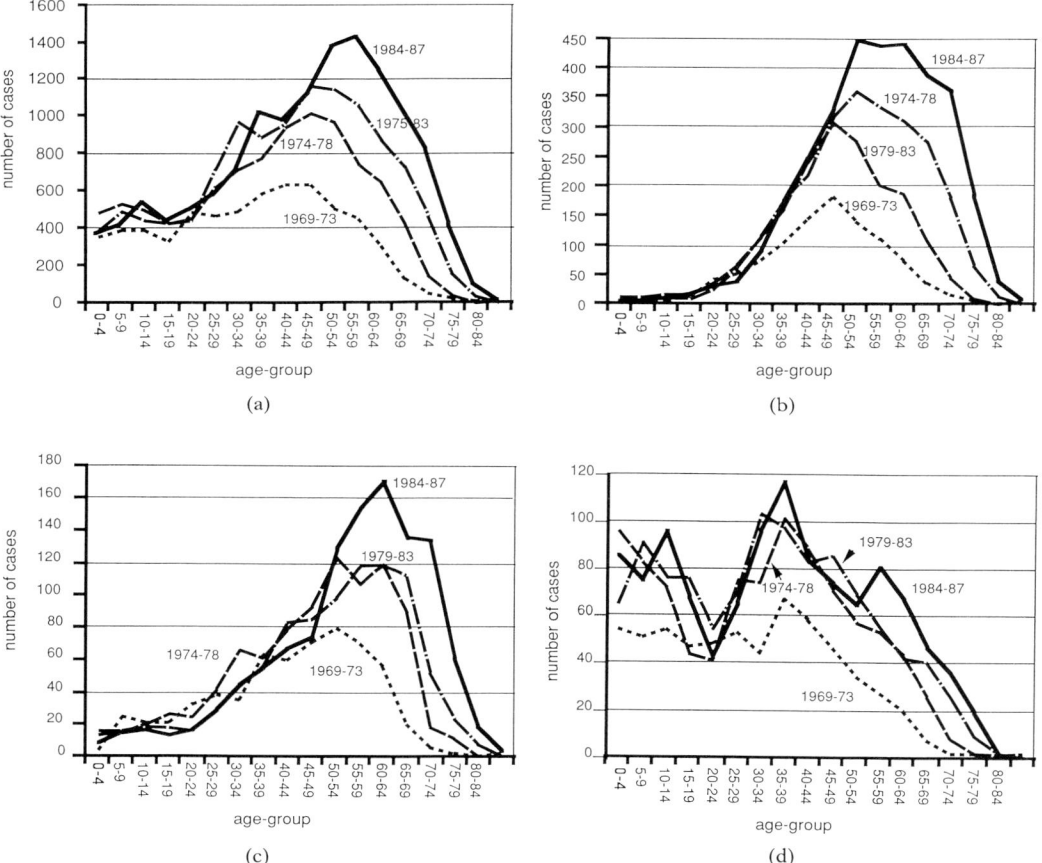

FIG. 5. Annual age distribution for each registry year
  a) All primary brain tumor patients. b) Meningioma patients. c) Glioblastoma patients. d) Astrocytoma patients.

TABLE III. Frequency of Various Types of Tumor by Anatomical Site

Site	Giobl (%)	Oligo (%)[a]	Epend (%)[a]	Astro (%)[a]	Medullo (%)
Frontal lobe	1,449 (35.2)	442 (50.5)	89 (11.1)	2,111 (32.8)	10 (1.0)
Temporal lobe	1,002 (24.4)	105 (12.0)	45 (5.6)	1,101 (17.2)	9 (0.9)
Parietal lobe	793 (19.3)	114 (13.0)	74 (9.2)	831 (12.9)	5 (0.5)
Occipital lobe	219 (5.3)	22 (2.5)	27 (3.4)	172 (2.7)	—
Chiasma region	11 (0.3)	2 (0.2)	7 (0.9)	120 (1.9)	4 (0.4)
Third ventricle	27 (0.7)	23 (2.7)	47 (5.8)	148 (1.5)	2 (0.2)
Lateral ventricle	52 (1.2)	85 (9.9)	148 (17.2)	137 (2.1)	5 (0.5)
Corpus callosum & septum pellucidum	105 (2.6)	33 (3.8)	2 (0.2)	121 (1.9)	3 (0.3)
Rostral brain stem & basal ganglia	194 (4.7)	21 (2.4)	6 (0.7)	304 (4.7)	—
Cerebellar vermis	24 (0.6)	3 (0.3)	34 (4.2)	292 (4.5)	651 (67.6)
Cerebellar hemisphere	64 (1.6)	4 (0.5)	20 (2.5)	518 (8.1)	90 (9.3)
Fourth ventricle	6 (0.1)	—	267 (33.3)	61 (0.9)	138 (14.3)
Caudal brain stem	79 (1.9)	4 (0.5)	14 (1.7)	277 (4.3)	14 (1.5)
Optic nerve	1 (0.0)	2 (0.2)	—	72 (1.1)	—
Others	87 (2.1)	16 (1.8)	23 (2.9)	163 (2.5)	32 (3.3)
Total	4,113 (100.0)	876 (100.0)	803 (100.0)	6,428 (100.0)	963 (100.0)

Abbreviations: astro, astrocytoma; oligo, oligodendroglioma; epend, ependymoma; giobl, glioblastoma; medullo, medulloblastoma.
[a] Anaplastic type is included in each category.

TABLE IV. Cumulative Survival Rate for 5 Years (1984–1987)

	Case 1[a]	Case 2[b]	1-Year	2	3	4	5
Astrocytoma	921	46	85.9	73.4	67.6	64.4	61.1
Malignant astrocytoma	559	16	67.8	43.2	32.4	25.4	22.7
Oligodendroglioma	144	4	96.3	91.4	84.2	81.9	70.8
Malignant oligodendroglioma	18	2	82.9	63.7	56.2	56.2	56.2
Ependymoma	103	7	89.5	81.1	75.8	72.6	64.4
Malignant ependymoma	33	2	77.8	50.7	42.9	37.2	9.3
Glioblastoma	983	55	50.1	20.5	11.4	8.7	7.1
Medulloblastoma	149	10	82.9	60.8	52.2	48.1	38.6
Neurinoma	1,055	69	97.3	96.8	95.9	95.1	94.1
Von Recklinghausen's disease	38	2	97.2	94.0	94.0	94.0	94.0
Meningioma	2,678	71	96.4	94.9	93.1	92.1	90.8
Malignant meningioma	57	2	84.5	82.2	77.3	67.3	58.3
Germinoma	277	9	93.5	88.4	87.9	85.1	83.1
Non-functioning pituitary adenoma	581	38	97.7	96.7	96.2	95.7	95.5
PRL producing pituitary adenoma	459	24	96.6	94.0	94.0	92.9	92.9
All pituitary adenomas	1,875	148	99.3	99.3	99.3	99.3	99.3
Craniopharyngioma	385	20	92.6	90.2	87.9	85.1	82.3
Primary tumors (total)	10,980	834	87.3	79.7	76.0	73.8	71.8
Metastatic tumors (total)	2,210	371	36.0	18.1	13.1	9.9	8.2

[a] Number of cases living more than 30 days.
[b] Number of cases dying within 30 days, which was excluded for survival rate analysis.

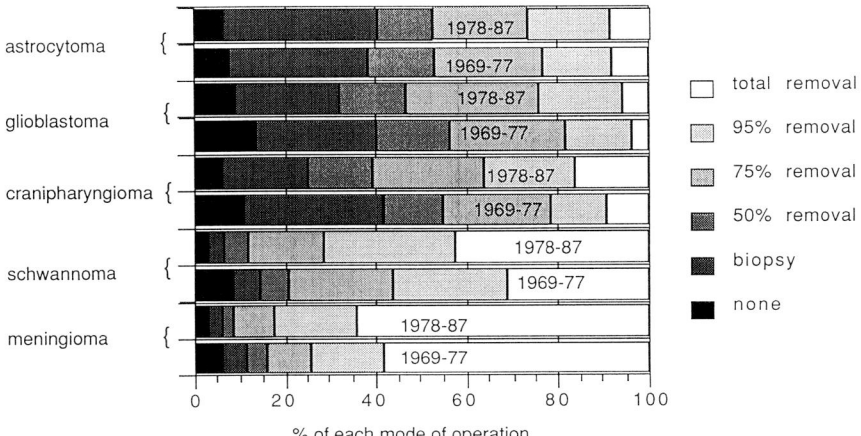

FIG. 6. Rates of types of surgery during the two periods, 1969–77 and 1978–87 for each type of tumor

TABLE V. Mode of Operation and Survival Time: Supratentorial Astrocytoma (1978–87)

Mode of operation	Case 1[a]	Case 2[b]	1-Year	2	3	4	5
PAT1 biopsy	554	25	84.7	68.4	59.3	56.1	54.8
PAT2 50% resected	178	10	89.4	78.1	69.7	59.3	56.7
PAT3 75% resected	344	13	86.1	76.4	69.0	62.6	57.6
PAT4 95% resected	283	8	90.8	83.1	79.0	74.1	70.8
PAT5 total removal	158	7	94.9	88.5	86.5	84.1	82.1

PAT: abbreviation of treatment for statistical analysis.
Mantel Chi-Square Test: PAT1; 4, 5 PAT2; 5 PAT3; 5 ($p < 0.001$), PAT2, 4 PAT4; 5 ($p < 0.05$) PAT3, 4 ($p < 0.01$).
[a,b] See the legend of Table IV.

TABLE VI. Mode of Operation and Survival Time: Supratentorial Malignant Astrocytoma (1978–87)

Mode of operation	Case 1[a]	Case 2[b]	1-Year	2	3	4	5
PAT1 biopay	255	8	56.6	36.3	28.1	21.7	19.3
PAT2 50% resected	121	6	65.4	42.3	28.8	23.7	20.5
PAT3 75% resected	275	7	74.4	49.2	34.7	28.5	25.8
PAT4 95% resected	179	1	76.4	54.6	43.0	34.9	32.4
PAT5 total removal	61	0	90.3	67.2	55.8	51.5	51.8

Mantel Chi-Square Test: PAT1; 3 ($p < 0.01$) PAT2; 4 PAT4; 5 ($p < 0.05$) PAT1; 4, 5 PAT2; 5 PAT3; 5 ($p < 0.001$).
[a,b] See the legend of Table IV.

TABLE VII. Mode of Operation and Survival Time: Glioblastoma (1978–87)

Mode of operation	Case 1[a]	Case 2[b]	1-Year	2	3	4	5
PAT1 biopay	454	33	41.7	15.3	8.2	7.0	5.4
PAT2 50% resected	277	20	43.8	19.7	10.3	6.8	—
PAT3 75% resected	558	23	52.9	20.4	12.7	10.3	9.0
PAT4 95% resected	354	12	68.2	33.2	22.6	15.8	11.9
PAT5 total removal	109	4	74.7	42.5	32.5	22.6	23.0

Mantel Chi-Square Test: PAT1; 3, 4, 5 PAT2; 4, 5 PAT3; 4, 5 ($p < 0.001$) PAT4; 5 ($p < 0.05$).
[a,b] See the legend of Table IV.

TABLE VIII. Survival Time of Glioblastoma Patients Treated with Operation with and without Radiation (1978–1987)

Mode of treatment	Case 1[a]	Case 2[b]	1-Year	2	3	4	5
PAT1 ope.; biopsy+R	386	3	47.9	17.7	9.3	7.3	5.3
PAT2 ope. alone; biopsy	121	35	19.5	7.8			
PAT3 ope.; 75% resected+R	660	1	54.7	22.1	12.8	10.0	8.4
PAT4 ope. alone; 75% resected	175	42	29.7	11.4	7.2		
PAT5 ope.; 100% removal+R	377	3	71.9	36.8	25.5	17.3	14.1
PAT6 ope. alone; 100% removal	86	13	56.8	25.6	18.0	13.1	
PAT7 ope. (all cases)+R	1,423	7	57.4	24.8	15.2	11.3	9.1
PAT8 ope. alone (all cases)	382	90	32.4	13.4	8.8	6.3	4.8

Abbreviations: ope, operation; R, radiation therapy.
Mantel Chi-Square Test: PAT1; 2, 4, 8 PAT2; 3, 5, 6, 7 PAT3; 4, 8 PAT4; 5, 6, 7 PAT 5; 7, 8 PAT7; 8 ($p < 0.001$), PAT1; 5 PAT6; 8 ($p < 0.01$), PAT5; 7 ($p < 0.05$).
[a,b] See the legend of Table IV.

55–59 years in 1984–1987 (Fig. 5a). This shift was particularly marked in patients with meningiomas, whose age distribution peak was 45–49 years in 1969–1973, while that in 1984–1987 showed a plateau extending across the age groups of 50–54, 55–59, and 60–64 years (Fig. 5b). In glioblastoma patients, the age distribution peak was observed at 50–54 years in 1969–1973, but at 60–64 in 1984–1987 (Fig. 5c). The peak in astrocytoma patients revealed the same ages of 35–39 in 1969–1973 as in 1984–1987, although the number of cases increased in the ages between 55–59, which made a third peak in the line of data between 1984–1987 (Fig. 5d).

Results of Treatments for Primary Brain Tumors

1. *General survival rates for brain tumors (Table IV)*

The five-year survival rates according to type of brain tumor between 1984–1987 are shown in Table IV. Meningioma, pituitary adenoma, and schwannoma showed high survival rates reflecting good treatment results, while those for glioblastoma and malignant astrocytoma suggest that they remain devastating in spite of aggressive treatments including surgery, radiation, and chemotherapy.

2. *Effect of type of surgery*

The rates of types of surgery during the two periods 1969–1977 and 1978–1987 for each type of tumor are shown in Fig. 6. For so-called benign brain tumors such as schwannoma and meningioma, the rate of total or more than 95% removal of the tumor was increased during the latter period. However, the type of surgery for gliomas like astrocytoma and glioblastoma showed little change between these two periods.

3. *Rate of survival after surgical removal of gliomas*

The mode of operation and survival time for supratentorial astrocytoma are shown in Table V; the survival time was strongly related to the extent of removal. Surprisingly, patients who underwent total tumor removal (macroscopic observations) showed a 5-year survival of 82.1%. Ninety-five to 100% removal of supratentorial malignant astrocytoma and even glioblastoma also showed higher survival rate than those who underwent 50% tumor resection (Tables VI and VII).

4. Radiation therapy and survival

The effect of radiation therapy for glioblastoma under the tumor removal conditions shown in Table VIII was analyzed. For all the modes of operation, patients who also received combined radiation showed higher survival rates than those who did not.

Discussion

The general demographic features of primary brain tumor have changed greatly, particularly in terms of the frequencies of various types (Fig. 2). The incidence of meningioma and pituitary adenoma has increased gradually but substantially since 1975, the year in which CT scanning was introduced on a large scale in Japan. This year also marked the development of a simple method of analysis of various pituitary hormones which facilitated the detection of pituitary adenoma in Japan, resulting in gradual increase of the incidence of this tumor until 1979 and a subsequent plateau. The change in the frequency of pituitary adenoma has also been influenced by the introduction of microsurgery and its technical development in Japan. The gradual decrement in the rate of pituitary adenoma since 1983 indicates the effect of introduction of bromocriptin to treat microadenoma, especially for prolactinoma. The contrasting decline in the frequency of glioma of all primary brain tumors must be considered in relation to the increased rate of detection of these two tumors.

The frequency of glioma in Japan (33.8%) is slightly lower than that reported in China (42.9%) (6, 11), the United States (4) (49.3%), and Germany (12) (44.4%). Twenty-four percent of all gliomas were found in children, and glioma constituted 61% of all pediatric brain tumors. These percentages are almost the same as those reported in the other countries (1).

On the other hand, craniopharyngiomas, 29% of which were seen in children (11% of all pediatric tumors), accounted for 4.5% of all brain tumors. The frequencies of craniopharyngioma in China (5.0%), reported by Wen-Quing *et al.* (11), and Japan are higher than those reported in Western countries (2, 13). In Japan, the ratio of the frequency of craniopharyngioma in children to that in adults is 3.1.

The reported frequency of germinoma is quite high in Japan (8.5%) compared to that elsewhere (0.4–0.7%). This study also revealed that the frequency of germinoma as a percentage of all brain tumors (2.3%) is particularly high in male children.

The location of a brain tumor is an important factor in the diagnosis of its type. The frequencies of representative gliomas are shown in Table III; other representative locations for brain tumors, which are not shown herein, are the pituitary fossa and chiasmal regions. In these regions, pituitary adenoma is most frequent, followed by craniopharyngioma. The cerebello-pontine angle is a specific site for schwannoma. Medulloblastoma is frequently located in the cerebellar vermis (67.6%) and IVth ventricle (14.3%) (data not shown).

The classification of tumors as either supra- or infratentorial is well known to indicate differences in frequency between adults and children. In addition, children under one year or over 8 years of age show supratentorial tumors at much higher rate than infratentorial tumors, while the reverse is observed in children between the age of 2 and 7 years. Our findings for tumors classified based on the location in relation to the tentorium are almost the same as those in previous reports (Fig. 3).

The analysis of the sex distribution of the 46,002 patients with primary brain tumors of all ages revealed that 22,130 occurred in males, with a male/female ratio of 0.93. The male/female ratio for patients with brain tumors including children has long been larger than 1.0 in registry studies, and the present analysis therefore indicates a great difference from the earlier registry findings. This difference is due to the increase in the rates of meningioma and pituitary adenoma (Fig.2), which are much more likely to occur in females. However, there is still a preponderance of males among children with brain tumor.

The age distribution peak shifted by about 10 years to the older group in the latter period of 1984–1987 (Fig. 5a, 5b). This shift may be due to the increased aged population for this period, although some reports have suggested that the increase in the incidence of both meningioma and glioblastoma cannot be accounted for only by the development of diagnostic tools (*3, 5, 7, 9*). In any case, when the aged have a brain tumor it is frequently meningioma or glioblastoma, which are typical tumors in that age group.

The analysis of treatment results for benign brain tumors, such as meningioma, schwannoma, and pituitary adenoma indicate that total tumor removal is frequently curative. The rate of total tumor removal has increased gradually each year (Fig. 6). There has been little change in the mode of operation for gliomas, especially in total removal of the tumor and the low incidence of curative treatment by operation alone. These results may indicate that glioma is frequently not diagnosed until it is too late to treat by operation alone. The data also indicate that even patients with malignant astrocytoma or glioblastoma can be expected to live longer if the tumor is removed totally or subtotally (95% removal) (Tables VI and VII). Although de Tribolet and Frankhauser have reported that the goal of surgery should be the radical removal of the tumor and that partial resection does not seem to offer any benefit to a patient (*10*), the registry statistics indicate that even 75% removal is more effective than lesser percentage removal in lengthening the survival period. The registry data also clearly show that the survival of patients after all types of surgery is increased by the addition of radiation therapy (Table VIII).

Acknowledgments

The committee members of the Brain Tumor Registry of Japan would like to express their appreciation to Drs. Naohito Yamaguchi and Shaw Watanabe (Cancer Information and Epidemiology Division) for their thoughtful advice and suggestions on the statistical analysis, and to Mr. T. Yoshida for his help in the computer analysis.

This work was partially supported by a Cancer Research Grant from the Japanese Ministry of Health and Welfare and the Japan Brain Foundation. The enthusiastic cooperation of neurosurgeons in the registered hospitals all over the country is also gratefully acknowledged.

REFERENCES

1. Behrend, R.C. Epidemiology of brain tumors. *In* "Tumors of the Brain and Skull," ed. P.J. Vinken and G.W. Bruyn, pp. 56–88 (1974). North-Holland, Amsterdam/Elsevier, New York.
2. Cushing, H. "Intracranial Tumors," (1932). Thomas, Springfield.
3. Desmeules, M., Mikkelsen, T., and Mao, Y. Increasing incidence of primary malignant tumors: influence of diagnostic methods. *J. Natl. Cancer Inst.*, **84**, 442–445 (1992).
4. Grant, F.C. A study of the results of surgical treatment in 2326 consecutive patients with brain tumor. *J. Neurosurg.*, **13**, 479–488 (1956).
5. Greig, N.H., Ries, L.G., Yancik, R., and Rapoport, S.I. Increasing annual incidence of primary malignant brain tumors in the elderly. *J. Natl. Cancer Inst.*, **82**, 1621–1624 (1990).
6. Hwang, S.L. and Hwong, S.L. An analysis of brain tumors in south Taiwan. *Kao Hsiung I Hsueh Ko Hsueh Tsa Chin (Taiwan)*, **8**, 656–664 (1992).
7. Preston-Martin, S., Mack, W., and Henderson, B.E. Risk factors for gliomas and meningiomas in males in Los Angeles County. *Cancer Res.*, **49**, 6137–6143 (1989).
8. Statistics and Information Department, Minister's secretariat, Ministry of Health and Welfare. Vital Statistics of Japan, 1969–1986, Japan. Volume 3 of each year.
9. Takeuchi, K., Sano, K., and Nomura, K. An epidemiological study of brain tumours in the elderly. *Neurol. Res.*, **13**, 21–24 (1991).
10. de Tribolet, N. and Frankhauser, H. Surgery in the treatment of malignant glioma: Current status and future perspectives. *In* "Glioma, Principles and Practice in Neuro-oncology," ed. A. Karim and E. Laws, pp. 93–103 (1991). Springer-Verlag, Berlin.
11. Wen-Quing, H., Shi-Ju, Z., Quing-Sheng, T., Jian-Quing, H., Yu-Xia, X., Quing-Zhong, L., Zi-Jun, L., and Wen-Cui, Z. Statistical analysis of central nervous system tumors in China. *J. Neurosurg.*, **56**, 555–564 (1982).
12. Zülch, K.J. (ed.). *In* "Brain tumors. Their Biology and Pathology," 3rd ed., pp. 85–114 (1986). Springer-Verlag, New York.
13. Zülch, K.J. (ed.). Germ cell tumors. *In* "Brain Tumors. Their Biology and Pathology," 3rd ed., pp. 414–425 (1986). Springer-Verlag, New York.

THE JAPAN CHILDREN'S CANCER REGISTRY: OUTLINE, RESULTS, AND PERSPECTIVES

The Committee of the Japan Children's Cancer Registry*

Between 1969 and 1992 the Japan Children's Cancer Registry recorded 29,804 cases of malignant neoplasms and related conditions in children under 15 years at their first visit to hospital. Annual entries numbered around 1,200, which presumably reflected about half the cases occurring throughout Japan. The collected data included identification of hospitals and patients, patho-histological diagnosis, past medical history, major complications, family history of X-ray exposure, pregnancy course and delivery, and pedigree chart for cancers among relatives, *etc*. Thus the Registry can be of great advantage to genetic/epidemiological studies in cancer research, as well as providing an applicable means of knowing actual morbidity and distribution of cancers in Japan.

Many investigators have access to the Registry database, and the Registration Committee implemented rules which carefully guard the privacy of both the patient and the attending physician. Many investigations on cancer research in children have been made using the database: differences in environmental factors of registered cases of leukemia and solid tumor; childhood neuroectodermal tumors after maternal ovulation induction, detailed analysis of neurofibromatosis type 1 and childhood cancer; germ cell tumors and Down syndrome. Newspapers, journals, and other media have also utilized the database. Future planned use of the Registry includes: 1) a survey on the prognosis of children's cancer cases, multiple cancer and secondary cancer investigations; 2) measures for social rehabilitation following completion of treatment; and 3) measures for periodic health management after treatment.

Rapid progress in molecular biology has demonstrated the mechanism of carcinogenesis at the DNA and chromosome level. However, these findings on cytological and molecular changes in cancer cells have no direct relation to a given type of cancer in an individual, or to clinical onset of cancer in a patient. It is precisely here that a hospital-based registry is of value, because if there is such a relation it could be determined by the detailed analysis of a great number of clinical cases accumulated in the registry.

---

* Manuscript was prepared by Masako Tanimura, Ichiro Matsui, Department of Child Ecology, National Children's Medical Research Center, 3-35-31 Taishido, Setagaya-ku,Tokyo 154, Japan; Noboru Kobayashi, National Children's Hospital, 3-35-31 Taishido, Setagaya-ku, Tokyo 154, Japan; Ikuo Okabe, Department of 1st Surgery, Nihon University, 30-1 Oyaguchikami-cho, Itabashi-ku, Tokyo 173, Japan; Masaru Yokoyama, Department of Pediatrics, Hirosaki University, 5 Zaifu-cho, Hirosaki 036, Japan; and Kohei Hashizume, Department of Pediatric Surgery, Japan Red Cross Medical Center, 4-1-22 Hiroo, Shibuya-ku, Tokyo 150, Japan

The Children's Cancer Association of Japan was established in November 1968 and designated that the Japan Children's Cancer Registry be started. This was done in January, 1969, by a Registration Committee organized by the Cancer Committee of the Pediatric Association of Japan and the Cancer Committee of the Pediatric Surgeons Association of Japan. The Committee of Retinoblastoma of Japan, part of the Japan Association of Ophthalmology, has also worked in close cooperation with the Registry since 1984. The Registry has been financed primarily by the Children's Cancer Association of Japan, with partial support from the Ministry of Health and Welfare, Japan.

The program of the Registry is to undertake an annual nationwide survey as a means of clarifying the status and analyzing the risk and causative factors of childhood malignancy. As in other developed countries, childhood malignancy is not a common disease but remains the second leading cause of death among children in Japan; accidents are the first. The rates and trends obtained from an analysis of death statistics reflect only limited information on the recent marked progress in treatment for cancer in children. The Children's Cancer Registry, by patho-histological cancer diagnosis, provides a relevant means of revealing the actual morbidity and the distribution of this disease in Japan.

Most cases of children's cancer are of unknown cause, and the period until onset is extremely short. Virtually half of the cases of childhood cancer develop between the time of birth and 4 years of age, in contrast to adult cancer which requires several decades to develop. It might be inherent that individual intrinsic and genetic factors have a predominant role in childhood cancer, as compared to environmental exposure and extrinsic factors in adult cancer. It is in this sense that a registry of children's cancer can be of great advantage to genetic/epidemiological studies in cancer research.

In this report we wish to outline the registration system used and show the results from our Registry, what kind of research information it can provide on childhood malignancy, and to discuss future problems.

Registration System

All 47 prefectures of Japan are included in seven zones from north to south according to the actual distribution of hospitals (2). Each zone has its own Regional Registration Center to handle the registrations within that zone. The annual data collected at each Regional Center are sent to the Central Registration Office which since 1985 has been located in the Department of Child Ecology, at the National Children's Medical Research Center, Tokyo. Registered data gathered since the beginning of the Registry are entered in the database in the Central Office. Figure 1 presents the system and function of the Children's Cancer Registry, which is a hospital-based registry containing a variety of medical and social information.

Nearly 30,000 cases of childhood malignancy have been registered to date, with the cooperation of more than 500 various institutions all over Japan; 65% of the registered cases are from pediatrics departments, 15% from pediatric surgery, 8% from brain surgery, 7% from hematology/oncology, 5% from ophthalmology, and the rest from other departments, including orthopedic surgery, gynecology, urology, otolaryngology, internal medicine, and clinical laboratories.

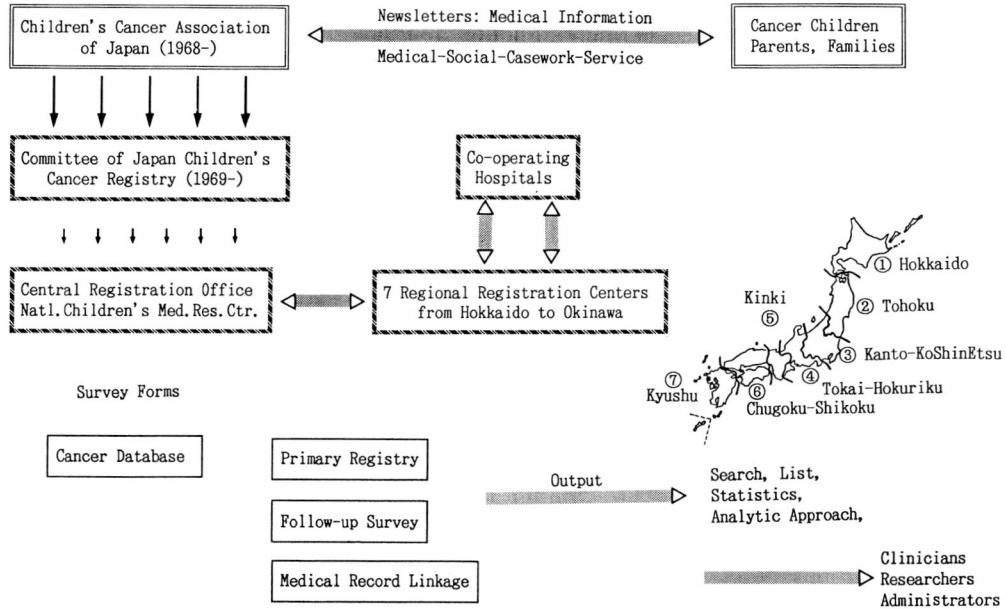

FIG. 1. System of the Japan Children's Cancer Registry

The overall reporting rate of the registry is estimated to be around 50% of the total children's cancers in Japan.

Survey Forms and Classification of Diseases

Major items in the survey include: 1) identification code (ID) for hospital and patient, personal information on patients, 2) diagnosis, date of first visit to the hospital, 3) past medical history, 4) major complications and detailed medical examination, 5) family history of X-ray exposure, pregnancy course and delivery, and 6) pedigree chart for cancers among relatives (2). The Registry seeks to include all malignant neoplasms and related conditions observed in children under 15 years at the time of their first visit to the hospital.

A specially designed patho-histological code number (4-digit code) is employed. In 1985 the survey forms were revised to include leukemia classification of the FAB (French-American-British) study group, and some malformation syndromes as specific items to be checked. Along with these detailed descriptions of the diagnosis in cancer, an extra one-digit code number was added. The International Classification of Diseases, revisions 8 and 9 (ICD-8 and ICD-9), are also coded in each registered case in order to discuss international differences or to compare with cancers at adult ages.

Gross Statistics of Childhood Malignancies in the Registry

1. *Annual trends in registered cases*

Since the Registry began in 1969, basic statistics on registered cases in a fixed

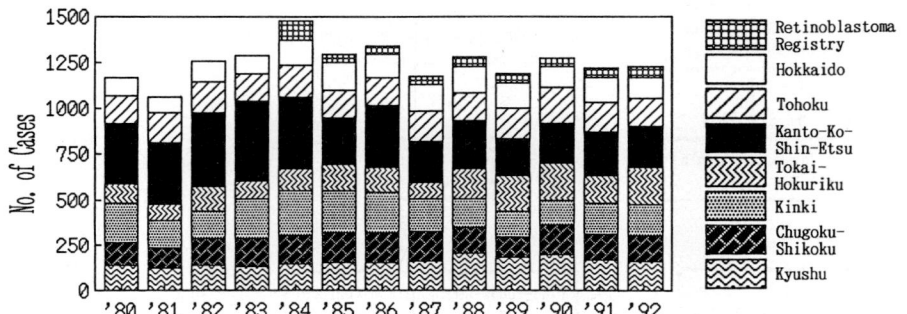

FIG. 2. Number of registered cases by year and region

TABLE I. Area-specific Incidence Rate per Million Child Population in the Registry

	Hokkaido	Tohoku	Kanto-Ko-Shin-Etsu	Tokai-Hokuriku	Kinki	Chugoku-Shikoku	Kyushu	Total
Location of office	Sapporo	Sendai	Tokyo	Nagoya	Osaka	Hiroshima	Fukuoka	(Tokyo)
No. of prefectures	1	6	10	7	6	9	8	47
No. of cases—1992	117	148	227	198	175	143	160	1,168
Incidence rate—1992	108.9	77.0	28.7	59.8	46.3	63.4	69.6	51.8
Incidence rate—1991	128.5	83.8	30.0	45.9	44.9	61.6	74.8	54.2
Annual average for 1980–1992	121.9	83.9	37.5	42.6	49.1	64.3	69.2	55.4
Population (×10^3)	5,670	9,750	43,670	17,228	20,392	11,997	14,546	123,253
Child population (×10^3)	1,074	1,921	7,896	3,311	3,782	2,255	2,299	22,538

Population: from vital statistics of Japan, 1989. Child population: under 15 years.

format have been issued every year, providing an up-to-date picture/overview of childhood cancer in Japan (published in the Japanese Journal "Shonigan" (Children's Cancer)).

Annual trends of the registered cases for the past 13 years are shown in Fig. 2 by the seven regional zones including the Retinoblastoma Registry. The number of registered cases has remained stable at around 1,200 annually for the last decade, although cases registered at each Regional Center may have changed or fluctuated during this period.

Table I indicates the incidence per million of the child-under-15 years at the seven Regional Centers in 1992, 1991 and the average annual number during 1980–1992. Although the incidence rate for total cases per million population for 1992 was 54.4, the rates in the Kanto-Ko-Shin-Etsu (Tokyo and surroundings) and Kinki (Osaka and surroundings) are far lower. The same tendency was observed with the average rate over the last decade at each Regional Registration Center. This may well reflect the difficulties in collecting survey forms from the many hospitals in the Metropolitan Tokyo and Osaka areas.

The northernmost prefecture of Japan, the island of Hokkaido, however, is quite a different case from that of other Regional Centers in that it is a single prefecture with fewer hospitals than other regions, most of which cooperate with the Registry. It thus reports the highest incidence rate. We view the actual mean incidence of childhood cancer in Japan as being rather close to the figure obtained by the Hokkaido

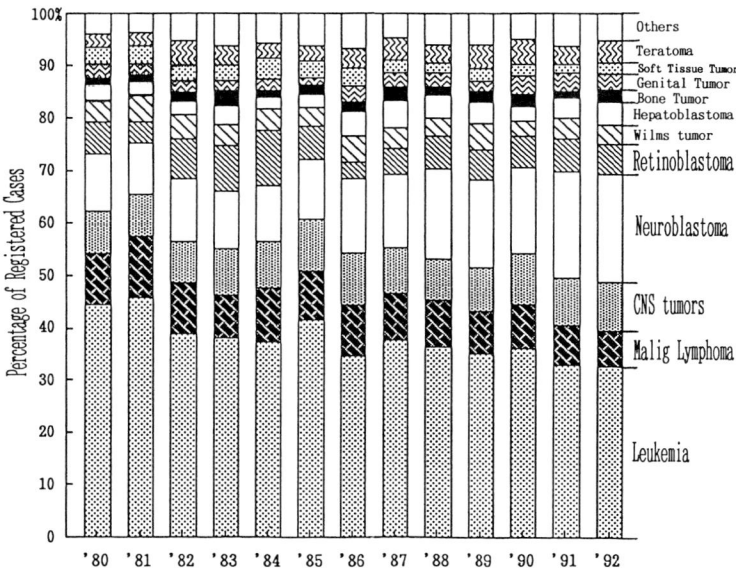

FIG. 3. Time trend in histological distribution of registered childhood cancer

Regional Center. Based on the assumption that the Hokkaido incidence of children's cancer is roughly the same as that for Japan as a whole, one may project that the national Registry reflects about half the cases occurring in the entire country.

2. *Major childhood malignancies in the Registry*

Figure 3 shows the percentage distribution of the types of malignancy in cases registered from 1980 to 1992. Leukemia was the most frequent (*ca.* 35%), followed by neuroblastoma (*ca.* 20%), brain tumor, malignant lymphoma, retinoblastoma, Wilms' tumor, and others. The percentage for neuroblastoma was about 10% before the 1985 introduction of a nationwide government-supported mass-screening program for this condition using urine samples for elevated vanillylmandelic acid (VMA) and homovanillic acid (HVA); it increased rapidly and has now doubled. A detailed discussion of the epidemiologic study on neuroblastoma in Japan is found elsewhere (7). Tumors in the central nervous system (CNS) appear to be less frequent in our series than in the United States (8), because our Registry has limited contact with neurosurgery departments where brain tumors are usually diagnosed in children in Japan. This also holds true of some orthopedic surgery departments, where the bone and soft tissue tumors of children are usually diagnosed. Thus the figures of our Registry of tumor rates at these sites are low and do not reflect the correct information.

Investigative Application of the Database

The Children's Cancer Registry database has the greatest amount of information on this subject in the world, not only clinical data but also genetic and environmental data and offers many facts on cancer etiology.

1. Differences in specific features of registered cases with leukemia and solid tumor

We compared the rates of parental exposure to irradiation, chemicals, and drugs taken by a mother during pregnancy and also of maternal smoking and drinking habits during pregnancy in cases of leukemia and solid tumors (*3*). The rates were statistically high in some blastomas (*e.g.*, retinoblastoma, neuroblastoma, hepatoblastoma, or osteosarcoma), in which loss of heterozygosity of the genes has been reported (*9*). On the other hand, there is no significant correlation with these factors in leukemia and malignant lymphoma, in which a high incidence of specific translocations has been reported (*5*). These differences between leukemia and other cancers suggest that the etiological mechanism of leukemia and malignant lymphoma differs from that in a group of blastomas like retinoblastoma and neuroblastoma.

2. Childhood neuroectodermal tumors after maternal ovulation induction

Encouraged by the suggestion of White *et al.* (*10*) on the possible association between assisted conception and neuroectodermal tumors in children, we used the database of our Registry to review the mother's drug history prior to pregnancy in 6,236 cases of childhood malignant diseases diagnosed from 1985 to 1989 (*4*). We clearly identified 4 cases of neuroblastoma in children born to mothers who underwent ovulation induction with statistically significant increase. Moreover, 1 Burkitt's lymphoma, 1 malignant lymphoma, 1 malignant fibrous histiocytoma, and 1 malignant fibrous histiocytoma (suspected) were found. No instance of maternal ovulation induction was found in children with leukemia or other malignant diseases.

These facts support the possibility of an association between the specific subset of tumors and ovulation induction.

3. Neurofibromatosis type 1 and childhood cancer

It is well known that patients with neurofibromatosis type 1 (NF1) are prone to develop malignancy, particularly malignant schwannoma in adult life. To assess the risk of childhood malignancy in NF1, we reviewed 26,084 patients with cancer in our Registry from 1969 to 1990 and compared the incidence of NF1 in each type of cancer with that in the Japanese population (*6*).

Fifty-six children with cancer had NF1 in the national Registry (Table II). The incidence of NF1 (0.21%) was 6.45 times that of the expected estimated rate of 1 per 3,000 in the Japanese population. These tumors tended to be type and site specific. The NF1 incidence was extremely high in optic nerve glioma (12.5%), and malignant schwannoma (31.4%). For nonneural tumors, NF1 incidence was increased in rhabdomyosarcoma (1.36%) and myelogenous leukemia (0.27%). The NF1 gene seems to increase the risk not only for neural tumors but also for some nonneural tumors in an age-specific, organ-dependent pattern of carcinogenesis.

4. Germ cell tumors and Down syndrome

The association of Down syndrome (DS) and cancer, particularly myelogenous leukemia, is well documented, but such association is not known for other types of cancer except leukemia. We reviewed 29,804 cancer cases entered in our Registry from 1969 to 1992.

Some 232 DS cases (0.78%) associated with particular types of childhood cancer

TABLE II. NF1 Rate in Childhood Malignancies

Tumors associated with NF1:		
Brain tumors	16/2,356	0.68%**
Optic glioma	6/48	12.50%**
Meduloblastoma	2/330	0.61%*
Astrocytoma	4/344	1.16%**
Unspecified glioma	4/399	1.00%**
Other	0/1,235	
Peripheral nerve	14/2,946	0.48%**
Neuroblastoma	3/2,876	0.10%
Malignant schwannoma	11/35	31.42%**
Other	0/35	
Ganglioneuroma	3/126	2.38%**
Leukemia	12/10,761	0.11%
ALL	4/6,086	0.07%
AML	2/2,674	0.08%
Juvenile CML	2/118	1.70%**
Adult CML	1/98	1.02%
AMMoL	1/71[a]	1.41%*
MDS	2/28[a]	7.14%**
Other leukemia	0/1,686	
Soft tissue tumor	10/826	1.21%**
Rhabdomyosarcoma	8/590	1.36%**
Fibrosarcoma	1/58	1.72%*
Leiomyosarcoma	1/24	4.17%**
Other	0/154	
Malignant teratoma	1/158	0.63%
Tumors not associated with NF1:		
Malignant lymphoma	2,177	
Spinal tumor	34	
Eye	1,899	
Urinary	1,149	
Gastrointestinal tract	814	
Respiratory	133	
Bone	400	
Male genital organ	335	
Female genital organ	274	
Skin	29	
Endocrine glands	141	
Other	1,526	
Total	56/26,084	0.21%*

NF1: Neurofibromatosis type 1; ALL: acute lymphocytic leukemia; AML: acute myelocytic leukemia; CML: chronic myelogenous leukemia; AMMoL: acute myelomonocytic leukemia; MDS: myelodysplastic syndrome.
[a] Data between 1985–1989.
* $p < 0.05$, ** $p < 0.01$.
(Compared with NF1 prevalence in the general population (0.03%)).

were found. This reflected a significant increase in DS as compared to the incidence (0.1%) reported by the Birth Defects Monitoring System, Tokyo in the years 1980–1988 (1). Of the various types of childhood cancer in the Registry, the number of leukemia cases, brain tumors, retroperitoneal tumors (malignant and benign), and genital tumors were significantly increased in DS. Major types of leukemia associated with DS were acute myelogenous leukemia, particularly M7 (FAB classification), which developed in neonatal or infancy periods, and acute lymphatic leukemia with common surface antigen, which developed in children with DS from infancy to school age in cases reported after 1985, when a more detailed classification of leukemia was begun in the Registry.

Nineteen solid tumors were associated with DS including 2 nonglioma-type teratomas out of 4 brain tumors, 7 retroperitoneal teratomas (malignant and benign), 4 fetal cancers of testis, 1 germ cell tumor of ovary, and 1 benign coccygeal teratoma. These facts indicate that, in addition to leukemia, there is a high risk of germ cell tumors in DS. Detailed data will be published in the near future.

Other Contributions and Database Perspectives

1. Information supply to children's cancer researchers

Since data processing for the Registry was proactively introduced in 1985, the stored data have become even more useful tools for cancer research as well as being an information center for children's cancer. Many investigators have access to data from the Registry, and the Registration Committee has implemented strict rules for carefully guarding the privacy of both patient and attending physician.

Ten to fifteen requests for data come in each year, are screened by the Committee and the decision for the use of data from the Registry is reported to the researcher from the Registration Center. Most of them seek information to present at conferences or for publication. This has encouraged communications among researchers and/or clinicians studying/treating the same kind of rare cancer. The media, including newspapers and journals, have also sought access to the database.

2. Toward an overall social approach to children's cancer

Because of the high cost of treatment and the need for an oncologist, children's cancer cannot be treated at just any hospital. The Registry helps to increase the number of facilities where this disease can be treated by surveying the institutions specializing in its treatment and by obtaining mutual cooperation.

Fortunately, the treatment and care of children's cancer have vastly improved in recent years. Thus, measures must now be taken from a societal standpoint to cover the long-term survivors of this disease. Just as in medical research, the database should be used for various purposes: 1) survey of the prognosis in cases of children's cancer, multiple cancer, and secondary cancer; 2) measures for social rehabilitation following completion of treatment; and 3) measures for periodic health management after treatment.

Acknowledgments

The Committee appreciates the great support provided by the Children's Cancer Association of Japan and pediatricians and pediatric surgeons with an interest in oncology and hematology, and for their cooperation with and generous support to the Japan Children's Cancer Registry. The role of local registration centers is highly appreciated, and the following doctors are representative committee members in each district: S. Matsumoto, J. Uchino, Y. Hata, Hokkaido University; T. Takeda, Sapporo National Hospital; T. Konno, S. Tsuchiya, R. Ohi, Y. Hayashi, Tohoku

University; M. Yanagisawa, F. Bessho, Y. Tsuchida, K. Yokomori, University of Tokyo; K. Watanabe, K. Horibe, Nagoya University; A. Masaoka, F. Hara, Nagoya City University; S. Okada, A. Tawa, Osaka University; N. Nagahara, T. Nakamura, Osaka City Medical Center; K. Ueda, H. Ueda, T. Yokoyama, E. Hiyama, Hiroshima University; K. Ueda, A. Matsuzaki, A. Suita, Y. Zaizen, Kyushu University. The following Scientific Advisors are also appreciated: T. Hirayama, S. Miyazaki, Y. Sera, S. Tominaga, S. Watanabe, K. Iwata, K. Ohmi, K. Yamamoto, and Y. Hanawa.

A part of this work was supported by a grant-in-aid for cancer research from the Ministry of Health and Welfare, Comprehensive 10-year Strategy for Cancer Control, and by grants-in-aid for Cancer Research from the Ministry of Education, Science and Culture of Japan.

REFERENCES

1. Congenital Malformations Worldwide: A report from the International Clearing House for Birth Defects Monitoring Systems. pp. 157–162 (1991). Elsevier Science Publishers, New York.
2. Japan Children's Cancer Registry Center. Japan Children's Cancer Registry, Vol. 3 (1979–1983) (1987). Children's Cancer Association of Japan, Tokyo.
3. Kobayashi, N. Contribution of Japan Children's Cancer Registry to Medical Research and Care of Childhood Leukemia and Related Conditions. *In* "Childhood Leukemia: Present Problems and Future Prospects," ed. N. Kobayashi, T. Akera, and S. Mizutani, pp. 107–117 (1991). Kluwer Academic Publishers, London.
4. Kobayashi, N., Matsui, I., Tanimura, M., Nagahara, N., Akatsuka, J., Hirayama, T., and Sato, K. Childhood neuroectodermal tumors and malignant lymphoma after maternal ovulation induction. *Lancet,* **338**, 955 (1991).
5. Look, A.T. The cytogenetics of childhood leukemia: clinical and biologic implications. *Pediatr. Clin. North Am.,* **35**, 723–741 (1988).
6. Matsui, I., Tanimura, M., Kobayashi, N., Sawada, T., Nagahara, N., and Akatsuka, J. Neurofibromatosis Type 1 and childhood cancer. *Cancer,* **72**, 746–754 (1993).
7. Matsui, I., Tanimura, M., Kobayashi, N., Sawada, T., Hashizume, K., and Yokoyama, M. Epidemiological study on neuroblastoma in Japan. *In* "Third International Symposium on Neuroblastoma Screening; Proceedings," ed. T. Sawada, T. Matsumura, and Z. Kizaki, pp. 3–11 (1994). Kyoto Prefectural University of Medicine, Kyoto.
8. Robinson, L.L. General principles of the epidemiology of childhood cancer. *In* "Principles and Practice of Pediatric Oncology," 2nd Ed., ed. P.A. Pizzo and D.G. Poplack, pp. 3–10 (1993). J.B. Lippincott, Philadelphia.
9. Strong, L.C. Mutational models for cancer etiology. *In* "Genetics in Clinical Oncology," ed. R.S.K. Chaganti and J. German, pp. 39–59 (1985). Oxford University Press, New York.
10. White, L., Giri, N., Vowels, M.R., and Lancaster, P.A.L. Neuroectodermal tumors in children born after assisted conception. *Lancet,* **336**, 1577 (1991).

APPENDIX

List of Hospitals Participating to the Registries

Abbreviations: H&N, head and neck, Eso, esophagus; STM, stomach; Col, colon and rectum; PLP, familial polyposis coli; Liv, liver; Bil, bile duct and gallbladder; Pnc, pancreas; Lng, lung; Bon, bone and soft part; SKN, skin; Brs, breast; Gyn, uterus and ovary; Bld, urinary bladder; Brn, brain.
●: participation to the registry. Departments, Divisions, and Sections are combined.

Hokkaido	H&N	Eso	STM	Col	PLP	Liv	Bil	Pnc	Lng	Bon	SKN	Brs	Gyn	Bld	Brn
Sapporo Railways Hospital					●	●						●		●	
NTT Sapporo Hospital															
Sapporo Medical College	●	●	●	●	●	●		●	●	●	●	●	●	●	●
Sapporo Municipal Hospital		●			●	●								●	
Sapporo Kosei General Hospital			●	●	●	●		●				●		●	
Tonan Hospital						●								●	
Sapporo Surgical Memorial Hospital					●										
Hokkaido University, School of Medicine	●	●		●	●	●	●	●		●	●	●	●	●	●
Hokkaido University, School of Dentistry	●														
Kinikyo Central Hospital					●										
National Sapporo Hospital	●	●		●	●					●		●		●	
Shiroishi Neurosurgery Hospital															●
Sapporo Tokushukai Hospital								●							
Self-Defense Force Sapporo Hospital			●		●										
Nakamura Neurosurgery Hospital															●
Kashiwaba Neurosurgery Hospital															●
National Sanatorium Nishi Sapporo Hospital						●			●						
Social Insurance Sapporo General Hospital				●								●			
Otaru Municipal Hospital						●				●		●		●	
2nd Otaru Municipal Hospital															●
National Hakodate Hospital		●	●			●						●			
Hakodate Municipal Hospital		●	●		●	●		●			●	●	●	●	●
Hakodate Kyoukai Hospital													●		
Hakodate Central Hospital						●									
Hakodate Goryokaku Hospital						●									
Kyoritsu Hospital															
Ebetsu Municipal General Hospital						●				●					
Iwamizawa Municipal General Hospital		●			●							●		●	
Bibai Rosai Hospital		●			●							●		●	●
Bibai Municipal Hospital		●	●												
Sunagawa Municipal Hospital															●
Fukagawa Municipal General Hospital					●										
Asahikawa Municipal Hospital		●			●	●				●				●	
Asahikawa Red Cross General Hospital															●
Karasawa Hospital				●											
Asahikawa Medical College	●	●	●		●			●		●	●	●	●	●	●
Asahikawa Kosei Hospital				●	●								●		
Shibetsu Municipal General Hospital					●										
Nayoro Municipal Hospital													●		
Muroran Municipal General Hospital		●	●									●	●		
NSC Muroran Hospital										●					
Nikko Memorial Hospital		●				●	●					●			
Ogawara Neurosurgery Hospital															●
Date Red Cross General Hospital		●	●									●		●	
Tomakomai Municipal General Hospital						●									
Tomakomai Oji General Hospital						●									
Social Work Association Obihiro Hospital			●												
Kushiro Rosai Hospital		●			●	●				●		●		●	●
Kushiro Red Cross General Hospital		●				●						●			
Kushiro Municipal Hospital													●		
Kushiro Medical Association Hospital						●					●				
National Teshikaga Hospital		●													
Abashiri Kosei Hospital													●		
Fujita Hospital										●					
Ezashi Hospital									●						
Wakkanai Municipal Hospital												●		●	
Rumoi Municipal Hospital														●	

APPENDIX

Aomori	H&N	Eso	STM	Col	PLP	Liv	Bil	Pnc	Lng	Bon	SKN	Brs	Gyn	Bld	Brn
Aomori Municipal Hospital		●	●	●		●		●						●	
Aomori Prefectural Central Hospital	●	●	●		●	●		●		●	●	●		●	●
Hirauchi Central Hospital						●									
National Hirosaki Hospital		●	●			●		●		●		●		●	●
Hirosaki University, School of Medicine	●	●		●	●	●		●		●	●	●	●	●	●
Aomori Rosai Hospital		●	●		●	●				●		●		●	
Hachinohe City Hospital		●	●							●		●		●	●
Hachinohe Red Cross Hospital		●				●						●		●	
National Health Insurance Kuroishi Hospital												●			
Namioka Municipal Hospital			●												
Natl Hlth Insur Goshogawara Munic Northwest Central Hosp						●								●	
Towada Municipal Central Hospital						●		●						●	
Mutsu General Hospital														●	
Misawa Municipal Hospital						●				●				●	
Iwate															
Iwate Medical University, School of Medicine	●	●		●		●	●	●		●	●	●	●	●	●
Morioka Yuai Hospital						●									
Iwate Prefectural Central Hospital	●	●				●				●	●	●		●	●
Kurihara Clinic	●														
Morioka Red Cross Hospital				●				●					●	●	
Iwate Rosai Hospital											●			●	
Iwate Prefectural Kitakami Hospital												●			
Iwate Prefectural Senmaya Hospital					●										
Iwate Prefectural Ofunato Hospital			●			●								●	
Iwate Prefectural Kamaishi Hospital			●			●		●						●	●
Iwate Prefectural Miyako Hospital		●	●		●	●		●				●			
Iwate Prefectural kuji Hospital														●	
Iwate Prefectural Ichinohe Hospital														●	
Goto Hospital														●	
Miyagi															
Kamaishi Hospital						●									
Tohoku University, School of Dentistry	●														
Tohoku University, School of Medicine	●	●	●	●	●	●	●	●		●	●	●	●	●	●
Tohoku Rosai Hospital	●	●	●	●		●	●	●				●		●	
Social Insurance Sendai Hospital												●			
Tohoku Kosai Hospital												●			
The Res Inst for Tuberculosis and Cancer, Tohoku University		●	●			●			●			●			
Sendai Railways Hospital														●	
NTT Tohoku Teishin Hospital	●														
Sendai Municipal Hospital	●				●									●	
Sendai Red Cross General Hospital			●	●		●								●	
National Sendai Hospital	●	●	●	●	●	●		●		●		●	●		●
Miyagino Hospital												●			
Sendai Medical Center Sendai Open Hospital				●	●									●	
Ishinomaki Red Cross Hospital				●								●			
Miyagi Prefectural Cancer Health-Screening Center				●											
Saka General Hospital						●									
Shiogama Ekisaikai Hospital					●										
Furukawa Municipal Hospital												●		●	
Kesennuma General Hospital		●	●			●						●		●	
Karita General Hospital												●			
Oizumi Memorial Hospital									●						
The Center for Adult Diseases, Miyagi		●				●						●			
Akita															
Kazuno Union Hospital						●								●	
Odate Municipal Hospital														●	●
Akita Rosai Hospital												●			

Akita	H&N	Eso	STM	Col	PLP	Liv	Bil	Pnc	Lng	Bon	SKN	Brs	Gyn	Bld	Brn
Yonaizawa General Hospital															
Health Insurance Minsei Hospital														●	
Yamamoto Union General Hospital		●												●	
Akita Red Cross Hospital		●				●		●				●		●	●
Nakadori Hospital						●									●
Akita Union General Hospital		●	●			●						●		●	
Akita Municipal General Hospital						●		●						●	
Akita Prefectural Cerebral Vascular Research Center															●
Akita University School of Medicine	●	●	●	●	●	●	●	●		●		●	●	●	●
Uri Union General Hospital			●		●	●						●		●	●
Hiraka General Hospital		●				●		●				●		●	
Ogachi Central Hospital					●									●	●
Yamagata															
Yamagata Prefectural Central Hospital				●	●	●		●			●		●	●	●
Yamagata Municipal Hospital, Saiseikan						●		●						●	
Shinoda General Hospital			●									●	●		
Yamagata University, School of Medicine	●				●	●		●		●	●	●	●	●	●
Yamagata Prefectural Kahoku Hospital														●	
Yamagata Prefectural Shinjyo Hospital		●				●		●						●	●
Shinoda General Hospital														●	
Sakata Municipal Hospital		●	●			●	●							●	
Honma Hospital					●										
Tsuruoka Municipal Shonai Hospital			●			●								●	●
Nagai Municipal General Hospital						●		●					●	●	
Yonezawa Municipal Hospital														●	●
Sanyukai Hospital					●										
Fukushima															
Ohara General Hospital			●			●			●		●		●		
Fukushima Medical College	●	●	●	●	●	●	●	●		●	●	●	●	●	●
Fujita General Hospital															●
Social Insurance Fukushima Nihonmatsu Hospital													●		
National Koriyama Hospital															●
Ota Memorial Hospital		●				●						●		●	●
Jyusendo General Hospital		●				●						●		●	
Otanishinouchi Hospital															●
Iwase Hospital						●									
Shirakawa Kosei General Hospital						●						●		●	
Fukushima Prefectural Aizu General Hospital		●			●	●						●		●	●
Takeda General Hospital			●		●	●					●	●		●	●
Soma Hospital													●		
Fukushima Rosai Hospital			●			●		●				●		●	
Iwaki Municipal Iwaki Kyoritsu General Hospital		●				●	●	●				●		●	●
Kureha General Hospital						●									
Ibaraki															
National Mito Hospital			●			●		●		●			●	●	●
Mito Red Cross Hospital						●								●	●
Mito Kyodo General Hospital				●		●								●	
Suifu Hospital	●														
Mito Saiseikai General Hospital					●										
Ibaraki Prefectural Central Hospital					●								●	●	●
Ibaraki Prefectural Nishi Hospital					●								●		
Hitachi General Hospital			●	●								●	●	●	●
Kashima Rosai Hospital															●
Toride Kyodo General Hospital														●	●
National Kasumigaura Hospital				●	●	●		●		●		●	●	●	
Tsuchiura Kyodo General Hospital					●	●		●					●		
Miura Central Hospital					●										

APPENDIX

Ibaraki	H&N	Eso	STM	Col	PLP	Liv	Bil	Pnc	Lng	Bon	SKN	Brs	Gyn	Bld	Brn
Tokyo Medical College, Kasumigaura Hospital			●	●		●								●	●
University of Tsukuba, School of Medicine	●	●			●	●	●	●		●	●	●	●	●	●
Tsukuba Gakuen Hospital												●			
Tsukuba Memorial Hospital															●
Shimodate Municipal Hospital												●			
National Sanatorium Seiranso Hospital									●						
Tochigi															
Saiseikai Utsunomiya Hospital					●	●		●						●	●
National Tochigi Hospital		●	●	●	●	●		●		●		●	●	●	●
Jichi Medical School, School of Medicine	●			●	●	●	●	●		●	●	●	●	●	●
Tochigi Cancer Center Hospital				●		●	●	●	●	●					
Kamitsuga General Hospital		●				●						●		●	
Dokkyo University School of Medicine	●	●		●	●	●	●	●		●	●	●	●	●	●
Dokkyo University, School of Dentistry	●														
Oyama Municipal Hospital														●	
Shioya Hospital					●										
Otawara Red Cross Hospital					●									●	
Sano Kosei General Hospital			●			●									
Ashikaga Red Cross Hospital				●	●	●		●		●		●		●	●
Gunma															
Gunma University School of Medicine	●	●			●	●		●		●	●	●		●	●
Maebashi Prefectural Hospital															
Maebashi Red Cross Hospital						●								●	●
Geriatric Research Institute															●
Saiseikai Maebashi Hospital						●									
National Takasaki Hospital						●					●	●		●	●
Kiryu Kosei General Hospital		●	●			●	●				●	●	●		
Ota General Hospital												●			●
Isesaki Municipal Hospital						●		●						●	
Mihara Memorial Hospital															●
Gunma Cancer Center Hospital, Higashige	●	●	●	●	●	●	●	●		●		●	●	●	
Tomioka Kosei Hospital													●		
Motojima General Hospital			●									●			
National Sanatorium Nishi Gunma Hospital						●									
National Shibukawa Hospital		●										●			
Tano General Hospital															●
Usui Hospital															
Gunma Univ School of Medicine, Kusatsu Branch Hospital						●							●		
National Numata Hospital			●											●	
Tone Central Hospital															●
Tatebayashi Kosei Hospital													●		
Saitama															
Urawa Municipal Hospital						●	●								
Social Insurance Saitama Central Hospital	●	●	●	●		●	●	●		●		●		●	
Omiya Red Cross Hospital		●	●		●	●						●		●	●
Toda Central General Hospital						●									●
National Health Insurance Kawaguchi Municipal Hospital												●			●
Saiseikai Kawaguchi General Hospital					●	●									●
Kawaguchi Industrial General Hospital					●										
Saitama Kyodo Hospital	●					●									
Social Insurance Omiya General Hospital		●				●						●			
Hashimoto Hospital					●										
Higashi Omiya Hospital					●										
Saitama Cancer Center Hospital	●	●				●		●		●	●	●	●	●	●
Jichi Medical School, Omiya Medical Center						●	●	●							
National Saitama Hospital				●		●		●		●				●	●
Soka Municipal Hospital					●										

	H&N	Eso	STM	Col	PLP	Liv	Bil	Pnc	Lng	Bon	SKN	Brs	Gyn	Bld	Brn
Saitama															
Ikeda Hospital														●	
Meikai University, School of Dentistry	●														
Saitama Medical School	●	●		●	●	●	●	●		●	●	●		●	●
Saitama Medical School, Saitama Medical Center	●			●		●					●				
National Nishi Saitama Hospital						●						●			●
National Defense Medical College	●			●	●	●		●	●	●	●	●	●	●	●
Ogawa Red Cross General Hospital															
Chichibu Municipal Hospital															●
Toma Hospital													●		
Fukaya Red Cross Hospital						●								●	
Arai Hospital					●										
Kasukabe Municipal Hospital				●	●	●	●			●				●	
Saitama Prefectural Children's Medical Center															●
Koshigaya Municipal Hospital			●			●								●	
Dokkyo University School of Medicine, Koshigaya Hospital	●					●									
Higashi Saginomiya Hospital					●										
Chiba															
National Chiba Hospital		●				●								●	●
School of Medicine, Chiba University	●	●	●	●	●	●	●	●	●	●	●	●	●	●	●
National Institute of Radiological Sciences													●		
Chiba Municipal Hospital						●							●		
Kawasaki Steel Chiba Hospital		●				●									●
Chiba Cancer Center Hospital	●			●		●		●	●			●	●	●	●
Chiba Prefectural Emergency Medical Center						●									
The Center for Neurology and Psychiatry, Natl Kounodai Hosp		●												●	●
Kusakabe Hospital				●											
Juntendo University, School of Medicine, Urayasu Hospital	●					●									
National Sanatorium Matsudo Hospital						●			●						
Matsudo Municipal Hospital						●								●	●
Nihon University, School of Dentistry at Matsudo	●														
Tokiwadaira Central Hospital													●		
Narita Red Cross Hospital						●							●	●	
National Sakura Hospital						●							●		
Chiba Prefectural Sawara Hospital													●		
National Health Insurance Asahi Central General Hospital	●			●							●		●	●	●
Chiba Rosai Hospital		●				●							●	●	
Keiyoh Urological Clinic													●		
Tsudanuma Hospital													●		
Toho University School of Medicine, Sakura Hospital													●		
Teikyo University School of Medicine, Ichihara Hospital	●					●	●	●					●		
National Health Insurance Kimitsu Central General Hospital						●							●		
Kameda General Hospital						●						●	●	●	●
Social Insurance Funabashi Central Hospital						●				●			●		
Funabashi Municipal Medical Center										●					
Chiba Tokushukai Hospital															●
National Health Insurance Naruto Hospital													●		
National Kashiwa Hospital										●					
Fukamachi Hospital					●										
The Jikei University School of Medicine, Kashiwa Hospital	●												●		
National Narashino Hospital					●								●		
Tokyo															
Kudanzaka Hospital		●			●	●								●	
Tokyo Police Hospital					●	●			●			●	●		●
Hibiya Hospital															●
1st Hospital of Nippon Medical School		●		●	●	●		●		●	●	●	●		
Tokyo Teishin Hospital	●		●			●	●					●	●	●	●
The Institute For Adult Diseases Asahi Life Foundation						●									

APPENDIX

Tokyo	H&N	Eso	STM	Col	PLP	Liv	Bil	Pnc	Lng	Bon	SKN	Brs	Gyn	Bld	Brn
Sanraku Hospital					●	●								●	
Nihon University, School of Medicine, Surugadai Hospital	●	●			●	●	●	●		●		●	●	●	●
Mitsui Memorial Hospital	●			●		●	●					●	●	●	●
Kyoundo Hospital					●										
National Cancer Center Hospital	●	●	●	●	●	●	●	●	●	●	●	●	●	●	●
St. Luke's International Hospital						●						●		●	
Ginza Kikuchi Hospital					●										
The Institute of Medical Science, University of Tokyo		●		●		●						●			
Tokyo Senbai Hospital												●		●	
Saiseikai Central Hospital						●		●						●	●
The Kitasato Institute Hospital										●		●			
The Jikei University School of Medicine	●	●	●	●	●	●	●	●		●	●	●		●	●
Toranomon Hospital		●		●	●	●	●	●			●	●		●	
National Medical Center				●	●	●		●				●	●	●	●
Tokyo Kosei Nenkin Hospital					●	●	●					●	●	●	●
Tokyo Women's Medical College	●	●		●	●	●	●	●				●	●	●	●
School of Medicine, Keio University	●	●	●	●	●	●	●	●	●	●	●	●	●	●	●
Tokyo Metropolitan Okubo Hospital												●			
Tokyo Medical College	●	●	●	●	●	●	●	●	●	●	●	●	●	●	●
Social Insurance Central General Hospital		●		●	●									●	●
Faculty of Medicine, University of Tokyo, Branch Hospital	●	●			●	●		●				●	●	●	
Yamauchi Orthopedic Hospital										●					
Hikawa Setsurument Hospital					●										
Faculty of Medicine, University of Tokyo	●	●	●	●	●	●	●	●	●	●	●	●	●	●	●
Tokyo Medical and Dental University, School of Dentistry	●														
Tokyo Medical and Dental University, School of Medicine	●	●	●	●	●	●	●	●		●	●	●	●	●	●
Tokyo Metropolitan Komagome Hospital		●	●	●	●	●		●			●	●	●	●	●
Juntendo University, School of Medicine	●	●		●	●	●	●	●		●	●	●	●	●	●
Nippon Medical School	●	●		●	●	●		●		●	●	●	●	●	●
Eijyu General Hospital						●						●			
Tokyo Metropolitan Bokuto Hospital		●			●	●								●	●
Sanikukai Hospital					●							●			
Doai Memorial Hospital			●									●	●	●	
Koto Hospital						●							●		
Showa University, School of Dentistry	●														
Showa University School of Medicine, Toyosu Hospital	●			●		●						●			
Kanto Teishin Hospital	●	●	●	●	●	●	●	●		●		●	●	●	●
Social Insurance Tonan General Hospital			●			●		●					●		
Toshiba Central Hospital				●	●	●							●		
Showa University School of Medicine	●	●				●	●	●		●	●	●	●	●	●
Kosei Central Hospital	●		●	●	●							●			
Mishuku Hospital						●						●			
Tokyo Kyosai Hospital				●		●							●		
Toho University School of Medicine, Ohashi Hospital	●			●	●	●		●		●		●	●		
The 2nd Tokyo National Hospital		●	●	●		●		●				●	●	●	●
Jyonan General Hospital													●		
Toho University School of Medicine, Omori Hospital	●	●	●	●	●	●		●		●	●	●	●	●	●
Tokyo Metropolitan Ebara Hospital														●	●
Showa University, School of Dentistry	●														
Tokyo Rosai Hospital				●		●								●	●
Social Insurance Kamata General Hospital													●		
Ota Hospital				●											
National Children's Medical Research Center Hospital						●									
Self-Defense Force Central Hospital		●			●	●								●	●
Tokyo Metropolitan Matsuzawa Hospital				●											
Ito Hospital	●														
Kanto Central Hospital	●				●								●	●	

Tokyo	H&N	Eso	STM	Col	PLP	Liv	Bil	Pnc	Lng	Bon	SKN	Brs	Gyn	Bld	Brn
National Okura Hospital				●	●	●	●	●		●		●			
Kugayama Hospital														●	
JR Tokyo General Hospital	●	●	●											●	●
Tokyo Metropolitan Hiroo Hospital		●	●			●								●	●
Japan Red Cross Medical Center				●	●									●	●
Tokyo Metropolitan Aoyama Hospital														●	
Yoyogi Hospital															
School of Medicine, Tokai University, Tokyo Hospital	●													●	
Nakano General Hospital					●									●	
Kosei General Hospital		●	●	●	●							●	●		●
National Sanatorium Nakano Hospital									●						
Kawakita General Hospital												●			
Tokyo Metropolitan Otsuka Hospital			●		●							●		●	●
Japanese Foundation for Cancer Research Hospital	●	●	●	●	●	●		●	●	●		●	●	●	
Hiratsuka Stomach and Intestinalillness Hospital					●										
National Oji Hospital		●							●						
Kanachi Hospital	●														
Tokyo Women's Medical College, 2nd Hospital	●			●	●	●	●	●				●			●
Tokyo Metropolitan Geriatric Hospital													●		
Tokyo Metropolitan Toshima Hospital	●				●	●								●	
Nihon University, School of Medicine, Itabashi Hospital		●	●	●	●	●	●	●		●	●	●	●	●	●
Teikyo University School of Medicine				●	●	●		●		●	●	●	●	●	●
Nerima General Hospital														●	
Itabashi-ward Medical Association Hospital					●										
Tokyo Dental University, School of Dentistry	●														
Nishikubo Hospital														●	
Ogikubo Hospital														●	
Kokusai Shinzen Hospital														●	
Nagakubo Clinic														●	
The Jikei University School of Medicine, Aoto Hospital				●		●	●	●				●		●	
East Region Hospital						●								●	
Kasai Central Hospital					●										
Oume Municipal General Hospital					●	●									
Akito Hospital					●										
Minami Tama Hospital														●	
Hino Municipal Hospital														●	
Nippon Medical School, Tama Nagayama Hospital	●					●									
Inagi Municipal General Hospital														●	●
Machida Municipal Hospital					●										
Tokyo Metropolitan Fuchu Hospital					●		●						●	●	●
Tokyo Metropolitan Neurology Hospital															●
Jishu Hospital														●	
Tamagawa General Hospital					●										
The Jikei University School of Medicine, 3rd Hospital		●	●	●		●	●	●				●		●	
National Tachikawa Hospital					●							●			
Tachikawa Hospital		●		●	●	●						●		●	●
Japan Red Cross Musashino Hospital		●	●		●	●				●		●		●	●
Kyorin University, School of Medicine	●	●		●	●	●		●		●	●	●		●	●
Tanashi Hospital														●	
Sasa General Hospital														●	
Showa Hospital					●	●								●	
Gakuen Nishi Machi Hospital															
Tokyo Metropolitan Tama Geriatric Medical Center														●	
Tokyo Metropolitan Kiyose Children's Hospital						●									
Tokyo Metropolitan Cancer Health-Screening Center				●											
Orimoto Hospital						●									
Higashi Nihon Gakuen University, School of Dentistry	●														

Tokyo	H&N	Eso	STM	Col	PLP	Liv	Bil	Pnc	Lng	Bon	SKN	Brs	Gyn	Bld	Brn
Fussa Hospital						●									
Saiseikai Kanagawa Hospital						●								●	●
Higashi Yokohama Neurosurgery Hospital															●
Oguchi Higashi General Hospital														●	
Kanagawa															
Yokohama Municipal Kowan Hospital						●								●	
Yokohama Red Cross General Hospital		●				●								●	
Social Insurance Yokohama Central Hospital										●		●			
Keiyu General Hospital		●		●								●		●	●
Kanagawa Prefectural Children's Medical Center						●									●
Yokohama City University, School of Medicine	●				●	●	●	●		●	●	●	●	●	●
Saiseikai Yokohama Southern Region Hospital						●		●						●	●
Yokohama Municipal Hospital					●									●	
Yokohama Seamen's Insurance Hospital						●								●	
Kanagawa Cancer Center Hospital	●	●	●	●	●	●		●	●	●	●	●	●	●	●
St. Marianna Western Yokohama Hospital						●					●				●
Yokohama Minami Kyosai Hospital														●	●
Showa University School of Medicine, Fujigaoka Hospital	●			●		●	●	●			●			●	
National Yokohama Hospital		●	●		●					●	●	●			●
Yokohama Sakae Kyosai Hospital														●	●
Tsurumi University, School of Dentistry	●														
Kawasaki Municipal Hospital		●	●		●	●		●				●	●	●	●
Ota General Hospital														●	●
Health Insurance Kawasaki Central Hospital												●		●	
NKK Hospital		●			●	●				●				●	
Kawasaki Sachi Hospital					●										
Kanto Rosai Hospital		●	●		●	●	●	●				●		●	●
Kawasaki City Ida Hospital			●	●		●	●					●		●	●
St. Marianna University School of Medicine, Toyoko Hospital	●					●								●	
2nd Hospital of Nippon Medical School						●				●			●	●	
Toranomon Branch Hospital					●	●									
Takatsu Central General Hospital														●	
Teikyo University School of Medicine, Mizonokuchi Hospital	●			●		●	●			●				●	
St. Marianna University School of Medicine	●	●	●	●	●	●	●			●	●	●		●	●
Inada Noborito Hospital				●										●	
National Yokosuka Hospital				●										●	
Yokosuka Municipal Hospital															●
Yokosuka Kyosai Hospital		●				●						●		●	●
Kanagawa Dental College, School of Dentistry	●														
Northern Yokosuka Kyosai Hospital														●	
Hiratsuka Municipal Hospital		●				●								●	●
School of Medicine, Tokai University, Oiso Hospital															●
Fujisawa Municipal Hospital						●								●	●
Odawara Municipal Hospital														●	
National Sagamihara Hospital		●	●			●		●			●	●		●	●
Sagamihara Kyodo Hospital			●									●			
Social Insurance Sagamino Hospital														●	
School of Medicine, Kitasato University	●		●	●	●	●	●	●		●	●	●	●	●	●
School of Medicine, Kitasato University, East Hospital				●											
Kanagawa Prefectural Atsugi Hospital		●	●		●	●						●			
Kanagawa Rehabilitation Hospital						●									●
Kanagawa Prefectural Ashigarakami Hospital														●	
National Sanatorium Kanagawa Hospital				●		●									
Hadano Red Cross General Hospital														●	●
Isehara Kyodo General Hospital														●	
School of Medicine, Tokai University		●			●	●	●	●		●	●	●		●	●
Yamato Municipal Hospital														●	

Kanagawa	H&N	Eso	STM	Col	PLP	Liv	Bil	Pnc	Lng	Bon	SKN	Brs	Gyn	Bld	Brn
Chigasaki Municipal Hospital						●								●	
Niigata															
Niigata Teishin Hospital															●
Niigata Rinko Hospital				●	●										
Niigata Municipal Hospital	●					●		●						●	●
Niigata University, School of Medicine	●	●	●	●	●	●	●	●	●	●	●	●	●	●	●
Saiseikai Niigata Central Hospital						●								●	
The Nippon Dental University, School of Dentistry at Niigata						●									
Niigata University, School of Dentistry	●														
Niigata Cancer Center Hospital	●	●	●	●	●	●	●	●		●	●	●	●	●	
Niigata Prefectural Shibata Hospital		●	●			●				●		●		●	
Suibarago Hospital															●
Niigata Prefectural Yoshida Hospital						●								●	
Niigata Prefectural Kamo Hospital														●	
Sanjyo General Hospital										●				●	
Nagaoka Red Cross General Hospital		●				●				●		●		●	
Nagaoka Central General Hospital						●								●	
Tachikawa General Hospital														●	
Odiya General Hospital						●									
Yukiguni Yamato General Hospital					●										
Nakajyo Hospital						●									
Sado General Hospital															●
Niigata Rosai Hospital														●	●
Jyoetsu General Hospital															
National Takada Hospital											●				
Niigata Central Hospital				●										●	●
Toyama															
Toyama Prefectural Central Hospital		●				●		●	●			●		●	●
Toyama Red Cross Hospital				●		●						●			
Toyama Medical and Pharmaceutical Univ., Faculty of Medic	●	●		●		●		●	●			●		●	
Toyama Municipal Hospital						●	●					●			
Kurobe Municipal Hospital						●						●			
Takaoka Municipal Hospital						●						●			
Takaoka Hospital		●				●				●					●
Namerikawa Hospital					●										
Tonami Municipal General Hospital						●				●				●	
Hasegawa Hospital														●	
Hokuriku Central Hospital				●											
Himi Municipal Hospital														●	
Toyama Rosai Hospital						●								●	
Ishikawa															
Kanazawa Municipal Hospital														●	
Kanazawa Seirei General Hospital					●										
School of Medicine, Kanazawa University	●			●		●	●	●		●	●	●		●	
Kanazawa University Cancer Research Center						●		●							
National Kanazawa Hospital	●					●	●	●		●		●	●	●	
Hokuriku Hospital														●	
Uchida Hospital													●		
Jyohoku Hospital				●											
Social Insurance Naruwa General Hospital						●						●		●	
Ishikawa Prefectural Central Hospital	●				●	●				●		●	●	●	●
Hojyu Memorial Hospital														●	
National Health Insurance Komatsu Municipal Hospital			●			●				●		●		●	●
Keijyu Hospital						●								●	
Noto General Hospital															●
Kaga Central Hospital														●	
Ishikawa Central Hospital														●	

Ishikawa	H&N	Eso	STM	Col	PLP	Liv	Bil	Pnc	Lng	Bon	SKN	Brs	Gyn	Bld	Brn
Kanazawa Medical University	●	●		●	●	●	●		●	●			●	●	●
National Health Insurance Wajima Hospital			●										●		
Fukui															
Fukui General Hospital						●									
Fukui Prefectural Hospital		●		●	●	●	●					●	●	●	●
Fukui Red Cross Hospital						●		●				●	●	●	●
Fukui Saiseikai Hospital						●	●						●		
Fujita Memorial Hospital													●		
Fukui Medical School	●			●		●	●	●		●	●		●	●	●
Mikuni Municipal Hospital					●										
Tsuruga Municipal Hospital													●		
Obama Hospital						●							●	●	●
Yamanashi															
National Kofu Hospital		●			●							●		●	
Yamanashi Prefectural Central Hospital					●	●						●	●	●	●
Kofu Municipal Hospital	●					●						●	●		
Yamanashi Medical University	●			●		●	●	●		●	●		●	●	●
Yamanashi Kosei Hospital													●		
Miyagawa Kushigata Hospital					●										
Nagano															
Asama General Hospital														●	●
Saku General Hospital		●				●					●	●		●	●
Komoro Kosei Hospital						●									
National Toshin Hospital														●	●
Yodakubo Hospital														●	
Suwa Red Cross Hospital														●	
Okaya Municipal Hospital														●	
Health Insurance Okaya Shiomine Hospital	●														
Suwakohan Hospital															●
Ina Municipal Central General Hospital													●		
Showa Inan General Hospital		●										●		●	●
Iida Municipal Hospital													●		
Takamatsu Hospital	●														
Nagano Prefectural Kiso Hospital													●		
National Matsumoto Hospital	●					●				●		●	●	●	
Shinshu University, School of Medicine	●	●	●	●	●	●	●	●		●	●	●	●		●
Aizawa Hospital													●		
Omachi Municipal General Hospital													●		
Shinonoi Hospital													●		
National Nagano Hospital															●
Nagano Prefectural Suzaka Hospital					●										
Hokushin General Hospital					●	●								●	●
Matsushiro General Hospital													●		
Nagano Stomach and Intestinalillness Hospital			●												
Nagano Red Cross Hospital		●			●	●						●	●	●	●
Iiyama Red Cross Hospital	●														
Gifu															
School of Medicine, Gifu University	●	●	●	●	●	●	●	●		●	●	●	●	●	●
Gifu Prefectural Hospital			●			●						●		●	●
Gifu Municipal Hospital		●	●			●		●		●	●			●	●
Gifu Red Cross Hospital	●														
Asahi Univ, School of Dentistry, Murakami Memorial Hosp	●	●				●						●			
Tokai Central Hospital						●									
Gihoku General Hospital				●											
Ogaki Municipal Hospital		●	●	●	●	●	●					●		●	●
Asahi University, School of Dentistry												●			
Yawata Hospital						●									

Gifu	H&N	Eso	STM	Col	PLP	Liv	Bil	Pnc	Lng	Bon	SKN	Brs	Gyn	Bld	Brn
Gifu Prefectural Tajimi Hospital			●			●		●				●			●
Gifu Prefectural Gero Hot-Spring Hospital						●						●		●	
Manabe Hospital														●	
Takayama Red Cross Hospital					●	●								●	●
Kumiai General Hospital					●							●			
Shizuoka															
Shizuoka Prefectural Children's Hospital															●
National Shizuoka Hospital												●		●	
Shizuoka Municipal Hospital						●	●						●	●	
Shizuoka Red Cross Hospital		●			●	●	●	●				●		●	●
Shizuoka Kosei Hospital														●	
Shizuoka Prefectural General Hospital						●	●				●		●	●	●
Inasa Red Cross Hospital						●									
Saiseikai Shizuoka General Hospital		●	●			●						●			
Nakamura Hospital				●											
Hamamatsu University School of Dentistry	●														
Hamamatsu University School of Medicine	●			●	●	●				●	●	●		●	●
National Tenryu Hospital														●	
Hamaoka General Hospital														●	
Hamamatsu Rosai Hospital						●		●		●				●	●
Hamamatsu Red Cross Hospital					●									●	
Enshu General Hospital			●									●	●	●	
Social Insurance Hamamatsu Hospital														●	
Seirei Hamamatsu Hospital						●				●		●		●	●
Seirei Mikatahara Hospital														●	
Hamamatsu Medical Center	●	●		●	●		●	●		●		●		●	●
National Atami Hospital														●	●
Numazu Medical Association Hospital															
Sugiyama Hospital					●										
Juntendo University, School of Medicine, Izunagaoka Hospital										●					●
National Tosei Hospital						●				●			●	●	●
Numazu Municipal Hospital					●	●									
Fuji Municipal Central Hospital															●
Fujinomiya Municipal Hospital														●	●
Shimizu Kosei Hospital		●										●		●	●
Social Insurance Sakuragaoka General Hospital														●	
Kyoritsu Kanbara General Hospital												●	●		
Shimizu Municipal General Hospital														●	
Fujieda City Shida Hospital	●			●	●							●		●	
Yaizu Municipal General Hospital			●			●						●		●	●
Shimada Municipal Hospital				●		●		●			●		●	●	●
Haibara General Hospital					●									●	
Kyoritsu Kikukawa Hospital														●	
Kakegawa Municipal General Hospital						●						●		●	
Iwata Municipal General Hospital						●								●	
Fukuroi Municipal Hospital														●	
Kyoritsu Kosai General Hospital						●								●	
Aichi															
Aichi Gakuin University, School of Dentistry	●														
Aichi Cancer Center Hospital	●	●	●	●	●	●	●	●	●			●	●	●	
Nagoya Municipal Higashi Hospital			●			●						●		●	●
Nagoya Municipal Jyohoku Hospital														●	
Meitetsu Hospital						●								●	●
JR Tokai General Hospital		●				●									
Nagoya Municipal Jyosai Hospital														●	
Japanese Red Cross 1st Nagoya Hospital	●	●	●	●	●	●		●				●	●	●	●
National Nagoya Hospital				●		●	●	●		●	●	●	●	●	●

Aichi	H&N	Eso	STM	Col	PLP	Liv	Bil	Pnc	Lng	Bon	SKN	Brs	Gyn	Bld	Brn
NTT Tokai General Hospital						●								●	
Meijyo Hospital					●									●	
Nagoya University, School of Medicine	●	●	●	●	●	●	●	●		●		●	●	●	●
Japanese Red Cross 2nd Nagoya Hospital						●								●	●
Seirei Hospital						●								●	
Medical School, Nagoya City University		●	●	●	●	●	●	●		●	●	●	●	●	●
Kyoritsu General Hospital					●										
Nagoya Ekisaikai Hospital			●		●	●	●			●				●	●
Fujita Hlth Univ, School of Med, Banbuntane Hotokukai Hos	●					●				●					
Chubu Rosai Hospital						●								●	●
Social Insurance Chukyo Hospital	●	●	●		●	●								●	●
Daido Hospital						●						●			
Nagoya Municipal Moriyama Hospital														●	
Nagoya Municipal Midori Hospital					●	●									
Shinjo Municipal Hospital														●	
Nagaya Memorial Hospital						●									
National Toyohashi Hospital					●	●								●	●
Toyohashi Municipal Hospital						●								●	●
Narita Memorial Hospital														●	
Takikawa Hospital										●					
Okazaki Municipal Hospital		●	●		●	●						●		●	
Ichinomiya City Hospital	●													●	●
Daiyukai General Hospital					●	●						●			●
Daiyukai Daiichi Hospital			●									●		●	
Tosei Hospital			●			●								●	●
Fujita Health University School of Medicine	●	●		●	●	●	●	●		●		●		●	●
Aichi Medical University	●		●		●	●	●	●		●	●	●	●	●	●
Handa Municipal Hospital	●					●								●	●
Aichi Prefectural Colony Central Hospital for the Handicapped															●
Kasugai Municipal Hospital						●						●			
Toyokawa Municipal Hospital															●
Kariya General Hospital			●	●		●								●	
Kamo Hospital						●								●	
Toyota Hospital														●	
Kosei Hospital		●				●								●	●
Nishio Municipal Hospital															
Tokoname Municipal Hospital														●	
Tokai Industrial Medical Organization Central Hospital					●	●									
Komaki Municipal Hospital						●								●	
Mie															
Yamamoto General Hospital					●									●	
Mie Prefectural Shiohama General Hospital														●	
Okanami Hospital														●	
Hadu Hospital														●	
Kawamura Hospital					●										
Yokkaichi Municipal Hospital		●	●			●	●	●				●	●		●
Suzuka General Hospital								●						●	
Nogaki Hospital				●	●										
School of Medicine, Mie University	●	●	●	●	●	●	●	●		●	●	●	●	●	●
National Tsu Hospital			●			●	●							●	
Matsusaka Municipal General Hospital					●	●								●	
Saiseikai Matsusaka General Hospital		●	●		●	●								●	
Matsusaka Central General Hospital		●	●			●						●		●	●
Ise Keio Hospital															●
Ise Municipal General Hospital					●	●		●						●	
Yamada Red Cross Hospital		●				●		●						●	
Ueno Municipal Hospital														●	

Mie	H&N	Eso	STM	Col	PLP	Liv	Bil	Pnc	Lng	Bon	SKN	Brs	Gyn	Bld	Brn
Mie Prefectural Shima Hospital						●								●	
Owase General Hospital						●						●			
Shiga															
Otsu Municipal Hospital			●		●	●		●						●	●
Otsu Red Cross Hospital		●				●		●				●		●	●
Health Insurance Shiga Hospital														●	
Shiga University of Medical Science	●	●		●		●		●				●		●	●
The Center for Adult Diseases, Shiga		●	●			●									
Saiseikai Shiga Hospital			●			●								●	
Kouga Hospital								●							
Hikone Municipal Hospital					●			●						●	
Toyosato Hospital						●									
Nagahama Municipal Hospital						●									
Nagahama Red Cross Hospital														●	
Kohoku General Hospital						●	●								
Takashima General Hospital														●	
Kyoto															
Health Insurance Kurama Hospital														●	
Kyoto Prefectural University of Medicine	●	●	●	●	●	●		●		●	●			●	●
2nd Kyoto Red Cross Hospital	●			●		●				●		●	●	●	●
Nishijin Hospital														●	
Chest Disease Research Institute, Kyoto University									●	●					
Kyoto University, Faculty of Medicine	●	●	●	●	●	●		●		●	●	●		●	●
Kyoto Municipal Hospital					●	●		●					●	●	
Kyoto Prefectural Hospital		●										●			
1st Kyoto Red Cross Hospital		●		●	●	●	●			●			●	●	●
Yamashina Hospital														●	
National Kyoto Hospital		●	●	●	●	●	●					●		●	●
Iseikai Fujihara Hospital														●	
Kyoto Katsura Hospital						●									
Saiseikai Kyoto Prefectural Hospital		●	●			●									●
Mishina Urological Office														●	
Breast Diseases Kodama Clinic												●			
Uji Tokushukai Hospital						●									
Kidugawa Hospital															●
National Fukuchiyama Hospital					●										
National Maizuru Hospital		●			●	●									
Maizuru City Hospital						●									●
Maizuru Kyosai Hospital												●		●	
Osaka															
Osaka Teishin Hospital				●	●	●						●		●	
Osaka Saiseikai Nakatsu Hospital						●		●				●		●	
Kitano Hospital					●	●	●	●		●			●	●	●
Sumitomo Hospital					●	●		●						●	
Yukioka Hospital															●
Osaka Central Hospital						●						●		●	
Osaka Dental University, School of Dentistry	●														
Osaka University, School of Dentistry	●														
Osaka University Medical School	●	●	●	●	●	●	●	●	●	●	●	●	●	●	●
Osaka Kosei Nenkin Hospital		●			●	●		●				●		●	●
Kansai Electric Power Hospital		●	●			●						●		●	
Kita City Hospital														●	
National Osaka Hospital		●	●	●	●	●		●					●	●	●
Otemae Hospital		●	●			●								●	
Osaka Ekisaikai Hospital							●								
Tane General Hospital														●	●
Saiseikai Nissei Hospital		●				●	●			●		●		●	

APPENDIX

Osaka	H&N	Eso	STM	Col	PLP	Liv	Bil	Pnc	Lng	Bon	SKN	Brs	Gyn	Bld	Brn
Ono Hospital					●										
Osaka Seamen's Insurance Hospital						●								●	
Nakamura Hospital					●										
Osaka Red Cross Hospital		●	●		●	●	●	●				●	●	●	●
Osaka Municipal Momoyama Hospital					●										
Momoyama Municipal Hospital														●	
Osaka Police Hospital						●		●		●		●	●	●	●
Hayaishi Hospital					●										
Yukawa Stomach and Intestinalilllness Hospital					●										
Aizomebashi Hospital					●										
Tominaga Neurosurgery Hospital															●
Kaisei Hospital			●			●								●	
Nishi Osaka Hospital															●
Yodogawa Christian Hospital						●								●	●
The Center for Adult Diseases, Osaka		●		●	●	●		●	●	●		●	●	●	●
Osaka Municipal Children's Medical Health Center															●
Osaka Municipal Johoku City Hospital						●			●					●	
Bobath Hospital														●	
Saiseikai Noe Hospital						●						●		●	●
Osaka Railways Hospital						●		●						●	
Osaka City University, Medical School	●	●	●	●	●	●	●	●		●		●	●	●	●
Tanaka Surgery Hospital			●												
Osaka Prefectural Hospital	●	●	●	●		●				●		●		●	●
Hanwa Hospital														●	
Higashi Sumiyoshi Morimoto Hospital															●
3rd Yamamoto Hospital															●
Jyuso Municipal Hospital														●	
Sumiyoshi Municipal Hospital						●				●		●	●		
National Sanatorium Kinki Central Hospital						●			●						
Osaka Rosai Hospital		●	●		●	●	●					●		●	●
Otori Stomach and Intestinalillness Hospital					●										
Sakai Municipal Hospital		●	●			●						●		●	
Asakayama Hospital													●		
Mimihara General Hospital															●
Daiwa Hospital															●
Seikeikai Hospital															●
National Senhoku Hospital		●				●						●			●
Ikeda Municipal Hospital						●		●				●			
Minoo Municipal Hospital														●	●
National Sanatorium Toneyama Hospital						●			●						
Toyonaka Municipal Hospital					●	●		●				●		●	●
Nagahori Hospital						●									
Osaka Neurosurgery Hospital															●
Research Institute for Microbial Diseases, Osaka University				●		●		●				●	●		
Saiseikai Suita Hospital				●								●			
Shinsenri Hospital				●		●						●			
National Cardiovascular Center															●
Suita Municipal Hospital		●				●								●	●
Osaka Saiseikai Ibaraki Hospital														●	
Hokusetsu Hospital														●	
Osaka Medical College	●	●	●	●	●	●	●	●				●	●	●	●
Sankou Hospital														●	
Osaka Prefectural Mishima Emergency Center															●
Hoshigaoka Kosei Nenkin Hospital						●						●		●	●
Hirakata Municipal Hospital												●			
Kansai Medical University	●	●	●	●	●	●	●	●		●	●	●	●	●	●
Moriguchi Ikuno Hospital															●

Osaka	H&N	Eso	STM	Col	PLP	Liv	Bil	Pnc	Lng	Bon	SKN	Brs	Gyn	Bld	Brn
Matsushita Memorial Hospital		●	●			●		●		●		●		●	●
Higashi Osaka Central Hospital			●							●		●		●	
Yao Municipal Hospital						●						●		●	
Yao Tokushukai Hospital														●	●
Yao Hospital														●	
Osaka Prefectural Habikino Hospital									●						
Kinki University School of Medicine	●	●	●	●	●	●	●	●		●	●	●	●	●	●
PL Hospital						●								●	
National Osaka Minami Hospital			●			●	●					●		●	●
Izumi Municipal Hospital			●			●								●	●
Kishiwada Municipal Hospital						●				●				●	●
Yodogawa Christ Hospital														●	
Bobards Memorial Hospital														●	
Asakayama Hospital														●	
Kikkoukaitane General Hospital														●	
Ishinkai Yao Hospital														●	
Terada Manjyu Hospital					●										
Izumisano Municipal Hospital			●									●		●	
Matsubara Municipal Hospital															●
Meijibashi Hospital													●		
Hyogo															
Konan Hospital						●		●							
Kawasaki Hospital						●		●				●			
Yoshida Hospital															●
Kobe Nishi Municipal Hospital								●						●	●
Kobe Asahi Hospital						●									
Shinsuma Hospital															●
Hyogo Prefectural Children's Hospital						●									●
Kurihara Thyroide Diseases Clinic	●														
Suma Red Cross Hospital						●									
National Kobe Hospital						●		●						●	●
Manaboshi Hospital				●											
Social Insurance Kobe Central Hospital		●										●		●	●
Kobe Teishin Hospital								●							
Shinkou Hospital		●	●			●		●				●		●	
Kobe Rosai Hospital		●	●			●	●					●		●	
Kobe University School of Medicine	●	●		●	●	●	●	●		●	●	●	●	●	●
Kobe Red Cross Hospital						●									
Kobe Ekisaikai Hospital						●						●		●	●
Kuma Hospital	●														
Ogiwara Orthopedic Hospital										●					
Hara Genito Urinary Hospital														●	
Kobe Municipal Central Hospital			●			●		●		●			●	●	●
National Himeji Hospital							●							●	
Himeji Red Cross Hospital						●	●					●	●	●	
Himeji St. Maria Hospital						●								●	
Tsukazaki Hospital															●
Himeji Central Hospital					●	●									●
Himeji Cardiovascular Center						●									
Showa Hospital					●										
Hyogo Prefectural Tsukaguchi Hospital						●		●							●
Kanzaki General Hospital								●							
Hyogo Prefectural Amagasaki Hospital		●	●			●								●	
Kansai Rosai Hospital													●	●	
Hyogo Prefectural Nishinomiya Hospital						●	●		●			●		●	
Kosetsu Memorial Hospital															
Hyogo College of Medicine	●	●			●	●	●	●		●	●	●	●	●	●

APPENDIX

Hyogo	H&N	Eso	STM	Col	PLP	Liv	Bil	Pnc	Lng	Bon	SKN	Brs	Gyn	Bld	Brn
Nishinomiya Municipal Central Hospital		●	●	●	●	●		●				●		●	
Ashiya Municipal Hospital						●								●	
Itami Municipal Hospital		●	●			●		●				●		●	
Kawanishi City Hospital				●											
Mita Municipal Hospital								●							
National Akashi Hospital								●				●			
Akashi Municipal Hospital														●	
The Center for Adult Diseases, Hyogo		●	●	●		●				●			●	●	●
Hyogo Prefectural Kakogawa Hospital				●	●	●						●		●	
Nishiwaki Municipal Hospital						●								●	●
Takasago Municipal Hospital		●				●						●		●	
Shin Suma Hospital														●	
Kasai Municipal Hospital								●						●	
Yashiro General Hospital								●							
Akou Municipal Hospital								●						●	●
Toyooka Hospital		●	●		●			●				●	●	●	
Ooi Hospital															●
Izushi Municipal Hospital				●											
Youka Hospital								●							
Hyogo Prefectural Kashiwabara Hospital								●						●	●
Hyogo Prefectural Awaji Hospital					●	●								●	
Nara															
National Nara Hospital						●				●				●	●
Nara Prefectural Hospital						●								●	●
Takanohara Central Hospital														●	
Tenri Yorozu Sodanjyo Hospital	●	●	●			●		●					●	●	●
Tenri Municipal Hospital													●		
Takai Hospital														●	
Saiseikai Nara Hospital														●	
Social Insurance Yamato Koriyama General Hospital														●	
Nara Prefectural Mimuro Hospital						●								●	●
Nara Medical University	●	●		●		●	●	●		●	●		●	●	●
Hirao Hospital														●	
Saiseikai Chuwa Hospital														●	
Omiwa Hospital						●									
Haibara Municipal Hospital														●	
Nara Rehabilitation Center for the Handicapped														●	
Yamatotakada Municipal Hospital				●										●	
Yoshimoto Orthopedic Hospital										●					
Oyodo Municipal Hospital															●
Wakayama															
Social Insurance Kinan General Hospital	●					●		●						●	
Wakayama Medical College, Kihoku Branch Hospital					●	●									
Wakayama Medical College	●	●			●	●		●		●		●	●	●	
Wakayama Red Cross Hospital					●	●		●					●		●
Kinan General Hospital													●		
Saiseikai Wakayama Hospital									●						
Koyo Hospital													●		
Wakayama Rosai Hospital			●			●		●					●	●	●
National Health Insurance Hidaka General Hospital														●	●
National Tanabe Hospital	●		●			●				●					
Kushimoto Hospital															●
Shingu Municipal Hospital						●						●		●	●
Hibi Memorial Hospital															●
Tottori															
Tottori Red Cross Hospital						●				●				●	●
Tottori Seikyo Hospital															●

Tottori	H&N	Eso	STM	Col	PLP	Liv	Bil	Pnc	Lng	Bon	SKN	Brs	Gyn	Bld	Brn
Tottori Prefectural Central Hospital		●	●	●	●	●	●	●		●	●			●	●
Tottori Prefectural Kosei Hospital	●												●		
National Yonago Hospital			●			●						●		●	
Tottori University, Faculty of Medicine	●	●	●	●	●	●	●			●		●		●	●
Sanin Rosai Hospital						●	●			●				●	
Hakuai Hospital															
Saiseikai Sakaiminato General Hospital					●							●			
Shimane															
Matsue Municipal Hospital		●	●			●						●	●	●	
Matsue Red Cross Hospital		●				●	●					●		●	●
Matsue Seikyo General Hospital										●					
Unnan General Hospital										●					
Shimane Prefectural Central Hospital					●	●	●							●	●
Shimane Medical University	●	●		●		●	●			●	●			●	●
National Ota Hospital														●	
National Hamada Hospital						●						●		●	
Saiseikai Gotsu General Hospital					●										
Masuda Red Cross Hospital														●	
Okayama															
National Okayama Hospital			●			●	●			●		●	●	●	●
Okayama University, School of Dentistry	●														
Okayama University, Medical School	●	●		●	●	●	●	●	●	●	●	●	●	●	●
Okayama Rosai Hospital			●	●	●	●							●		
Okayama Municipal Hospital					●								●		
Okayama Saiseikai General Hospital		●			●	●	●	●				●	●	●	●
Kawasaki Medical School, Kawasaki Hospital	●	●	●		●	●	●					●	●	●	●
The Center for Heart Diseases Sakakibara Hospital					●										
Okayama Central Hospital													●		
Okayama Kyoritsu Hospital					●										
Tamura Urology Hospital														●	
The Center for Adaut Diseases, Kurashiki														●	
Kurashiki Central Hospital	●	●				●	●	●					●	●	
Kanko Hospital														●	
Ochiai Hospital														●	
Tsuyama Central Hospital														●	
Tamano Municipal Hospital														●	
Kawasaki Medical School	●	●	●	●	●	●	●	●		●	●			●	●
Oomoto Hospital				●		●									
Shigei Medical Research Hospital					●										
1st Okayama Red Cross General Hospital	●		●	●	●	●				●			●	●	
Mizushima Kyodo General Hospital													●		
Hiroshima															
Yoshida General Hospital					●										
Social Insurance Hiroshima Municipal Hospital		●			●	●	●					●	●	●	●
Japan Red Cross Hiroshima Atomic Bomb Hospital					●	●						●	●		
Hiroshima University School of Medicine	●	●		●	●	●				●	●	●		●	●
Res. Inst. for Nuclear Medical and Biology, Hiroshima Univ.				●											
Hiroshima University, School of Dentistry	●														
Hiroshima Prefectural Hospital	●	●	●			●		●				●	●	●	●
Chugoku Rosai Hospital						●				●				●	
National Kure Hospital		●		●		●	●				●	●		●	●
Kure Kyosai Hospital		●	●			●						●		●	●
Matsuda Hospital						●								●	
Hiroshima General Hospital						●				●				●	
National Sanatorium Hiroshima Hospital															
Mihara Red Cross Hospital						●								●	
Onomichi General Hospital		●			●	●							●	●	

Hiroshima	H&N	Eso	STM	Col	PLP	Liv	Bil	Pnc	Lng	Bon	SKN	Brs	Gyn	Bld	Brn
Mitsugi General Hospital														●	
National Fukuyama Hospital		●	●									●	●	●	●
Chugoku Central Hospital					●	●									
Futami Central Hospital														●	
Shobara Red Cross Hospital						●									
NKK Fukuyama Hospital														●	
Kosei General Hospital						●									
Harada Hospital										●					
Fukuyama Municipal Hospital						●									
Hiroshima Municipal Asa Hospital	●													●	
Tsuchiya General Hospital						●									
Onomichi Municipal Hospital						●				●				●	●
Saiseikai Hiroshima Hospital						●									
Yamaguchi															
National Shimonoseki Hospital						●								●	●
Saiseikai Shimonoseki Hospital														●	
Shimonoseki Kosei Hospital		●													●
Shimonoseki Municipal Central Hospital		●	●			●						●		●	●
National Iwakuni Hospital		●		●		●						●		●	●
Shuto General Hospital														●	
Social Insurance Tokuyama Central General Hospital			●			●						●		●	●
Ota Hospital															●
Yamaguchi Prefectural Central Hospital		●				●				●		●		●	●
Nagato General Hospital														●	
Yamaguchi Red Cross General Hospital						●				●		●	●		
Saiseikai Yamaguchi General Hospital															●
Yamaguchi University, School of Medicine	●	●	●		●	●	●	●		●	●			●	●
Ubekosan Central Hospital						●								●	●
Yamaguchi Rosai Hospital														●	
Onoda Municipal Hospital															●
Tokushima															
School of Dentistry, The University of Tokushima	●														
School of Medicine, The University of Tokushima	●	●	●	●	●	●	●	●		●	●	●	●	●	●
Tokushima Prefectural Central Hospital					●	●					●		●	●	●
Tokushima Municipal Hospital														●	
Tokushima Kensei Hospital						●									
Health Insurance Naruto Hospital						●								●	
Komatsusima Red Cross Hospital						●				●				●	●
Anan Medical Association Central Hospital					●									●	
Anan Kyoei Hospital						●									
Oe Kyodo Hospital						●									
Miki Hospital										●					
Tokushima Prefectural Miyoshi Hospital														●	
Kagawa															
Okawa General Hospital														●	
Kagawa Prefectural Central Hospital						●							●	●	●
Sakaide Kaisei Hospital														●	
Takamatsu Municipal Hospital						●								●	●
Takamatsu Red Cross Hospital						●			●			●	●	●	
Yashima General Hospital														●	
Social Insurance Ritsurin Hospital			●	●								●			
Kagawa Medical School	●			●	●	●	●			●			●	●	●
Takamatsu Heiwa Hospital					●										
Sakaide St. Marutin Hospital						●									
Kaisei General Hospital						●								●	
Kagawa Rosai Hospital					●	●									
Kishikawa Neurosurgery Hospital															●

Kagawa	H&N	Eso	STM	Col	PLP	Liv	Bil	Pnc	Lng	Bon	SKN	Brs	Gyn	Bld	Brn
National Zentsuji Hospital		●						●				●		●	
Mitoyo General Hospital						●									
Ehime															
Shikoku Central Hospital														●	
Ehime Rosai Hospital														●	
Jyuzen General Hospital						●		●						●	
Sumitomo Besshi Hospital		●			●	●								●	●
Shuso Hospital														●	●
Saiseikai Imabari Hospital														●	
Ehime Prefectural Imabari Hospital															●
Shikoku Cancer Center Hospital	●	●	●	●	●	●						●	●	●	
Matsuyama Red Cross General Hospital		●	●					●		●		●	●	●	●
Matsuyama Municipal Hospital														●	●
Sadamoto Hospital														●	
Ehime Prefectural Central Hospital		●			●	●				●				●	●
Takanoko Hospital														●	
Ehime University School of Medicine	●	●				●	●	●		●	●	●		●	●
Osu Municipal Hospital														●	
Yawatahama Municipal Hospital												●		●	
Uwajima Municipal Hospital				●		●									
Kochi															
Kochi Prefectural Central Hospital		●			●	●		●		●			●	●	●
Kochi Municipal Hospital		●	●			●		●				●	●	●	
Kochi Red Cross Hospital						●						●		●	
National Kochi Hospital			●									●			
Hosogi Hospital		●										●			
Kochi Takasu Hospital														●	
Kochi Medical School	●					●	●	●		●	●		●	●	●
Nakamura Municipal Hospital														●	●
Fukuoka															
JR Kyushu Hospital		●						●							
Kitakyushu Municipal Moji Hospital												●			
Moji Rosai Hospital															
Kyushu Dental College, School of Dentistry	●														
Kitakyushu Municipal Medical Center	●		●			●	●					●			
Shinkokura Hospital					●	●						●			●
Mihagino Hospital														●	
Kitakyushu Central Hospital						●									
Social Insurance Kokura Memorial Hospital		●	●	●	●	●						●		●	●
Kenwakai General Hospital														●	
National Kokura Hospital													●	●	
Kyushu Rosai Hospital			●			●				●					●
Kitakyushu Municipal Yahata Hospital						●						●		●	●
Saiseikai Yahata Hospital															●
NSC Yahata Hospital					●										
Kyushu Kosei Nenkin Hospital						●				●		●		●	●
University of Occupational and Environmental Health	●	●			●	●		●		●	●			●	●
Hara Hospital														●	
Kitakyushu Municipal Tobata Hospital														●	
National Fukuoka Central Hospital		●		●	●	●		●		●		●	●		
Fukuoka Teishin Hospital			●									●			
Saiseikai Fukuoka General Hospital					●	●						●		●	
Hamanomachi Hospital		●	●		●	●						●			●
Sata Hospital					●										
Hakuaikai Hospital	●														
Chidoribashi Hospital															●
National Kyushu Cancer Center Hospital	●			●		●		●	●	●		●	●		

APPENDIX

Fukuoka	H&N	Eso	STM	Col	PLP	Liv	Bil	Pnc	Lng	Bon	SKN	Brs	Gyn	Bld	Brn
Fukuoka Red Cross Hospital															●
Fukuoka Dental College, School of Dentistry	●														
School of Medicine, Fukuoka University	●	●	●	●	●	●		●		●		●	●	●	●
Sawara Hospital					●										
Faculty of Dentistry, Kyushu University	●														
Faculty of Medicine, Kyushu University	●		●	●	●	●		●		●	●	●	●	●	●
Chihaya Hospital						●									
Kashiibara Hospital					●										
Omuta Municipal Hospital		●										●		●	●
Yonenoyama Hospital						●									
National Fukuoka Higashi Hospital						●									
Self-Defense Forces Fukuoka District Hospital					●										
School of Medicine, Fukuoka University, Chikushi Hospital				●						●					
Iizuka Hospital												●			●
Tagawa Municipal Hospital						●									
Social Insurance Tagawa Hospital					●										
National Kurume Hospital							●			●				●	
Social Insurance 1st Kurume Hospital						●						●		●	
St. Maria Hospital					●										
Kurume University, School of Medicine	●	●		●	●	●	●	●		●	●	●	●	●	●
Fukuoka Prefectural Asakura Hospital														●	
Fukuoka Saiseikai HOspital														●	
Chikugo Municipal Hospital														●	
Takagi Hospital														●	
Fukuoka Prefectural Yanagawa Hospital														●	
Saga															
National Saga Hospital						●								●	
Saga Prefectural Hospital, Koseikan		●	●	●		●		●				●		●	●
Saga Medical School	●					●				●	●		●	●	●
Minamisato Urology Hospital														●	
Fujisaki Hospital														●	
Notomi Hospital														●	
National Ureshino Hospital						●						●		●	
Nagasaki															
Jyuzenkai Hospital														●	
Nagasaki Municipal Hospital					●		●					●		●	
Ekisaikai Nagasaki Hospital														●	
Nagasaki Memorial Hospital														●	
The Center for Adult Diseases, Nagasaki														●	
Nagasaki University, School of Medicine	●	●	●	●	●	●	●	●	●	●	●	●	●	●	●
Koseikai Hospital														●	
Nagasaki University, School of Dentistry	●														
Nagasaki Atomic Bomb Hospital		●	●		●	●						●	●	●	
Sasebo Kyosai Hospital		●	●							●				●	
Nagasaki Rosai Hospital														●	●
Self-Defense Forces Sasebo Hospital														●	
Sasebo Municipal General Hospital					●	●		●				●	●	●	
National Nagasaki Central Hospital						●		●		●				●	●
Omura Municipal Hospital		●			●									●	
National Sanatorium Kawadana Hospital															
Health Insurance Isahaya General Hospital														●	
National Obama Hospital															●
Goto Central Hospital						●								●	
National Tsushima Hospital			●												
Kumamoto															
Kumamoto Municipal Hospital				●		●		●					●	●	
Kumamoto University, Medical School	●	●	●	●	●	●	●	●		●	●	●	●	●	●

Kumamoto	H&N	Eso	STM	Col	PLP	Liv	Bil	Pnc	Lng	Bon	SKN	Brs	Gyn	Bld	Brn
Kumamoto Central General Hospital						●		●				●		●	
Kumamoto Red Cross Hospital														●	●
Kawano Hospital			●											●	
Takano Hospital				●											
National Kumamoto Hospital		●				●	●	●				●	●	●	
Saiseikai Kumamoto Hospital								●							●
Arao Municipal Hospital														●	
Yamaga Municipal Hospital														●	
Kumamoto Rosai Hospital						●						●		●	●
Yatsushiro General Hospital			●			●						●		●	
Minamata Municipal Hospital												●		●	
Hitoyoshi General Hospital														●	
Oita															
National Health Insurance Kokuho General Hospital					●										
National Beppu Hospital		●		●	●	●		●	●					●	
Medical Institute of Bioregulation, Kyushu University						●		●					●		
Shin Beppu Hospital															●
Beppu Nakamura Hospital														●	
Beppu Central Hospital														●	
Noguchi Hospital	●														
National Oita Hospital						●								●	
Oita Prefectural Hospital		●	●			●				●		●	●	●	●
Oita Red Cross Hospital		●	●			●		●				●		●	
Oita Medical Association Aimeruda Hospital														●	●
Oita Urology Hospital														●	
Furusawa Stomach and Intestinalillness Hospital					●										
Oita Memorial Hospital															
Oita Medical University	●	●		●		●		●		●	●			●	●
Miyoshi Urology Hospital														●	
National Health Insurance Koiki General Hospital														●	
Institute for Hot-Spring Cure, Kyushu University												●	●		
Nankai Hospital														●	
National Nakatsu Hospital		●										●		●	
Nakatsu 1st Hospital														●	
Nakatsu Neurosurgery Hospital															●
Miyazaki															
Miyazaki Prefectural Hospital						●		●	●			●		●	●
Social Insurance Miyazaki Konan Hospital						●									
Miyazaki Medical College	●				●	●	●	●		●	●	●		●	●
National Miyakonojyo Hospital		●	●			●	●					●		●	
Miyakonojyo Medical Association Hospital															●
Miyazaki Prefectural Nobeoka Hospital						●								●	●
Miyazaki Prefectural Nichinan Hospital		●	●					●						●	●
Kobayashi Municipal Hospital														●	
Kushima Municipal Hospital														●	
Kagoshima															
Kagoshima Municipal Hospital					●	●		●					●	●	●
Shimoinaba Hospital														●	
Faculty of Medicine, Kagoshima University	●	●	●	●		●	●	●		●	●	●	●	●	●
Kagoshima University, Dental School	●														
Nanpu Hospital						●									●
Imakiire General Hospital										●				●	
Atuji Neurosurgery Hospital															●
National Minami Kyushu Central Hospital						●									
National Ibusuki Hospital												●		●	
Kaseda Hospital															●
Izumi Municipal Hospital															

Kagoshima	H&N	Eso	STM	Col	PLP	Liv	Bil	Pnc	Lng	Bon	SKN	Brs	Gyn	Bld	Brn
Noda Municipal Hospital					●										
National Sanatorium Minami Kyushu Hospital									●						
Soh-gun Medical Association Hospital														●	
Kagoshima Prefectural Kanoya Hospital															
Kimotsuki County Doctor's Hospital														●	
Kagoshima Prefectural Oshima Hospital			●			●						●		●	
Southern Region Hospital				●											
Okinawa															
Okinawa Prefectural Nago Hospital														●	
Okinawa Prefectural Chubu Hospital		●				●						●	●	●	●
Nakagami Hospital														●	
Okinawa Red Cross General Hospital								●						●	
Naha Municipal Hospital														●	
Okinawa Prefectural Naha Hospital	●													●	
Minei Hospital															●
Urasoe General Hospital														●	
School of Medicine, University of the Ryukyus	●	●				●	●	●		●	●		●	●	●
Okinawa Prefectural Yaeyama Hospital														●	
Nakagami Hospital														●	

SUBJECT INDEX

Acral lentiginous melanoma 149
Actinic keratosis 147
Acute pancreatitis 109
Adjuvant chemotherapy 141, 162
Adoptive immunotherapy 152
Adriamycin 145
Alphafetoprotein 85
Ampullary cancer 98
Amputations 145
Amylase 110
Anaplastic astrocytoma 193
Anaplastic carcinoma 34
APC gene 77
Aspiration
  biopsy 162
  cytology 35
Astrocytoma 193
Auchincloss and Patey operation 162

Barrett's esophagus 46
Basal cell carcinoma 147
BCG instillation therapy 186
Benefits of registry 5
Beta-catenin 77
Bile duct cancer 98
Biliary tract cancer 97
Bilioenterostomy 100
Bladder cancer 181
Bone tumor 129
Bowen's disease 147
Brachytherapy 175
Brain tumor 191
Breast cancer 159
Breslow's thickness 152
Bromocriptin 199
Bronchoplasty 126

c-erbB-2 167
Carcinoembryonic antigen 110
CDV therapy 152
Children's cancer 203
Cholangiocarcinoma 83, 90
Choledochojejunostomy 100
Cholelithiasis 99, 109
Chondrosarcoma 131
Chordoma 193
Choriocarcinoma 178
Choroid plexus papilloma 193

Chronic alcoholism 109
Chronic diarrhea 109
Chronic pancreatitis 109
Cisplatinum 145
Citrovorum factor (CF) rescue 145
Clark's level 152
Clinical epidemiology 3
Clinical stage 13
Clinical trial 1
Colon cancer 57
Computed tomography (CT) 81, 99
Congenital hypertrophy of retinal
  pigment epithelium 77
Corpus cancer syndrome 173
Craniopharyngioma 193, 199
CT scan 37, 125
Cystadenocarcinoma 114

D1 dissection 54
D2 lymph node dissection 51
DAV therapy 152
Dermoid 193
Desmoid tumor 69, 76
Diabetes mellitus 109
Distal gastrectomy 50
Double primary carcinoma 40
Down syndrome 208
Dysgerminoma 175

E-cadherin 77
Early gastric cancer 48
Echography 162
Edmondson-Steiner classification 89
Embryocarcinoma 175
Endoscopic retrograde cholangio-
  pancreatography (ERCP) 99
Ependymoma 193
Epidermoid 193
Esophageal cancer 39
Esophagoscopic examination 40
Estrogen receptor 164
Etiologic factor 5
Ewing's sarcomas 131

Facial nerve paralysis 21
Familial adenomatous polyposis (FAP) 69
Family history 205

FIGO   175
Follicular carcinoma   31
Free flap transfer   16
French Surgical Association Survey   103

Gallbladder cancer   98
Gardner's syndrome   70
Gastric cancer   47
Germinoma   193, 199
Glioblastoma   193
Glioma   193
Glucose tolerance test   110
Growth pattern   88

Halsted operation   162
HB antigen carrier   95
HBs antigen   81, 95
Head and neck cancer   9
Hemangioblastoma   195
Hepatic cirrhosis   81
Hepatitis   81
Hepatoblastoma   77, 83, 208
Hepatocellular carcinoma   81
Hereditary non-polyposis colorectal cancer   69
Histological staging   50
Hormonal therapy   162
Hydatidiform mole   179

Ifosfamide   145
Ileal conduit   185
Immature teratoma   175
Immunotherapy   162
Interferon-β   152
Intracavitary radiation   172
Intractable cancer   6
Intraductal papilloma   167
Intrahospital registry   3
Iodine staining   40
Intravesical instillation therapy   186
Islet cell carcinoma   114

Japanese Joint Committee (JJC)   9
JSCCR   57
Juvenile polyposis   69

Larynx and hypopharynx   10
Law on Health and Medical Service for the Aged   167
Leeds Castle Polyposis Group   70
Lentigo malignant melanoma   149
Leukemia   208

Limb salvage operations   141
Lipase   110
Lipiodolization-transhepatic arterial embolization (TAE)   86
Lobular carcinoma   163
Local recurrence   54
Lung cancer   119

Magnetic resonance imaging   172
Major salivary glands   10
Malignant carcinoid   60
Malignant fibrous histiocytoma   131, 208
Malignant lymphoma   208
Malignant melanoma   147
Malignant schwannoma   208
Mammography   161
Mass screening   126, 167, 179
Mastectomy   162
Maxillary sinus   10
Medulloblastoma   193
Meningioma   193, 199
Mesopharynx   10
Methotrexate   145
Mitotic rate   141
Mixed carcinoma   83
Molecular diagnosis   77
Mucin-producing pancreatic cancer   114
Multiple primary cancers   6
Mycosis fungoides   147
Myelodysplastic syndrome   209

Nasal cavity   10
Nasopharynx   10
Neck dissection   36
Nephrostomy   185
Neuroblastoma   208
Neuroectodermal tumors   208
Neurofibromatosis   208
Nodular melanoma   149

Oligodendroglioma   193
Operative death rate   5, 41, 48, 60
Oral cavity   10
Organ-specific cancer registries   1
Orthotopic neobladder   185
Osteosarcoma   131, 208
Ovarian cancer   170

Paget's disease   144, 147
Pancreatectomy   112
Pancreatic cancer   107
Pancreatic cyst   109

Pancreatolithiasis 109
Pap smear test 170
Papillary carcinoma 31, 182
Paranasal sinuses 10
Parotid tumor 21
Past history 6
Pedigree chart 205
Pedigree map 70
Peptic ulcer 109
Percutaneus ethanol infusion therapy (PEIT) 86
Periampullary cancer 69
Peritoneal dissemination 55
Peutz-Jeghers syndrome 69
Pituitary adenoma 193, 199
Pituitary hormones 199
Population-based cancer registries 1
Portal vein invasion 88
Post-operative irradiation 175
Preoperative irradiation 175
Primary liver cancer 81
Procto-colectomy 75
Progesterone receptors 164
Prognosis 101, 116, 154
Prognostic factors 7, 64, 140
Prolactinoma 199
Proximal gastrectomy 51

Quality of life 167

Radionuclide scanning 37
Radiotherapy 162
Recurrence 55
Reconstructive surgery 16
Rectal cancer risk 75
Rectum
　cancer 57
　preserving surgery 75
Retinoblastoma 6, 208

Rhabdomyosarcoma 208

5-S-cystenyldopa 152
Sarcoma phyllodes 164
Schwannoma 193, 199
Serous cystadenocarcinoma 178
Solid tumor 208
Stage 62
　immigration 125
Stump cancer 173
Sulindac 76
Sunlight 150
Superficial bladder cancers 183
Superficial spreading melanoma 149

Teletherapy 175
Teratoma 193
Thyroid cancer 29
TNM committee 3
Total gastrectomy 51
Trophoblastic disease 178
TUC/TUR-Bt 184
Tumor markers 110

UICC 9
Ultrasonography 81, 99, 110
Ureterostomy 184
Urinary diversion 184
Urinary reservoir 185
Uterine cervical cancer 169
Uterine corpus cancer 170

Vulvar cancer 170, 178

Xero-radiography 162